Medical Product
Safety Evaluation
Biological Models and
Statistical Methods

Chapman & Hall/CRC Biostatistics Series

Shein-Chung Chow, Duke University of Medicine
Byron Jones, Novartis Pharma AG
Jen-pei Liu, National Taiwan University
Karl E. Peace, Georgia Southern University
Bruce W. Turnbull, Cornell University

For more information about this series, please visit: https://www.crcpress.com/go/biostats

Chapman & Hall/CRC Biostatistics Series

Medical Product Safety Evaluation

Biological Models and Statistical Methods

Jie Chen

Joseph F. Heyse

Tze Leung Lai

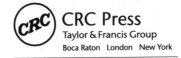

CRC Press
Taylor & Francis Group
Boca Raton London New York

CRC Press is an imprint of the
Taylor & Francis Group, an **informa** business

A CHAPMAN & HALL BOOK

CRC Press
Taylor & Francis Group
6000 Broken Sound Parkway NW, Suite 300
Boca Raton, FL 33487-2742

Jie: To my parents Yifan Chen and Shixia Wu for educating and inspiring me, and to my wife Hong Qi and my children Jessica, Jeffrey and Kyle for your love and support.

Joe: To my lovely wife Lillian and our two spirited daughters Angelina and Gabby as constant reminders of what is truly important in life.

Tze: To my wife Letitia for your love and support, and granddaughter Valerie for the joyful boost, brought by your birth when the book was near completion, to tackle the last set of hurdles.

Contents

List of Figures

List of Tables

Preface

The past decade witnessed a greatly increased focus on safety evaluation of medical products in the pharmaceutical and biotechnology industries. Safety data are routinely collected throughout preclinical *in-vitro* and *in-vivo* experiments (e.g., living cells and animal models), clinical development (e.g., randomized clinical trials), and post-licensure studies and monitoring. Whereas most clinical trials are designed to investigate the hypothesized efficacy of a compound, safety outcomes are usually not defined *a priori*, making the problem of quick detection of safety signals subject to prescribed upper bounds on the rates of false signals and false non-signals particularly challenging. Our book aims at addressing these challenges and presenting cutting-edge biological models and statistical methods that are tailored to specific objectives and data types for safety signal detection and benefit-risk assessment. Some frequently encountered issues and challenges in safety data analysis are discussed with illustrative applications and examples.

The two industry practitioners (Chen and Heyse) on our team began the book project by combining their extensive experience in this field with their long-term collaborator from academia (Lai) to develop short courses in professional meetings. This modest beginning quickly blossomed into an intensive effort to write up the material into the present book that can be used to teach not only short training programs and professional courses but also a one-semester graduate course in statistics and biomedical data science. The latter turned out to be very timely because of the current surge of interest in big data in universities all over the world. Whereas Chen and Heyse have used parts of the book to teach short courses and training programs, Lai and his colleagues at Stanford, National University of Singapore, Shanghai Jiao Tong University and Chinese University of Hong Kong in Shenzhen have used the book for data science courses. The website for the book can be found at https://sites.temple.edu/jiestat/publications/. We want to highlight in the book not only cutting-edge methods to analyze safety data, but also how these data are generated — from randomized clinical trials to observational studies. We also explain the regulatory background and biochemical models underlying these data and study designs. In addition to data science, the book also touches upon the closely related field of decision analysis, and in particular the benefit-risk assessment of medical products in their safety evaluation.

The authors want to thank Jing Miao, Lai's teaching assistant in the certificate program in health analytics of Stanford Center for Professional Development (SCPD), and Anna Choi, who co-taught courses with Lai on topics in data science at Stanford, the National University of Singapore, and Chinese University of Hong Kong in Shenzhen, for their timely help in organizing the material and preparing the final manuscript. They have also benefitted from helpful and stimulating discussions with their colleagues at Merck & Co., Inc. and Stanford: Larry Gould, Bill Wang, Sammy Yuan, Phil Lavori, and Ying Lu. Lai also acknowledges grant support by the National Science Foundation under DMS 1407828.

Merck & Co., Inc., Kenilworth, NJ, USA   *Jie Chen & Joseph F. Heyse*
Stanford University   *Tze Leung Lai*

1

Introduction

Strictly speaking, no medical product has zero risk; there are always safety concerns associated with the use of any medical product in a population of users under certain conditions. "A safe product is one that has acceptable risks, given the magnitude of the benefit expected in a specific population and within the context of alternatives available" (FDA, 2008b). A product may be relatively safe for short-term use by oral administration in adult patients with certain disorders. However, it may do more harm, as compared to the benefit of the product, for long-term use by different routes of administration in the same group of patients. In Section 1.1, we consider the probabilities of observing certain adverse events with various incidence rates, and give an overview of safety evaluation in product development that includes clinical trials and post-licensure observational studies. In this connection, we also provide a concise review of US medical product safety regulation. Section 1.2 briefly describes the concepts of adverse events and adverse drug reactions which are frequently encountered in the analysis, reporting, and dissemination of safety data. Section 1.3 describes commonly used coding standards for medical products (primarily drugs) and Section 1.4 reviews some widely used dictionaries for medical terminology. Section 1.5 gives an introduction to safety signals and serious adverse events. We discuss in Section 1.6 statistical strategies for medical product safety evaluation, and in this connection also give an overview of the other chapters of the book and provide suggestions on how the book can be used by different groups of readers. Supplements and problems are given in Section 1.7.

1.1 Expecting the unexpected

Before marketing authorization, a medical product is typically investigated thoroughly for therapeutic effects, i.e., safety and efficacy, through clinical trials with hundreds or thousands of somewhat homogeneous subjects (sampled from a population with pre-defined inclusion and exclusion criteria) for a relatively short period of time (2 to 5 years) with pre-specified route of administration and scheduled regimens. The number of

TABLE 1.1 Number of subjects needed for observing at least x events with $100(1-\alpha)\%$ confidence.

Incidence	$x = 1$		$x = 2$		$x = 3$	
rate	$\alpha = 0.05$	$\alpha = 0.01$	$\alpha = 0.05$	$\alpha = 0.01$	$\alpha = 0.05$	$\alpha = 0.01$
0.0001	29958	46052	47439	66383	62958	84060
0.0005	5992	9211	9488	13277	12592	16812
0.0010	2996	4606	4744	6639	6296	8406
0.0050	600	922	949	1328	1260	1682
0.0100	300	461	475	664	630	841
0.0500	60	93	95	133	126	169
0.1000	30	47	48	67	63	85

subjects to be enrolled in such a trial is usually determined by the objective of demonstrating efficacy (with exceptions discussed in the next subsection), with the consequence that rare adverse events may be unobservable in the trial. To illustrate, suppose that the occurrence of an adverse event follows a Poisson distribution. Then the minimum number of subjects (or observational time in person-years) needed in order to observe at least 1 reported case, with 95% confidence, of an adverse event with an incidence rate of 0.1% is approximately 2996; the number of subjects (or person-years) goes up to at least 4744 in order to observe at least two reported cases of the target adverse event with the same incidence rate; see Table 1.1 that lists the minimum number of subjects needed to observe at least $x = 1, 2$ or 3 cases of an adverse event with different incidence rates. The sample size needed to demonstrate efficacy, however, is much smaller. Moreover, there are additional inclusion and exclusion criteria for subject enrollment in clinical trials (e.g., the inclusion requirement of normal liver and renal functions and exclusion of disorders except for the health condition under investigation), which makes it difficult to observe adverse events that are associated with comorbidity discovered during such trials (Trontell, 2004).

Because of the aforementioned limitations of clinical trials, safety evaluation of medical products is usually carried out in post-licensure studies, either interventional or non-interventional, which may include phase IV randomized studies designed for comparative analysis of long-term risk and benefit, and epidemiologic observational studies (e.g., prospective cohort studies, case-control studies, case-series studies). The objectives of post-licensure safety studies are characterization of the safety profile of the product (e.g., confirmatory testing of a major safety concern), benefit-risk assessment, collection of information on rare adverse events with low incidence rates. Depending on the compound of interest and specific disease areas, these adverse events are called "special events of interest" or "designated medical events," such as pure red-cell aplasia, anaphylaxis (a severe allergic reaction to an antigen), toxic epidermal necrolysis, and Stevens-Johnson syndrome. A small number of reported cases of these events may trigger further investigation of the association between the adverse event and the product use (Trontell, 2004), and/or the revision of product label. In post-approval studies, a product is usually exposed to a much broader, possibly heterogeneous, population from whom long-term usage of the product and concurrent medical conditions or medications can be studied and safety issues such as chronic toxicity through long-term use may be revealed. In addition to these post-licensure studies, safety data are also routinely collected through spontaneous adverse event reporting systems such as the US FDA Adverse Event Reporting System (FAERS) (FDA, 2014a) and the World Health Organization's VigiBase (WHO, 2014); see Section 7.1.3.

1.1.1 A brief history of medical product regulation

Medical product safety has received much attention from government regulatory agencies in the past fifteen years. In response to the request of the Center for Drug Evaluation and Research (CDER) of the FDA in 2004, the Institute of Medicine (IOM) appraised and summarized the US drug safety system in its 2006 report, *The Future of Drug Safety: Promoting and Protecting the Health of the Public*, with 25 recommendations to strengthen the pre-licensure and the post-licensure process and to adopt a life-cycle approach to the investigation, regulation, and communication of the risks and benefits of medical products (Psaty and Burke, 2006; Burke et al., 2007). The report points out that the development and approval processes of medical products had focused on product efficacy and that safety had not been a primary concern in regulatory review and approval until the new millennium. Table 1.2 provides a brief history of important landmarks in FDA's medical product regulation (https://www.fda.gov/aboutfda/whatwedo/history/milestones/ucm128305.htm). It shows the evolution of regulatory principles and measures. To illustrate, the Prescription Drug User Fee Act (PDUFA) passed in 1992 and the subsequent FDA Modernization Act passed in 1997 by the US Congress banned the agency from spending the user fees on safety monitoring (Slater, 2005; Smith, 2007). The ban was not lifted until the PDUFA's third amendment in 2002 (Hennessy and Strom, 2007). The FDA Amendments Acts (FDAAA), signed into law in September 2007, empower the FDA to have greater control over drug safety, e.g., to make clinical trial operations and results more visible and transparent to the public, to require post-licensure studies, and to approve or reject drug marketing and labeling (FDAAA, 2007; Wechsler, 2007). In response to the IOM report, the FDA issued in May 2008 *The Sentinel Initiative: National Strategy for Monitoring Medical*

TABLE 1.2 Important landmarks in the history of US FDA medical product regulation.

Time period	Landmarks
1906	Establishment of the US FDA
1937	The Elixir Sulfanilamide crisis killing 107 persons, prompting the need to establish drug safety before marketing
1962	The Thalidomide tragedy, which caused severe birth defects of the arms and legs in thousands of babies born in Western Europe, stirred stimulating public support for stronger drug laws
1980's	The epidemic of AIDS prompting faster approval of (potentially lifesaving) therapies
1992	Prescription Drug User Fee Act (PDUFA) passed to improve FDA's efficiency in reviewing new drug applications
1997	FDA Modernization Act prohibiting spending user fees for safety monitoring
1998	The computerized Adverse Event Reporting System (AERS) introduced
2002	Amendments to the PDUFA to authorize the spending of user fees for selected drug safety activities
2004	The Center for Drug Evaluation and Research (CDER) at FDA asked the Institute of Medicine (IOM) to assess the US drug safety system
2005	FDA's Drug Safety Board formed to provide advice on drug safety issues and work with the agency in sharing safety information
2006	IOM report *The Future of Drug Safety: Promoting and Protecting the Health of the Public*
2007	The FDA Amendments Act (FDAAA) approved by the US Congress
2008	The Sentinel Initiative: National Strategy for Monitoring Medical Product Safety
2010	The Sentinel Initiative: Access to Electronic Healthcare Data for More Than 25 Million Lives
2012	Food and Drug Administration Safety and Innovation Act (FDASIA) authorizes FDA to collect user fees from industry for review of innovative drugs, medical devices, generic drugs, and biosimilar biological products

Product Safety, a national strategic safety blueprint calling for proactive safety surveillance and analysis through developing methods to obtain access to, and establish risk identification and analysis systems for, multiple data sources (FDA, 2008b). While introducing the concept of science of safety, *The Sentinel Initiative* stresses information technology enhancement and integration, as well as some key FDA activities in risk identification, assessment, and minimization. As a consequence, statistical methods play an increasingly important role in identification, investigation, validation, quantification, and monitoring of safety signals of biopharmaceutical products. Appropriate application of these methods and their integration into routine quantitative pharmacovigilance practice during the life cycle management of a product can achieve early detection of true safety signals, reduce the rate of false signals and false non-signals, and thereby protect the interests of both consumers and manufacturers.

Under the Sentinel Initiative, the FDA takes more steps to ensure the agency's potential capability to identify and evaluate in near real time safety issues that are not easily discovered by traditional passive monitoring systems. Examples are the expansion of FDA's access to (a) patient subgroups and special populations (e.g., the elderly), (b) long-term observational data and (c) adverse events occurring commonly in the general population (e.g., myocardial infarction, bone fracture) that tend not to be reported to the agency through its spontaneous reporting system. With the new vision for drug safety, the FDA coordinates internally among its Centers and collaborates with other US federal agencies to initiate safety projects, such as the SafeRx project for the development of active surveillance methods using Medicare data and innovative statistical approaches. The FDA also expands its partnership with academic or contractual research organizations in exploring the Sentinel Initiative's governance, stakeholder outreach, data, infrastructure, and scientific operations. One of the critical components in such partnership expansion is to determine the statistical methods that can best be employed within this framework to accurately, robustly, and flexibly detect safety signals (Nelson et al., 2009). Moreover, the FDA collaborates with the European Medicines Agency (EMA) on several fronts:

(a) To create a "network of excellence" consisting of research and medical-care centers, healthcare databases, electronic registries, and existing networks to strengthen post-marketing monitoring to facilitate the conduct of safety related post-licensure studies (European Network of Centers for Pharmacoepidemiology and Pharmacovigilance, ENCePP).

(b) To develop and validate tools and methods that will enhance adverse event data collection and signal detection.

(c) To develop standards for pharmacoepidemiologic studies and methods to integrate all data of relevant products for evaluation of benefit and risk.

(d) To design, develop, and validate computerized systems which are complementary to existing systems (e.g., EU-ADR) and which have more power but need less time to detect safety signals by using data from electronic healthcare records and biomedical databases.

The FDA is also in collaboration with the Canadian regulatory agency via the Drug Safety and Effectiveness Network (DSEN) to link researchers through a virtual network with a research agenda based on priorities identified by the national decision-makers, and to provide funding for research to assess the risks and benefits of marketed drug products. Moreover, the FDA teams up with Japanese Pharmaceuticals and Medical Devices Agency (PMDA) to secure access to their EMR (electronic medical records) databases, including claims data, to assess drug safety through adverse drug reaction (ADR) incidence surveys using pharmacoepidemiologic approaches (FDA, 2008b; Chakravarty, 2010).

Along the same line as the Sentinel Initiative, a Mini-Sentinel Program has been set up for academic and health research organizations to evaluate emerging methods in safety science and to develop and evaluate epidemiological and statistical methodologies for signal detection, signal validation, and association of identified adverse events with particular medical products; see (Platt and Carnahan, 2012) and (Ball et al., 2016). In particular, the statistical methodology research in the Mini-Sentinel Program develops

- frameworks for safety surveillance methods,

- regression methods and related approaches applicable to sequential surveillance programs,

- case-only methods (e.g., cross-over designs) utilizing time-varying covariates,

- enhanced methods for application of propensity score with confounder adjustment.

The preceding historical overview shows that in recent years there has been a remarkable global climate change in safety regulation of biopharmaceutical products. Following the regulatory agencies' initiatives, the pharmaceutical industry has taken proactive and collaborative actions worldwide , and has even assumed leading roles to propose and implement innovative measures to ensure safe products to be delivered to patients.

1.1.2 Science of safety

The science of safety is the study of all the aspects, including identification, quantification, mitigation, and prevention, of safety concerns. In response to the IOM's 2006 report in Table 1.2, the US FDA defines the science of safety as an emerging subject "combining the growing understanding of disease and its origins at the molecular level (including understanding of adverse events resulting from treatment) with new methods of signal detection, data mining, and analysis, enabling researchers to generate hypotheses about, and confirm the existence and causal factors of, safety problems in the populations using the products" (FDA, 2008b). This emerging science requires interdisciplinary collaborative efforts involving experts in basic sciences, toxicologists, clinical pharmacologists, clinicians, statisticians, epidemiologists, and informatics experts to assess safety problems during the entire life-cycle of a product from pre-clinical *in vitro* and *in vivo* testing, followed by the whole spectrum of clinical development (Phase I - Phase III), to post-licensure use by general populations. Shinde and Crawford (2016) describe the science of safety as an iterative process examining safety concerns along the life-cycle of prescribed drugs and biologics for target use among patients whose benefits are maximized constrained by risks that should be identified as quickly as possible, with envisioned objectives of providing more efficacious yet less toxic personalized medicines to diversified populations.

1.1.3 Differences and similarities between efficacy and safety endpoints

Even though almost all clinical trials are designed to demonstrate efficacy and safety, there are important differences in the treatment of efficacy and safety endpoints. First, unlike efficacy endpoints that are usually defined *a priori* in clinical development of a medical product, safety endpoints are rarely pre-determined when planning a clinical trial. For instance, whereas the overall survival and/or its surrogate endpoints (e.g., progression-free survival, tumor response rate) are the predefined primary efficacy endpoints for an oncology trial, and the incidence rate of a disease and/or immunogenicity endpoints (e.g., the titer of disease-specific antibodies) are the primary efficacy endpoints for a vaccine study, safety endpoints mostly remain unknown until the end of the study. Second, a clinical trial may have, say, up to 5 primary efficacy endpoints but more than 300 adverse event types reported from the study subjects. Third, an efficacy endpoint is a known benefit and it is usually believed that a high proportion of patients with a target disease can benefit from a product approved for treating the disease, but the proportion of patients experiencing a particular safety event is typically low. Fourth, the benefits of a product are usually established sooner than the adverse effects, and the relationship between benefit and risk may change over time, e.g., the risk may outweigh the benefit if a patient uses the product for more than 3 years.

On the other hand, there are similarities between efficacy and safety.

Both are relative measures and depend on factors, such as the medical condition and its prevalence rate, the population affected, and alternative options of treatment. In particular, a product may provide a better benefit than risk if it is used by a group of patients with a severe condition; a vaccine may provide a better protection to a population with a highly prevalent infectious disease that has fewer alternative options of preventive measures. Efficacy and safety are inseparable dual aspects of any medical product and are increasingly used in dynamic benefit-risk assessment for regulatory decision and life-cycle management, as will be discussed in Chapter 3.

1.1.4   Regulatory guidelines and drug withdrawals

The increasing focus on medical product safety in the past decade has led the FDA to update and issue its guidelines on safety, including the following:

- *Classifying Significant Postmarketing Drug Safety Issues* (August 2012)

- *Safety Reporting Requirements for INDs (Investigational New Drug Applications) and BA/BE (Bioavailability/Bioequivalence) Studies* (December 2012)

- *Safety Reporting Requirements for INDs and BA/BE Studies- Small Entity Compliance Guide* (December 2012)

- *Best Practices for Conducting and Reporting Pharmacoepidemiologic Safety Studies Using Electronic Healthcare Data Sets* (May 2013)

- *Risk Evaluation and Mitigation Strategies: Modifications and Revisions Guidance for Industry* (April 2015)

- *Safety Assessment for IND Safety Reporting Guidance for Industry* (December 2015)

- *Safety Considerations for Product Design to Minimize Medication Errors Guidance for Industry* (April 2016)

- *FDA's Application of Statutory Factors in Determining When a REMS Is Necessary Guidance for Industry* (September 2016).

A complete list of safety-related guidelines issued by the FDA can be found at `https://www.fda.gov/Drugs/`. The International Conference on Harmonisation (ICH) also has an inventory of guidelines with quite extensive coverage on safety aspects from preclinical research (S1-S11) to clinical development (E1-E3 & E9); see `http://www.ich.org/products/guidelines.html` for a complete list of the ICH safety guidelines.

A medical product may be withdrawn from the market if its serious adverse reactions are discovered after its marketing authorization. Qureshi et al. (2011) investigated market withdrawal of new molecular entities approved in the United States from 1980 to 2009 and found that safety was the primary reason for product withdrawal, accounting for approximately a quarter of total withdrawals. On the other hand, the time interval between product launch and the first report of adverse drug reaction or product withdrawal, due to serious safety concerns, has dropped dramatically over time. Rawson (2016) studied 462 medications that were discontinued for safety reasons from 1953 to 2009 and calculated three types of time intervals for these products. Table 1.3 shows that the medians of the three time intervals have dropped from 16-37 years in "pre-1961" to only 1-3 years in "1991-2013." After a systematic review and analysis, Onakpoya et al. (2016) also observed a similar trend in the time intervals between launch and worldwide withdrawal of medicinal products.

TABLE 1.3 Three types of time intervals, labeled 1,2,3, for four product launch periods.

Launch period	Interval*	Number of medicines	Median (years)	Interquartile range (years)
Pre–1961	1	187	20	932
	2	187	37	2757
	3	187	16	628
1961–1975	1	128[a]	8	315
	2	131	17	1022
	3	128[a]	5	111
1976–1990	1	75	3	25
	2	75	6	412
	3	75	2	06
1991–2013	1	69	1	04
	2	69	3	16
	3	69	1	02

* Interval 1 represents the time interval (in years) between launch year and the year in which an ADR (related to the reason for withdrawal) was first reported. Interval 2 represents the time interval between launch year and year of withdrawal. Interval 3 represents the time interval from the year in which an ADR (related to the reason for withdrawal) was first reported to the year of withdrawal.

Product withdrawal is a complex decision, relying on various sources of evidence on benefit or risk, and availability of alternative therapies. McNaughton et al. (2014) investigated drug products withdrawn from the European Union (EU) market due to safety reasons between 2002 and 2011 and the evidence used to support the withdrawn decision-making. They found that the level of evidence used to support drug withdrawal improved with increased use of case-control studies, cohort studies, randomized clinical trials, and well-designed meta-analyses during the study period.

1.2 Medical product safety, adverse events, and adverse drug reactions

A medical product is defined as a product that is used for the purpose of treatment, diagnosis, control, or prevention of a disease or a health condition. It may refer to a drug (chemical entity), a biologic (either therapeutic or preventive agent), or a medical device. Safety concerns depend on the type of product (drug, biologic, or medical device) and on the applications of the product. Even for the same type of product (e.g., drugs), the safety issues may vary from one kind of drugs to another. For example, a drug treating diabetes mellitus may cause safety problems that are different from those associated with a drug treating non-small cell lung cancer. Moreover, the threshold of tolerating side effects for cancer patients treated with an anti-cancer agent could be higher than that for asthma patients treated with an anti-allergic product, and the tolerability to a drug treating a sick condition is generally higher than that for a preventive product as the latter is usually applied to healthy populations.

1.2.1 Adverse events versus adverse drug reactions

The World Health Organization (WHO) defines an adverse event as "any untoward medical occurrence that may present during treatment with a medicinal product but which does not necessarily have a causal relationship with this treatment," and defines an adverse drug reaction as "a response that is noxious and unintended and that occurs at doses normally used in humans for the prophylaxis, diagnosis, or therapy of disease, or for the modification of physiological function" (WHO, 1992). Hence, an adverse event refers to any unwanted health condition or harm that occurs to a patient after taking a medical product, and the occurrence of the event may or may not be caused by the product. On the other hand, an adverse drug reaction usually refers to an adverse event that is suspected to be caused by the medical product. For regulatory reporting purposes, an adverse event is spontaneously reported, even if the relationship between the event and a product is unknown or unstated (ICH, 2003). Statistical analyses of adverse event data can provide the strength of evidence to support the justification of whether an adverse event is truly an adverse drug reaction caused by a product. However, in most cases the evidence of a causal relationship between a product and an adverse event comes from sources that include the molecular structure of a chemical compound, pharmacophysiological and toxicogenomic plausibility, and statistical and epidemiologic analyses. Chapter 6 gives details of causal inference from post-marketing safety data.

1.2.2 Safety data coding

When reporting and analyzing safety data, there are at least two kinds of terms—terms for relevant medical products and terms for adverse events—that should be standardized across therapeutical areas, product types, and geographical regions. Standardization of these terms is important for the transfer, exchange, pooling, tabulation, comparison, and analysis of safety data to help decision making for regulatory concerns. The collection of these standardized terms or terminologies, either for drugs or for adverse events, is commonly called a *dictionary*. Important considerations in coding medical products for such dictionaries are routes of administration, therapeutic and pharmacological categories, chemical structures, types of formulation, dosages, manufacturers, proprietary names, countries or regions where the products are approved. There are different coding standards used by different organizations for different purposes. The next two sections introduce some commonly used international coding standards for drugs and for adverse events.

1.3 Drug dictionaries

This section describes some widely used drug dictionaries.

1.3.1 WHO Drug Dictionary

The WHO (World Health Organization) Drug Dictionary (WHO-DD) originated from the WHO Programme for International Drug Monitoring, established in 1968 and managed by the Uppsala Monitoring Centre (UMC). As an international consolidated reference source of drug names and related information, the WHO-DD was developed to provide the information on drug products with a hierarchical structure. It uses the WHO drug number system and the anatomical-therapeutic-chemical (ATC) classification (see the next subsection) for chemical structure and therapeutic indications to allow for easy and flexible data retrieval and analysis at different levels of precision. The WHO-DD has evolved to meet the needs of various users, such as drug safety monitoring centers in individual countries, pharmaceutical companies, regulatory agencies, and clinical research organizations (WHO, 2012b). The WHO-DD and

TABLE 1.4 Metformin in the ATC classification.

Code	Term and Level
A	Alimentary tract and metabolism (1st level, anatomical main group)
A10	Drugs used in diabetes (2nd level, therapeutic subgroup)
A10B	Blood glucose lowering drugs, excl. insulins (3rd level, pharmacological subgroup)
A10BA	Biguanides (4th level, chemical subgroup)
A10BA02	metformin (5th level, chemical substance)

its subsequent enhanced versions contain the following product types: medicinal product, herbal remedy, vaccine, dietary supplement, radio-pharmaceutical, blood product, diagnostic agent. For each product type, further product identification information is supplied. For example, a medicinal product identifier can be a vector consisting of medicinal product name, name specifier, marketing authorisation holder, country, pharmaceutical form (dosage form), strength, and drug code as its components (WHO, 2012b).

It is worth noting that products added to the WHO-DD in the 1990's and 2000's also contain drug products from 1968 onwards, including those that had been withdrawn from market. In addition, the dictionary lists a large number of drug products used in countries participating in the Programme, and a new version of the dictionary called WHO-DD Enhanced was created in 2010 to have a much broader coverage in terms of geographic regions and product scope.

1.3.2 Anatomical-Therapeutic-Chemical classification

In the anatomical-therapeutic-chemical (ATC) classification, active substances are divided into different groups according to their therapeutic, pharmacological, and chemical characteristics, and the organ or system of the human body on which these substances act. Products are grouped into five different levels, namely, main anatomical groups with one letter as the first level, therapeutic subgroups with two digits as the second level, pharmacological subgroups with one letter as the third level, chemical subgroups with one letter as the fourth level, and the chemical substance with two digits as the fifth level. The second, third, and fourth levels are often used to identify the subgroups via a hierarchical approach (WHO, 2013) as illustrated in Table 1.4.

Medicinal products are classified according to the primary therapeutic use of the main active ingredient, with only one ATC code for each route of administration. Immediate-release and slow-release tablets normally have the same ATC code. However, a product can be given more than one ATC code if it is available in two or more strengths, or routes of administration with different therapeutic indications (WHO, 2013).

1.3.3 NCI Drug Dictionary

The NCI (National Cancer Institute) Drug Dictionary contains technical definitions and synonyms for drugs or agents used to treat patients with cancer or conditions related to malignancy. Each drug entry includes links to check for clinical trials reported in the NCI's List of Cancer Clinical Trials. The NCI Drug Dictionary contains technical definitions, alternative names, and links to related information for about 4,000 single agents and over 3000 combination therapies in clinical treatment and prevention trials, or for cancer drugs used in supportive care. Each entry includes a link to a more detailed entry in the NCI Thesaurus with an ontology-like cancer-centric terminology, which provides links to open clinical trials in NCI's List of Cancer Clinical Trials; see Sioutos et al. (2007) and https://www.cancer.gov/publications/dictionaries/cancer-drug.

1.4   Adverse event dictionaries

Adverse event dictionaries are standardized terminologies for coding adverse clinical manifestations, outcomes, experiences, and/or abnormal test and diagnostic results. This section introduces several commonly used adverse event dictionaries, each of which has a slightly different focus.

1.4.1   Medical Dictionary for Regulatory Activities

The Medical Dictionary for Regulatory Activities (MedDRA) provides an international terminology of medical information developed under the auspices of the International Conference on Harmonisation (ICH) of Technical Requirements for Registration of Pharmaceuticals for Human Use (MedDRA-MSSO, 2015). Since its inception in 1994, MedDRA has been widely used by many regulatory agencies for reporting, tabulation, and communication of medical information relevant to medicinal and biological products (Brown et al., 1999; Brown, 2004b). It has become the dominant dictionary for safety data reporting, analysis, comparison and communication, and for regulatory decisions. While primarily encompassing medical, health-related, and regulatory concepts pertaining to the development of medicinal and biologically derived products for human use, MedDRA also addresses health effects and malfunction of medical devices (MedDRA-MSSO, 2015). It can be used for recording and analyzing adverse events and medical history in clinical trials and in expedited submissions of safety data to government regulatory authorities. Its terminology may be used in constructing standard product information such as summaries of product characteristics, and in documentation to support applications for marketing authorization. After licensure of a medicine, it may be used in the planning and conduct of pharmacovigilance activities such as safety data entry and expedited or periodic reporting of adverse drug reactions. MedDRA is a hierarchically structured vocabulary, covering the following categories of terms: signs, symptoms, diseases, diagnoses, therapeutic indications, names and qualitative results of investigations (e.g., increased, decreased, normal, abnormal, present, absent, positive, and negative), medication errors, product quality terms, surgical and medical procedures, and medical/social/family history. Only terms relevant to pharmaceutical regulatory processes are included in MedDRA, which does not contain terms covering study design, patient demographics, or qualifiers such as those describing disease severity or frequency (http://www.meddra.org/).

MedDRA's five-level hierarchy of terminology consists of (from the lowest to the highest hierarchy) lowest level terms (LLTs), preferred teams (PTs), high level terms (HLTs), high level group teams (HLGTs), and system organ classes (SOCs), as shown in Table 1.5. The LLTs constitute the lowest level of terminology and each LLT is linked to one PT. In addition to facilitating data entry and promoting consistency by decreasing subjective choices, the LLTs can also be used for data retrieval without ambiguity because they are more specific than the PTs. A PT is a distinct descriptor for the symptom, sign, disease, diagnosis, therapeutic indication, surgical or medical procedure, and medical, social, or family history characteristic. The descriptors represent clinical, pathologic, etiologic qualifiers of specificity at the PT level. A PT must have at least one LLT linked to it, must be linked to at least one SOC, and must have a primary SOC under which the PT appears in data outputs. As subordinates of HLTs, PTs are linked to HLTs by anatomy, pathology, physiology, etiology, or function. HLTs are intended for the purpose of data retrieval and presentation at a group level. Each HLT must be linked to at least one SOC through one of HLGTs which group the HLTs, and each HLGT must be linked to at least one HLT and to at least one SOC, which is the highest level in the hierarchy. SOCs are formed by etiology, manifestation site, body functional structure, and purpose. An exception from this categorization is the social circumstances SOC containing information about a person, not adverse events, which provides grouping of factors giving insights into personal matters that may impact the event being reported (MedDRA-MSSO, 2015).

Although MedDRA has been widely used in regulatory activities for reporting, analysis, tabulation, and communication of safety information

TABLE 1.5 MedDRA's five-level hierarchy of terminology (version 19.0).

Level (Abbreviation)	Number of Codes	Examples
System Organ Class (SOC)	27	Vascular disorders, Cardiac disorders
High Level Group Term (HLGT)	335	Vascular hypertensive disorders, Congenital cardiac disorders
High Level Term (HLT)	1,732	Hypertension complications, Congenital cardiovascular disorders
Preferred Term (PT)	21,920	Hypertension, Cardiac failure
Lowest Level Term (LLT)	75,818	Blood pressure high, Cardiac insufficiency

related to biopharmaceutical products, some deficiencies were perceived regarding its specificity of terms and capability of data retrieval and electronic data submission. With the joint effort of the Council for International Organizations of Medical Sciences (CIOMS) and the MedDRA Maintenance and Support Services Organization (MSSO), the Standardised MedDRA Queries (SMQs) Working Group was established in 2002 to develop SMQs, which are groups of terms at the PT level from one or more MedDRA SOCs that can help the identification and retrieval of potentially relevant individual safety information from clinical trials and post-marketing studies in multiple therapeutic areas. They have been used for periodic safety reporting, safety signal detection (using multiple SMQs), case retrieval for suspected or known safety issues, and standardized communication of safety information (Mozzicato, 2007).

1.4.2 Common Terminology Criteria for Adverse Events

Originated from the Common Toxicity Criteria (CTC) developed by the Cancer Therapy Evaluation Program (CTEP) of the National Cancer Institute in 1983, the Common Terminology Criteria for Adverse Events (CTCAE) aid the description and grading of adverse events that occur during cancer treatment using drugs, biologics, radiotherapy, or surgery. CTCAE terms are grouped by MedDRA primary SOCs, and within each SOC, AEs are listed and accompanied by a description of severity (grade of AEs). An AE is a term that represents uniquely a specific event used for medical documentation and scientific analyses, and each CTCAE term is a MedDRA LLT. Each AE term is graded according to its severity, and there are five grades, from Grade 1 to Grade 5, with unique clinical descriptions of severity for each; see Table 1.6. In general, Grade 1 refers to mild AEs, Grade 2 moderate AEs, Grade 3 severe AEs, Grade 4 life threatening or disabling AEs, and Grade 5 death-related AEs; see `http://evs.nci.nih.gov/ftp1/CTCAE/About.html` and NCI (2009). Although it was initially designed for use in oncology clinical trials, the CTCAE grading system has been widely used also in non-oncology clinical trials for classifying adverse events and their associated severity. It is often used to guide medical decisions in routine health care, including drug dosing and supportive care interventions (Kuderer and Wolff, 2014). CTCAE also provides a tool not only for monitoring and documentation of AEs commonly encountered in medical practice and research, but also for documentation of the severity of treatment-related harm to facilitate comparison of the toxicity profiles among different treatments (Niraula et al., 2012; Kubota et al., 2014).

TABLE 1.6 Definitions of CTCAE Grades (version 4.0).

Grade	Definition
Grade 1	Mild; asymptomatic or mild symptoms; clinical or diagnostic observations only; intervention not indicated.
Grade 2	Moderate; minimal, local, or noninvasive intervention indicated; limiting age-appropriate instrumental ADL[1].
Grade 3	Severe or medically significant but not immediately life-threatening; hospitalization or prolongation of hospitalization indicated; disabling; limiting self care ADL[2].
Grade 4	Life-threatening consequences; urgent intervention indicated.
Grade 5	Death related to AE.

[1] Instrumental ADL refers to preparing meals, shopping for groceries or clothes, using the telephone, managing money, etc.
[2] Self care ADL refers to bathing, dressing and undressing, feeding self, using the toilet, taking medications, and not bedridden.

1.4.3   WHO's Adverse Reaction Terminology

Another widely used dictionary for adverse events is the World Health Organization's Adverse Reaction Terminology (WHO-ART), which was created in 1962 and maintained by the Uppsala Monitoring Centre. The WHO-ART has been used by regulatory agencies and pharmaceutical companies in many countries for monitoring adverse drug reactions and has been translated into multiple languages (e.g., French, Chinese, Spanish, and Portuguese). Similar to MedDRA, the WHO-ART is hierarchically structured with four levels starting from system organ class (SOC) as the highest level of the hierarchy, high level terms (HLTs), preferred terms (PTs), and included terms (ITs). The PTs are mainly used to describe adverse drug reactions reported to the WHO system while the ITs help point to the closest preferred term in case of uncertainty. The HLTs are grouped PTs for qualitatively similar but quantitatively different conditions and are mainly used for data summarization. The SOCs are groups of adverse reaction PTs pertaining to the same system-organ (Sills, 1989; Nahler, 2009). Until 2008 when MedDRA was implemented, WHO-ART was the only available dictionary for coding adverse drug reactions. Although it is no longer actively maintained, it is still used by some countries. The Uppsala Monitoring Centre is actively seeking collaboration with the ICH and the MSSO towards a global standard terminology solution for pharmacovigilance activities (https://www.who-umc.org/vigibase/services/learn-more-about-who-art/).

1.4.4 ICD and COSTART

The International Classification of Diseases (ICD) is an international diagnostic classification which was originally developed to classify causes of mortality as recorded at the registration of death and was later extended to include diagnoses in morbidity. It can be used to classify diseases and other health-related problems from many types of health records and vital signs. The ICD contains a wide variety of signs, symptoms, abnormal findings, complaints, and social circumstances in health-related records (WHO, 2012a). ICD version 10, endorsed in May 1990, has been used by more than 100 countries and translated into 43 languages. The usage includes monitoring of the incidence and prevalence of diseases, reimbursements and resource allocation trends, together with safety and quality guidelines. It also includes enumeration of deaths as well as diseases, injuries, symptoms, investigation of the reasons for encounter, factors that influence health status, and external causes of disease (www.who.int/whosis/icd10/).

The Coding Symbols for a Thesaurus of Adverse Reaction Terms (COSTART) was developed by the FDA and is primarily used for coding, filing, and retrieving post-marketing adverse drug and biologic experience reports (FDA, 1995). COSTART is organized into body systems with pathophysiology hierarchies, and contains a separate fetal/neonatal category of fewer than 20 terms. COSTART has been superseded by the MedDRA; see https://www.nlm.nih.gov/research/umls/sourcereleasedocs/current/CST/ and Brown (2004a).

1.5   Serious adverse events and safety signals

According to the FDA guideline on safety reporting requirements (FDA, 2010a), an adverse event or suspected adverse reaction is considered "serious" if "it results in any of the following outcomes: death, life-threatening, inpatient hospitalization or prolongation of existing hospitalization, persistent or significant incapacity or substantial disruption of the ability to conduct normal life functions, or congenital anomaly/birth defect." In addition, "important medical events that may not result in death, be life-threatening, or require hospitalization, may also be considered serious when, based upon appropriate medical judgment, they may jeopardize the subject who may require medical or surgical intervention to prevent one of the outcomes listed in this definition. Examples of such medical events include allergic bronchospasm requiring intensive treatment in an emergency room or at home, blood dyscrasias or convulsions that do not result in inpatient hospitalization, or the development of drug dependency or drug abuse." An adverse event or a suspected adverse reaction is considered "life-threatening" if, in the view of either the investigator or sponsor, "its occurrence places the patient or subject at immediate risk of death. It does not include an adverse event or suspected adverse reaction that, had it occurred in a more severe form, might have caused death." If either the sponsor or the investigator believes that an adverse event is serious (or life-threatening), the event must be considered serious (or life-threatening) and evaluated by the sponsor for expedited reporting (FDA, 2010a).

Serious adverse events are a primary focus during clinical trials and post-marketing surveillance. They are responsible for a substantial proportion of early termination of late-stage clinical trials (Williams et al., 2015) and post-marketing withdrawal (Onakpoya et al., 2016). Some well-designed clinical trials with pre-defined safety events incorporate statistical monitoring tools for safety monitoring and safety signal detection (Heyse et al., 2008; Mehrotra and Adewale, 2012; Yao et al., 2013; Davis and Southworth, 2016; Odani et al., 2017, and the references therein). A safety signal in this case refers to reported information on possible causal relationship between an adverse event and a medical product, the relationship being unknown *a priori*. A safety signal detection program is usually designed to monitor rare adverse events of special interest, serious adverse events of more common occurrence, and/or serious laboratory abnormalities. If a detected safety signal is a serious concern, a thorough investigation must be performed to determine whether the signal is a true drug-related adverse effect and a decision must be made according to a clinically sound risk management plan; the decision may include discontinuation of the clinical development program or post-marketing withdrawal of the product.

1.6 Statistical strategies for safety evaluation and a road map for readers

Post-marketing safety concerns of medical products after phase III trials have traditionally been handled through clinical review of individual reported cases by the manufacturer and the regulatory agency until a decision is reached on whether the product might cause certain serious adverse events. Statistical science has much to offer for improving the efficiency and quality of these decisions and supporting data analysis and collection, as the subsequent chapters will show. In particular, Chapter 6 gives an overview of causal inference that is inherently related to the aforementioned decision on whether use of a medical product might be the cause of serious adverse events. Clearly a medical product is worthless if it has little benefit. Hence, methodologies for benefit-risk assessments are of particular importance for deciding whether a medical product with safety concerns should be withdrawn from the market. These methodologies are described in Chapter 3, which also introduces multi-criteria statistical decision theory in this connection.

1.6.1 Safety data collection and analysis

For a medical product, safety data collection begins with pre-clinical studies of *in-vitro* and *in-vivo* toxicities. Chapter 2 gives an introduction to these studies and the statistical methods for analyzing the associated safety data. It also describes the underlying biological models of toxicity and efficacy, which also paves the way for the discussion on benefit-risk evaluation in Chapter 3. Regulatory approval of the product requires clinical trial data. Chapter 4 discusses dose-escalation methods in phase I clinical trials to determine a safe effective dose, and safety considerations in the design of phase II and phase III clinical trials. It also describes statistical methods and regulatory requirements in the analysis of the safety data from these trials. Chapter 6 considers post-marketing safety data, first from phase III clinical trials and then from spontaneous adverse event reporting. The latter poses many challenging statistical issues, and Chapters 5 and 6 develop statistical methods to address them.

One issue is related to multiplicity because the range of possible adverse effects in clinical trials of a medical product that gains regulatory approval can be very large and new unanticipated effects are also possible when administered to a large population. This creates the potential for drawing false positive conclusions. Although recent advances in multiple testing can control the false positive rate, applying such control may delay the detection of serious adverse reactions to the product. Chapter 5 reviews these advances and highlights an empirical Bayes approach that combines domain knowledge about the pharmacological profile of the product and the physiologic categorization of adverse events with statistical modeling to strike a good balance between false alarm rate and wrong non-detection rate of true adverse reactions to the product. It also points out the major differences in hypothesis formulation and multiple testing between multiplicity considerations for efficacy and those for safety.

Another issue is that when post-marketing safety data come from non-experimental sources (as in spontaneous reporting rather than phase III randomized trials), there may be confounding covariates that cause the adverse events, and adjustments have to be made for causality analysis. Chapter 6 describes methods for such adjustments, including matching, stratification, and reweighting, together with recent developments in propensity scores and instrumental variables.

1.6.2 Safety databases and sequential surveillance in pharmacovigilance

Safety evaluation of a medical product proceeds beyond clinical trials and observational studies. Chapter 7 gives an introduction to pharmacovigilance based on large databases of adverse events, separately for drugs and vaccines, and health insurance claims databases. The methods in Chapters 3, 5, and 6 are extended and modified to develop statistical methods for the analysis of these data and for pharmacovigilance. Timely detection of adverse effects of medical products can result in regulatory measures to rectify the situation and prevent repeated harmful occurrences. Chapter 8 gives an overview of sequential detection and diagnosis and refinement of these methods for post-marketing safety surveillance. In particular, it is shown how propensity scores and other adjustments for confounding can be used to modify traditional sequential methods in the presence of confounding covariates.

1.6.3 An interdisciplinary approach and how the book can be used

As the preceding road map of the book has shown, medical product safety evaluation is a multifaceted subject that involves different disciplines, from pharmacology and medicine to data science and statistics, and which traverses industry, government, and academia. This book, whose authors come from both industry and academia, tries to capture such character. The authors combine their diverse professional experiences to put together what they believe to be the core of the subject for the target audience, whom we will describe below. The book is organized in such a way that different groups of readers can focus on different self-contained groups of chapters.

We first consider the target audience of students, from advanced undergraduates to Ph.D. students. A one-semester course giving an introduction to clinical trials and regulatory biostatistics can be taught out of Chapters 4, 5 and 8. Another one-semester course on data science and decision analytics has been taught out of Chapters 2, 3, 6 and 7. The book covers a wide range of areas in biostatistics, some of which are not included in the usual curriculum. Accordingly we have provided basic background material in the supplements at the end of each chapter, where we also include exercises for course assignments and team projects. For these courses, the book attempts to strike the delicate balance between methodological developments, especially those at the cutting edge of statistical science, and practical insights into how the methods work in practice and relate to data.

We next consider biostatisticians and data scientists in industry who have graduate degrees in these disciplines and who want to learn more about cutting-edge methodologies for safety evaluation and regulatory requirements. The book can become part of their arsenal of reference materials. Short courses and professional training programs which the authors have given provide important material that has been used as some of the building blocks of the book. As the regulatory underpinnings and methodological innovations may change over time, we use the website of the book to update the changes and advances and to continue enriching the training programs and professional short courses.

1.7 Supplements and problems

1. The science of safety is an interdisciplinary subject that requires experts with different professional backgrounds (basic science, clinical science, regulatory science, data science, statistics and epidemiology) to work together for planning and execution of a safety evaluation program, and for interpretation and communication of safety concerns at different levels (namely, compound level, program level, project or study level). Statisticians play a critical role throughout the process of safety evaluation and decision making regarding regulatory approval, product label, use restriction, and/or product withdrawal. The roles and responsibilities of a statistician can be defined at different levels listed below; see Crowe et al. (2009) and Chuang-Stein and Xia (2013) for related discussions.

(a) Trial level: A trial statistician should be familiar with the safety information of the compound, including safety data collected in preclinical studies and early-phase clinical trials, safety information of similar compounds in the same disease area, and safety requirements by regulatory agencies. Working with the trial team, the statistician plays an important role to define unambiguously major safety concerns, if any, that may be anticipated during the clinical trial and to analyze the safety data related to serious adverse events, non-serious adverse events, and adverse events of special interest. The statistician also contributes to the statistical sections of the Data and Safety Monitoring Committee charter for the trial.

(b) Program level: A compound may be studied in multiple clinical trials for a single disease or for diseases with similar etiologies and/or clinical manifestations. In addition to the safety information compiled from individual trials, the program statistician develops the strategies and statistical methods to combine safety data from multiple studies, e.g., methods for meta-analysis and how to interpret the results of the combined analysis. Before regulatory approval, the program statistician works with the program team to finalize the safety profile of the product.

(c) Compound level across multiple disease areas: When the compound has multiple indications across different disease areas, the compound statistician or lead program statistician is responsible for the collection, summarization, analysis, and communication of all the safety information relevant to the compound and provides necessary support for the safety profile update, regulatory commitment, and other related activities (e.g., new development program).

2. Several aspects need to be considered to characterize the *safety profile* of a product. In the product insert, safety information typically covers:

(a) referenced data sources and analysis methods: data sources used in the product label and statistical analysis methods used in safety data analysis;

(b) serious adverse events: summary of serious adverse events and their incidence rates, clinical explanations on possible association of the serious adverse events with the product;

(c) observed treatment-emergent adverse events: summary of treatment-emergent adverse events (TEAEs) and their incidence rates and confidence intervals on the incidence rates;

(d) drug-drug interactions: potential drug-drug interactions based on the chemical structure of the compound and literature reports on similar products;

    (e) special warnings and precautions for use, which are issued on the basis of biological outcome pathways of the compound in order to reduce the chance of adverse experience by the user, e.g., serious infections, immunosuppression, hypersensitivity;

    (f) abnormal laboratory results for hematology, hepatic transaminases, bilirubin, urinary testing;

    (g) adverse impact on special body systems and functions, including the reproductive system, renal function, and hepatic function;

    (h) use in vulnerable populations such as pediatric and geriatric populations, pregnant women, or women in lactation;

    (i) recommended treatment in case of overdose, and symptoms observed among overdosed patients;

    (j) nonclinical safety findings from *in vivo* and *in vitro* studies, especially those linked to acute toxicity, carcinogenicity, mutagenesis, impairment of fertility;

    (k) other pharmacophysiologiccal findings related to drug toxicity.

See Crowe et al. (2013) and FDA (2015a) for further discussion.

3. Chakravarty et al. (2016) discuss large-scale clinical trials for regulatory decision making, and give examples on how a trial can be designed to evaluate safety, saying: "For a trial designed to evaluate safety, the trial objective is typically to rule out some amount of excess risk by comparing the upper bound of the 95% confidence interval (CI) (two-sided) against some pre-specified risk margin." They argue that the risk margin should be set as the maximum acceptable risk which incorporates the background incidence of the adverse event, prior safety information of the investigational product, and public health impact of the adverse events and that "the choice of the risk margin is most commonly based on risk/benefit considerations, feasibility considerations, and/or past precedence." They also point out that "most clinical trials designed to evaluate safety are event-driven, meaning that the statistical information that determine the size of the trial is the number of events." This can be translated into the number of subjects if the background (or control group) event rate is available, for which a low incidence rate often results in a large clinical trial; see Vesikari et al. (2006).

4. *Exercise.* Consider a two-arm clinical trial with a fixed sample size to compare a treatment group with a control group in terms of a pre-specified event. The trial has an $r : 1$ randomization ratio, i.e., for every one subject randomized to the control group, there are r subjects randomized to the treatment group. Suppose that a logrank test is used to test the null hypothesis $H_0 : \phi = 1$ against $H_1 : \phi = \phi_1$ at

a significance level $\alpha = 0.05$ (two-sided), where ϕ is the hazard ratio between treatment and control and ϕ_1 the pre-defined hazard ratio at the alternative hypothesis. Read Schoenfeld (1983) for the background of logrank tests and their applications to censored survival data.

(a) Calculate the total number of events for both treatment and control groups that are required to achieve 90% power at $\phi_1 = 2, 4, 8$.

(b) Let λ_0 be the incidence rate of the event in the control group. Suppose that the trial has a one-year enrollment time followed by a one-year follow-up period during which 20% enrolled subjects are censored. Calculate the number of subjects that are required in (a) for $\lambda_0 = 20\%, 50\%$ per patient-year.

2

Biological Models and Associated Statistical Methods

The development of adverse drug reactions (ADRs) induced by xenobiotics and other substances is a complex process starting from initial interactions with chemical or biological agents, via pharmacological and physiological pathways, to early biological and pathological effects, and then to clinical effects and events. Park et al. (1998) classified ADRs, from clinical and pharmacopathological perspectives, into five types based on their mechanisms, frequency, predictability, and pharmacological actions. Type A includes ADRs that are predictable from known pharmacology, often representing an aggregation of primary and/or secondary pharmacological effects of an agent. These ADRs are usually dose-dependent and can be alleviated through dose reduction or removal of the agent, with hemorrhage caused by anticoagulants as one such example. Type B consists of ADRs which are believed to be metabolically and/or immunologically mediated and for which individual susceptibility factors that have not been fully understood may play an important role. These reactions are less common than those in Type A, and usually tend to be more serious, and account for many drug-induced mortalities, e.g., anaphylaxis, halothane hepatitis. Type C consists of ADRs whose biological characteristics can be predicted from the structure of the agent including its metabolites, as in acetaminophen (paracetamol) hepatotoxicity. Type D consists of ADRs that occur many years after initial interaction with the agent; examples include secondary tumors induced by chemotherapeutic agents and teratogenic effects (e.g., thalidomide with limb abnormalities and malformations of other organs including congenital heart disease). ADRs of type E, though uncommon, are drug withdrawal effects, e.g., myocardial ischemia after β-blocker withdrawal.

The majority of ADRs belonging to the above types can be predicted by the knowledge of dose exposure, pharmacokinetics-pharmacodynamics (PK-PD) models, the etiology of the ADR, human genetic susceptibility, etc.; see Helma (2005a) for the growing field of predictive toxicology which uses information about chemical structures and biological systems in mathematical and statistical models for prediction of toxic effects. With the goal of providing reliable, reproducible, time-saving and cost-effective approaches for assessing adverse effects that might be observed at late-stage drug development, predictive toxicology is built upon advances of multiple scientific disciplines including molecular, cellular, biological, and computational sciences, reflecting a complete shift from assessing adverse effects observed at experimental and clinical stages toward identifying and avoiding toxicity pathways at the molecular level (Helma et al., 2001; Mannhold et al., 2014). However, because of the complexity of biological interactions and unknown biochemical mechanisms, quantitative biological models that give more precise and accurate prediction of clinical adverse effects of an agent are yet to be developed in predictive toxicology (Fielden and Zacharewski, 2001; Suter et al., 2004; Knudsen et al., 2015; Benigni, 2016). Recent developments and applications can be found in Wilson (2011), Mannhold et al. (2014) and Benfenati (2016). In addition, a sixth type of ADRs has been added to include unexpected failures of treatments caused by inappropriate dosages (Hartigan-Go and Wong, 2000; Edwards and Aronson, 2000).

This chapter introduces biological models that connect chemical characteristics (e.g., structure, transport properties, metabolites, etc.) and biological systems (biomarkers, -omics, etc.) with ultimate clinical manifestation of adverse outcomes and statistical models to delineate the relationship between chemical structures and biological outcomes. The concepts, tools, and some regulatory framework of predictive toxicology are also discussed. We begin by describing in Section 2.1 the biological models and statistical methods to develop *quantitative structure-activity relationships*, which play a fundamental role in predictive toxicology when the (biological) "activity" is associated with toxicity of the compound. Toxicity endpoints and molecular descriptors are introduced, and modern statistical/machine learning methods for high-dimensional regression and classification, gradient boosting and deep learning, together with model validation, are described for such applications. Section 2.2 focuses on pharmacokinetic-pharmacodynamic models to quantify responses of human body to a drug, followed by Section 2.3 on statistical and machine learning methods for the analysis of preclinical safety data, particularly from carcinogenicity and reproductive and developmental toxicity studies, and then by Section 2.4 on predictive cardiotoxicity models and analyses. Section 2.5 gives an introduction to toxicogenomics and its role in predictive toxicology and Section 2.6 continues with regulatory guidelines for safety biomarker qualification and for models and data in predictive toxicology. Supplements and problems are given in Section 2.7.

2.1 Quantitative structure-activity relationship

Under the general principle that chemical features of a molecule define its biological behavior and that molecules with similar chemical structures produce similar biological activities, quantitative structure-activity relationships (QSAR) combine interdisciplinary knowledge of compounds (from chemistry, physics, biomedicine) with mathematical-statistical modeling for the prediction of biological activities (responses or endpoints) of molecules based on their chemical attributes and/or physiochemical properties (descriptors). The mathematical formulation of a QSAR model for a response Y has the form

$$Y = f(\mathbf{x}; \boldsymbol{\theta}), \tag{2.1}$$

where x is a vector of explanatory variables (descriptors) characterizing the chemical features of a compound that are believed to correlate with Y, and $\boldsymbol{\theta}$ is a vector of parameters representing the direction and magnitude of effect of x on Y. QSAR models enable one to predict the biological activities of a new or untested chemical and have many applications in toxicology (Perkins et al., 2003; Yousefinejad and Hemmateenejad, 2015). In drug development, they have played important roles in (a) the prediction of responses of structurally similar compounds including toxicity prediction, (b) reduction in the use of experimental animals, (c) screening of compounds for drug potential, (d) structural optimization of lead molecules to design purpose-specific chemicals, and (e) structural refinement of synthetic target molecules (Roy et al., 2015). Depending on the nature of the response variable Y, the QSAR is also called a quantitative structure-property relationship (QSPR) if Y represents a physiochemical property or quantitative structure-toxicity relationship (QSTR) if Y is associated with toxicity.

2.1.1 Toxicity endpoints

Some representative endpoints in QSAR predictive toxicology analysis comprise hepatotoxicity, nephrotoxicity, cardiotoxicity, developmental toxicity, carcinogenicity, genotoxicity, inhalation toxicity, dermal toxicity, eye irritation, and skin corrosion (Roy et al., 2015). Similar to clinical safety data, the data types of toxicity endpoints measured as biological activities of chemical compounds can be continuous, ordinal, categorical or dichotomous. For instance, IC50 (the concentration of a chemical at which the response or binding is reduced by half) and LC50 (the lethal concentration required to kill 50% of the target organism) are measured as continuous response variables, and carcinogenicity, mutagenicity and skin sensitization are measured as dichotomous response variables.

There is a large number of endpoints, including molecular initiating event (MIE), cellular response, and organ-specific response to clinical adverse outcomes for toxicity measures in the adverse outcome pathways (AOPs). The AOP framework is based on the concepts of "mechanism of action" (MoA) and "toxicity pathways" and facilitates integration of all types of information at different levels (from molecular to cellular, organ, organism, and population) of biological organization for prediction of adverse outcomes (Ankley et al., 2010). Willett et al. (2014), Villeneuve et al. (2014a), Vinken (2013) and Wittwehr et al. (2017) describe the principles and recent developments of the AOP framework and how it can be implemented in toxicology from research to regulation.

Villeneuve et al. (2014a) discuss three primary components of an AOP: MIE, key events (KEs), and adverse outcomes (AOs). The MIE defines the starting point at which a chemical directly interacts with biomolecules to produce a perturbation at molecular level. Ligand-receptor interactions and binding to proteins and nucleic acids are examples of MIE (Vinken, 2013). The KE is a measurable change in biological state that is essential to trigger progression from biological perturbation toward an AO of regulatory and public health concern and thus represents nodes in an AOP diagram. Vinken (2013) illustrates an AOP for chemical-induced liver steatosis in which the activation of liver X receptor serving as the MIE induces a number of intermediate transcriptional changes at the molecular level, e.g., activation of the expression of carbohydrate-response binding protein. All together, these intermediate changes drive the accumulation of triglycerides KE, which in turn evokes cytoplasm displacement, distortion of the nucleus and mitochondrial disruption, and ultimately leads to the appearance of fatty liver cells at cellular level and changes at the organ level (other KEs), and further to clinical liver steatosis at the individual organism level (AO). AOs should correspond to clinically meaningful and regulatorily concerned endpoints. Figure 2.1 illustrates AOPs from exposure to a toxicant, molecular interaction events, key events, or responses at cellular and organ levels, and adverse outcomes at the organism and population levels; see Ankley et al. (2010). Villeneuve et al. (2014a,b) introduce strategies and principles for AOP development and considerations for best practice in developing an AOP. Perkins et al. (2015) give examples on how an AOP can be developed from hypothesis-based and discovery-based approaches, and practical and regulatory applications of AOPs.

2.1.2 Molecular descriptors

Molecular descriptors of chemicals, which constitute a key component of the QSAR equation (2.1), are numerical values extracted by a well-defined algorithm for representation of a complex system, namely, the molecule; these numerical values carry specific information that is associated with

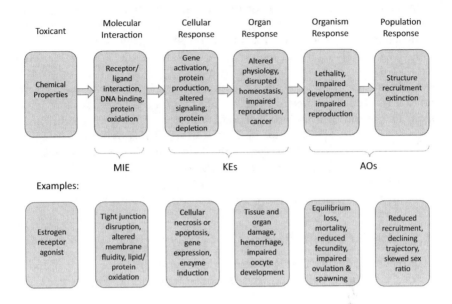

FIGURE 2.1 Illustration of adverse outcome pathways from exposure to a toxicant, molecular interaction event (MIE), key events (KEs) and adverse outcomes (AOs).

chemical or biological activities. The molecular descriptors are derived from chemistry, graph theory and information theory, discrete mathematics and topology, and are further processed using statistics, chemometrics, and chemoinformatics for use in QSAR and its variants. There are some desired properties of derived molecular descriptors, such as invariance to labeling of atoms and roto-translation, relevance to a broad class of compounds, structural interpretation of induced biological responses, etc. (Roy et al., 2015; Mauri et al., 2016).

There are several types of molecular descriptors reflecting various aspects of a chemical compound and different levels of its structural representation. Descriptors can be physicochemical (hydrophobic, steric, or electronic), structural, topological, or geometric, and are classified into three broad categories based on dimension, namely 1D, 2D and 3D descriptors. Descriptors derived from a partial list of structural fragments in a molecule are called 1D molecular descriptors, e.g., fragment counts, fingerprints. 1D descriptors can be easily calculated and interpreted, but hardly represent the topology of the chemical structure. 2D descriptors are the most popular descriptors derived from a two-dimensional topological representation of a molecule including connectivity of atoms in a molecule. 3D descriptors are derived from molecular geometric representation which adds the spatial information about atom positions to atom connectivity and in which every atom in a molecule is represented in terms of its three-dimensional coordinates. Examples of 3D descriptors are molecular volume, density, and surface area. Additional representation of a molecular structure can include dynamic properties (e.g., trajectory information of a molecule to reflect electron distribution and interactions), yielding 4D descriptors. Roy et al. (2015) provide summaries of the definition, classification, representation, and derivation of molecular descriptors as well as their roles in QSAR/QSTR modeling; T in QSTR refers to toxicological activity. More detailed information can be found in Todeschini and Consonni (2008, 2009) and Mauri et al. (2016).

2.1.3 Statistical methods

The purpose of QSAR/QSTR modeling is to quantify the impact of molecular descriptors on the measured response (endpoint) and then to use it to predict the toxicity effect or to screen compounds with similar molecular structures. Statistical methods for QSAR/QSTR modeling can be divided into two broad categories: regression-based methods for quantitative (continuous) endpoints and classification-based methods for qualitative endpoints; see Liaw and Svetnik (2015). With increasing availability of large amounts of data from clinical trials, spontaneous reporting databases, electronic healthcare records, and pharmacogenomics data, machine learning methods have become popular in safety data analysis. Here and in Section 2.7 we give an overview of these methods and their applications in QSAR/QSTR modeling. Machine learning methods can be broadly divided into three categories: *supervised learning, unsupervised learning*, and *reinforcement learning*. In supervised learning, a set of safety data with explanatory and outcome variables are provided to develop a functional relationship describing how the outcome variables are related to the explanatory variables. In unsupervised learning, the data contain no outcome variables and the aim is to cluster the objects (e.g., patients) based on their characteristics, as in cluster analysis, density estimation, discriminant analysis, and multidimensional scaling. Reinforcement learning is carried out sequentially with the aim of maximizing the total reward or minimizing the overall expected loss by continual learning and adaptation, as in Markov decision processes (Feinberg and Shwartz, 2002), multi-stage treatment optimization (Chakraborty and Moodie, 2013; Wallace et al., 2016), sequential experimentation in clinical trials, adaptive treatment strategies, and biomarker-guided personalized medicine (Lai and Liao, 2012; Lai et al., 2013; Bartroff et al., 2013). In the reminder of this section, we focus on recent developments in supervised learning. Supplement 2 in Section 2.7 describes other methods in machine learning.

Regularized high-dimensional linear regression. Multiple linear regression is one of the most commonly used methods in QSAR/QSTR modeling because of its ease of implementation and conceptual simplicity in relating the response Y_i to the molecular descriptors x_{ij} via

$$y_i = \beta_0 + \sum_{j=1}^{p} \beta_j x_{ij} + \epsilon_i; \tag{2.2}$$

see Benigni et al. (2000), Cash (2001), Helma (2005b), Mannhold et al. (2014) and Benfenati (2016) for concrete examples. The parameter vector $\beta = (\beta_0, \dots, \beta_p)^T$ can be easily estimated from a training sample $\{(\mathbf{X}_i, Y_i) : 1 \leq i \leq n\}$ by the method of least squares. When p is large, as is usually the case in toxicology studies, partial least squares (PLS), which assumes Y to be related to $\mathbf{X}$ through a much smaller number of latent factors, is often used to circumvent the difficulty; see Supplement 2 in Section 2.7, Geladi and Kowalski (1986), Wold et al. (2001), Roy and Roy (2009), Paliwal et al. (2010), Vinzi et al. (2010) and Hug et al. (2015). In the case $p \gg n$, the problem appears hopeless at first sight since it involves many more parameters than the sample size. The past two decades, however, have witnessed major advances in this problem, beginning with the observation that the regression function $f(x_1, \dots, x_p) = \beta_0 + \beta_1 x_1 + \dots + \beta_p x_p$ may still be estimable if the regression model is "sparse" and that many applications indeed involve sparse regression models. There are two major issues with estimating $\beta = (\beta_0, \dots, \beta_p)^T$ when $p \gg n$. The first is singularity of $\mathbf{X}^T \mathbf{X}$, noting that the n values $\beta^T \mathbf{x}_1, \dots, \beta^T \mathbf{x}_n$ cannot determine the p-dimensional vector β uniquely for $p > n$, where $\mathbf{X} = (x_{tj})_{1 \leq t \leq n, 1 \leq j \leq p}$ and $\mathbf{x}_i^T$ is the ith row vector of $\mathbf{X}$. Assuming the ϵ_i to be i.i.d. normal and using a normal prior $\beta \sim N(0, \lambda I)$ can remove such singularity since the posterior mean of β is the ridge regression estimator $\widehat{\beta}^{\text{ridge}} = (\mathbf{X}^T \mathbf{X} + \lambda I)^{-1} \mathbf{X}^T \mathbf{Y}$, where $\mathbf{Y} = (y_1, \dots, y_n)^T$. The posterior mean minimizes the penalized residual sum of squares $\|\mathbf{Y} - \mathbf{X}\beta\|^2 + \lambda \|\beta\|^2$, with the L_2-penalty $\|\beta\|^2 = \sum_{j=1}^{p} \beta_j^2$ and regularization parameter λ. The second issue with estimating β when $p \gg n$ is sparsity. Although the number of parameters is much larger than the sample size, one expects for the problem at hand that most of them are small and can be shrunk to 0. While the L_2-penalty does not lead to a sparse estimator $\widehat{\beta}^{\text{ridge}}$, the L_1-penalty $\sum_{j=1}^{p} |\beta_j|$ does. The minimizer $\widehat{\beta}^{\text{lasso}}$ of $\|\mathbf{Y} - \mathbf{X}\beta\|^2 + \lambda \sum_{j=1}^{p} |\beta_j|$, introduced by Tibshirani (1996), is called lasso (*least absolute shrinkage and selection operator*) because it sets some coefficients to be 0 and shrinks the others toward 0, thus performing both subset selection and shrinkage. Unlike ridge regression, $\widehat{\beta}^{\text{lasso}}$ does not have an explicit solution unless $\mathbf{X}$ has orthogonal columns, but can be computed by convex optimization algorithms. Zou and Hastie (2005) introduce the elastic net estimator $\widehat{\beta}^{\text{enet}}$ that minimizes a linear combination of L_1- and L_2-penalties:

$$\widehat{\beta}^{\text{enet}} = (1 + \lambda_2) \arg \min_{\beta} \left\{ \|\mathbf{Y} - \mathbf{X}\beta\|^2 + \lambda_1 \|\beta\|_1 + \lambda_2 \|\beta\|^2 \right\}, \qquad (2.3)$$

where $\|\beta\|_1 = \sum_{j=1}^p |\beta_j|$. The factor $(1 + \lambda_2)$ above is used to correct the "double shrinkage" effect of the naive elastic net estimator, which is Bayes with respect to the prior density proportional to $\exp\left\{-\lambda_2 \|\beta\|^2 - \lambda_1 \|\beta\|_1\right\}$. Note that (2.3), which is a compromise between the Gaussian prior (for ridge regression) and the double exponential prior (for lasso), is still a convex optimization problem. The choice of the regularization parameters λ_1 and λ_2 in (2.3), and λ in ridge regression or lasso, is carried out by k-fold cross-validation; see Section 2.1.4 and Hastie et al. (2009) for details. The R package glmnet can be used to compute $\widehat{\beta}^{\text{lasso}}$ and $\widehat{\beta}^{\text{enet}}$ and perform k-fold cross validation.

Since the non-convex optimization problem of minimizing

$$\left\{ \|\mathbf{Y} - \mathbf{X}\beta\|^2 + \lambda \sum_{j=1}^{p} I_{(\beta_j \neq 0)} \right\}, \qquad (2.4)$$

which corresponds to the L_0-penalty, is infeasible for large p, lasso is sometimes regarded as an approximation of (2.4) by a convex optimization problem. Ing and Lai (2011) recently introduced a fast stepwise regression method, called the *orthogonal greedy algorithm* (OGA), and used it in conjunction with a *high-dimensional information criterion* (HDIC) for variable selection along the OGA path. The method, which provides an approximate solution to the L_0-regularization problem, has three components. The first is the forward selection of input variables in a greedy manner so that the selected variables at each step minimize the residual sum of squares after ordinary least squares (OLS) is performed on it together with previously selected variables. This is carried out by OGA that orthogonalizes the included input variables sequentially so that OLS can be computed by component-wise linear regression, thereby circumventing matrix inversion; OGA is also called *orthogonal matching pursuit* in signal processing. The second component of the procedure is a stopping rule to terminate forward inclusion after K_n variables are included. The choice $K_n = O((n/\log p)^{1/2})$ is based on a convergence rate result reflecting the bias-variance trade-off in the OGA iterations, under the assumption $p = p_n \to \infty$ such that $\log p_n = o(n)$. The third component of the procedure is variable selection along the OGA path according to

$$\text{HDIC}(J) = n \log \hat{\sigma}_J^2 + \#(J) w_n \log p, \qquad (2.5)$$

where $J \subset \{1, \ldots, p\}$ represents a set of selected variables, $\hat{\sigma}_J^2 =$

$n^{-1} \sum_{i=1}^{n} (y_i - \hat{y}_{i;J})^2$ in which $\hat{y}_{i;J}$ denotes the fitted value of y_i when $\mathbf{Y}$ is projected into the linear space spanned by the column vectors $\mathbf{X}_i$ of $\mathbf{X}$, with $j \in J$, and w_n characterizes the information criterion used (e.g., $w_n = \log n$ for HDBIC, and $w_n = c$ for some constant c that does not change with n for HDAIC). Letting $\hat{J}_k = \{\hat{j}_1, \ldots, \hat{j}_k\}$ denote the set of selected variables up to the kth step of OGA iterations, Ing and Lai (2011) choose $\hat{k}_n = \arg\min_{1 \le k \le K_n} \mathrm{HDIC}(\hat{J}_k)$ and eliminate irrelevant variables $\hat{j}_l$ along the OGA path if $\mathrm{HDIC}(\hat{J}_{\hat{k}_n} - \{\hat{j}_l\}) > \mathrm{HDIC}(\hat{J}_{\hat{k}_n})$, $1 \le l \le \hat{k}_n$. The procedure is denoted by the acronym OGA+HDIC+Trim, which they showed to have the *oracle property* of being equivalent to OLS on an asymptotically minimal set of relevant regressors under a strong sparsity assumption.

AdaBoost and modified gradient boosting. AdaBoost was introduced by Freund and Schapire (1995) in the computational learning literature to combine "weak" learner from training data into much better performing classifiers, and immediately attracted much attention because of its superior performance over classification trees and other methods available those days. It spurred subsequent developments by the statistical learning community, leading to Breiman's bagging predictors and arcing classifiers (Breiman, 1996, 1998), Friedman, Hastie and Tibshirani's additive logistic regression approach to boosting (Hastie and Tibshirani, 1990), and Friedman's gradient boosting approach to function estimation (Friedman, 2001), which was motivated by applications to trees and other additive models in regression and classification. In high-dimensional nonlinear regression problems where the number of candidate base learners can be much larger than the sample size, the gradient boosting algorithm can be viewed as a stage-wise basis selection procedure, which uses steepest-descent minimization to handle nonlinearities in the basis functions so that each iteration of the algorithm selects a base learner that has the highest correlation with the current gradient vector.

Although convergence and consistency properties of AdaBoost and gradient boosting have been an active area of research in machine learning and high-dimensional regression, major convergence issues, particularly when to terminate the iterative algorithm, still remain to be addressed and a comprehensive theory is lacking. Gradient boosting in linear regression problems with squared error loss is called L_2-boosting by Bühlmann and Yu (2003), who study the bias-variance tradeoff as the number m of iterations increases when $(\mathbf{x}_1, y_1), \ldots, (\mathbf{x}_n, y_n)$ are i.i.d. Zhang and Yu (2005) prove the convergence of the population version of the boosting algorithm and use it to derive the convergence of an appropriately terminated sample version under certain sparsity and moment conditions. Bühlmann (2012) refines the argument further for the case $p = \exp(O(n^\xi))$ with $0 < \xi < 1$ and shows that for linear regression the conditional mean squared prediction error

$$\text{CPE} = E\left\{ \left[f(\mathbf{x}) - \hat{f}^m(\mathbf{x}) \right]^2 \mid y_1, \mathbf{x}_1, \ldots, y_n, \mathbf{x}_n \right\}, \qquad (2.6)$$

in which $\mathbf{x}$ is independent of $(\mathbf{x}_i, y_y)$ and has the same distribution as $\mathbf{x}_i$, converges in probability to 0 if $m = m_n \to \infty$ sufficiently slowly, but does not provide results on how slowly m_n should grow. Bühlmann and Hothorn (2007) consider several criteria for the choice of m_n, including cross-validation, a corrected version of AIC, and a gMDL criterion that bridges AIC and BIC, whereas Yao et al. (2007) propose another stopping rule. Thus, even in the simple case of linear regression with squared error loss, there are still no definitive results on the stopping rule of the iterative procedure. Lai et al. (2017) note that for linear regression models in which gradient boosting is also called a "pure greedy algorithm" (PGA) or "matching pursuit", a major difference between OGA and PGA is that at each iteration OGA selects a new input variable whereas PGA can select the same input variable in multiple iterations. Thus termination of OGA after m_n iterations implies inclusion of m_n regressors in the linear regression model whereas the number of regressors included in PGA after m_n iterations is unclear other than that it cannot be greater than m_n, contributing to the difficulties in analyzing PGA. For OGA, Ing and Lai (2011) have shown that optimal bias-variance tradeoff in high-dimensional sparse linear models entails that m_n should be $O((n/\log p_n)^{1/2})$, suggesting termination of the OGA iterations with $K_n = O((n/\log p_n)^{1/2})$ input variables, as we have already explained. This is followed by backward trimming along the OGA path by a high-dimensional information criterion (HDIC) to eliminate irrelevant variables that have entered in the forward greedy inclusion of variables, thereby coming up with an optimal rate of convergence of the overall procedure.

Central to the derivation of this optimal convergence rate result is a semi-population version of OGA that uses the same sequential variable selection procedure but assumes the corresponding parameters to be known. Another important tool used by Ing and Lai (2011) is an upper bound on the conditional mean squared prediction error (2.6) for weak orthogonal greedy algorithms due to Temlyakov (2000) that can be applied to analyze the semi-population version of OGA. By making use of moderate deviation bounds for the least squares estimates of the unknown regression coefficients in the sample version of the procedure, Ing and Lai (2011) derive the desired convergence rate from that of the semi-population version. For PGA, there is a corresponding Temlyakov bound for the semi-population version, which has been used in the aforementioned works of Bühlmann and Yu (2003) and Zhang and Yu (2005). However, because the same input variable can be used repeatedly in the PGA iterations, there are inherent difficulties in determining the number of iterations and deriving the convergence rate of PGA from the Temlyakov bound for the semi-population version of PGA. These difficulties become even more intractable for gradient boosting in regression models with nonlinear parameters in the basis functions. Lai et al. (2017) have recently modified Friedman's gradient boosting algorithm to circumvent these difficulties in additive expansion model $f(\mathbf{x}) = \alpha + \sum_{k=1}^{p} \beta_k \phi_k(\mathbf{x}; \mathbf{b}_k)$, in which ϕ_k is a basis function that involves a nonlinear parameter vector $\mathbf{b}_k \in \Gamma$ and is linearly associated with a regression coefficient β_k, and for general loss functions $L(Y_i, f(\mathbf{x}_i))$.

Friedman (2001) assumes $\alpha = 0$ and $\phi_k = \phi$ and his gradient boosting algorithm can be summarized by the following steps: (1) $\hat{f}^0(\mathbf{x}) = 0$; (2) for $k = 1, \ldots, m$, let (a) $\hat{u}_i^{k-1} = -\partial L/\partial f(Y_y, \hat{f}^{k-1}(\mathbf{x}_i))$, $i = 1, \ldots, n$, (b) $\hat{\mathbf{b}}_k = \arg\min_{\mathbf{b} \in \Gamma, \beta \in \mathbb{R}} \sum_{i=1}^{n} \left[\hat{u}_i^{k-1} - \beta\phi(\mathbf{x}_i, \mathbf{b}) \right]^2$, (c) $\hat{\beta}_k = \arg\min_\beta \sum_{i=1}^{n} L(Y_i, \hat{f}^{k-1}(\mathbf{x}_i) + \beta\phi(\mathbf{x}_i; \hat{\mathbf{b}}_k))$, (d) $\hat{f}^k(\mathbf{x}) = \hat{f}^{k-1}(\mathbf{x}) + \hat{\beta}_k\phi(\mathbf{x}; \hat{\mathbf{b}}_k)$; (3) output $\hat{f}^m(\cdot)$. Given the current estimate $\hat{f}^{k-1}$, Step 2(b) of gradient boosting adds a new basis function $\phi(\cdot; \hat{\mathbf{b}}_k)$ so that $\phi(\mathbf{x}_i; \hat{\mathbf{b}}_k)_{1 \le i \le n}$ is as close as possible to the negative gradient vector $(-\partial L/\partial f(Y_i, \hat{f}^{k-1}(\mathbf{x}_i)))_{1 \le i \le n}$, which represents the steepest descent direction. Step 2(c) chooses a step size $\hat{\beta}_k$ in this direction to minimize the loss $\sum_{i=1}^{n} L(Y_i, \hat{f}^{k-1}(\mathbf{x}_i) + \hat{\beta}_k\phi(\mathbf{x}_i; \hat{\mathbf{b}}_k))$. For the more general model $f(\mathbf{x}) = \alpha + \sum_{j=1}^{p} \beta_k\phi_k(\mathbf{x}; \mathbf{b}_k)$, Lai et al. (2017) first center $\mathbf{x}_i$ by $\mathbf{x}_i - \bar{\mathbf{x}}$, where $\bar{\mathbf{x}} = n^{-1} \sum_{i=1}^{n} \mathbf{x}_i$ and then modify Steps 2(b) and (c) to

$$(\hat{j}_k, \hat{\mathbf{b}}_k) = \arg \min_{1 \le j \le p, \mathbf{b} \in \Gamma, \beta \in \mathbb{R}} \sum_{i=1}^{n} \left[\hat{u}_i^{k-1} - \hat{\alpha}_{k-1} - \beta\phi_j(\mathbf{x}_i; \mathbf{b}) \right]^2, \quad (2.7)$$

$$(\hat{\alpha}_k, \hat{\beta}_k) = \arg \min_{\alpha, \beta \in \mathbb{R}} \sum_{i=1}^{n} L\left(Y_i, \hat{f}^{k-1}(\mathbf{x}_i) + \alpha + \beta\phi_{\hat{j}_k}(\mathbf{x}_i; \hat{\mathbf{b}}_k) \right), \quad (2.8)$$

and modify Step 2(d) to $\hat{f}^k(\mathbf{x}) = \hat{f}^{k-1}(\mathbf{x}) + \hat{\alpha}_k + \hat{\beta}_k\hat{\phi}_{\hat{j}_k}(\mathbf{x}; \hat{\mathbf{b}}_k)$, in which (2.8) first chooses the step size $\hat{\beta}_k$ with $\hat{\alpha}_{k-1}$ fixed as in (2.7) and then chooses the intercept α with β fixed at $\hat{\beta}_k$ Another important innovation by Lai et al. (2017) is in the application of "weak greedy algorithms" introduced by Temlyakov (2000), which they use to derive the stepwise selection procedure. Because backward elimination of variables following the OGA procedure of Ing and Lai (2011) entails re-computation of the minimization steps (2.7) with fewer variables and is therefore computationally expensive, Lai et al. (2017) incorporate the spirit of backward elimination into their modified gradient boosting (MGB) algorithm as follows. Basically the HDIC for linear regression used in backward elimination can be viewed as maximization of the likelihood up to a margin specified by the information criterion (IC), with preference given to models with fewer parameters within that IC margin. This suggests replacing the minimization definition of $(\hat{j}_k, \hat{\mathbf{b}}_k)$ in (2.7) by a weak greedy algorithm that chooses

$(\hat{j}_k, \hat{\mathbf{b}}_k)$ with the smallest number of iterations up to step $k-1$ among the $1 \leq j \leq p_n$ and $\mathbf{b} \in \Gamma$ that are within ϵ times the maximum squared correlation of $(\hat{u}_i^{k-1} - \hat{\alpha}_{k-1})_{1 \leq i \leq n}$ and $\phi_j(\mathbf{x}_i; \mathbf{b})_{1 \leq i \leq n}$.

As in OGA, the first stage of MGB stops at stage m when K_n distinct $\hat{j}_k$'s are included in the basis expansion. The second stage MGB continues the preceding procedure with j restricted to the K_n distinct $\hat{j}_k$'s until loss minimization in (2.8) is achieved with some tolerance. Lai et al. (2017) have developed an asymptotic theory of MGB, using the ideas of Ing and Lai (2011) and a reformulation of weak greedy algorithms together with an extension of Temlyakov's bound (Temlyakov, 2000) for the reformulation; central to this analysis is a semi-population version of MGB. Note that the basis functions $\phi_k(\mathbf{x}; \mathbf{b})$ feature in regression and classification trees and in neural networks. Gradient boosting has become a popular machine learning algorithm in building predictive QSAR / QSTR models. Svetnik et al. (2005) use it for predicting a compound's biological activity based on a quantitative description of the compound's molecular structure. Martin et al. (2006) develop robust classification rules by using stochastic gradient boosting for toxicity screening of hepatotoxic potential of human pharmaceutical compounds. Lampa et al. (2014) use a boosted regression tree to uncover complex interaction effects of toxicity, and Basant et al. (2016) use gradient boosting to develop decision tree models from a database comprising toxicity endpoints and relevant structural features of 334 chemical compounds for prediction of reproductive toxicity potential of diverse chemicals.

Neural networks. In artificial (machine) intelligence, neural networks (NN) refer to a computational architecture derived from a simplified concept of biological neural networks in which a number of nodes, called neurons, are interconnected. For QSTR applications, a typical NN consists of at least three layers: an input layer (molecular descriptors x_i), an output layer (toxicological endpoint y) and hidden layers between the input and output layers. The number of hidden layers and the number of neurons in each hidden layer are determined by the complexity of a particular problem under investigation. Each neuron is interconnected with other neurons in the next layer and the information passing through the neurons is determined by the weights that are calculated by algorithms that will be described later. Figure 2.2 illustrates a feedforward NN in which there is one input layer comprising x_1, x_2, x_3 and x_4, n hidden layers consisting of neurons $h_{11}, \ldots, h_{16}$ in the first hidden layer and $h_{n1}, \ldots, h_{n4}$ in the nth hidden layer, and one output layer with two output variables y_1 and y_2. In the feedforward NN, information for each neuron passes to every neuron in the next layer and then moves forward all the way to the output layer. We illustrate with a simple example using a training sample of size n, which consists of J descriptors in the input layer x_{ij}, one response variable y_i in the output layer and one hidden layer with H

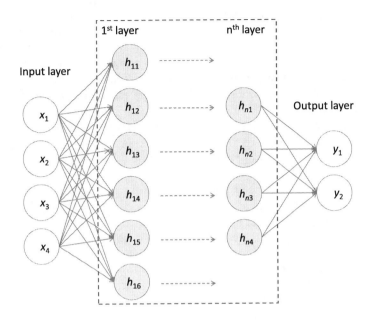

FIGURE 2.2 Illustration of feedforward neural network with n hidden layers.

neurons for the ith sample, $i = 1, \ldots, n; j = 1, \ldots, J$. The feedforward NN represents output y_i as a function of the input information x_{ij}

$$y_i = f\left(a_0 + \sum_{h=1}^{H} w_h f_h \left(a_h + \sum_{j=1}^{J} w_{hj} x_{ij}\right)\right) \qquad (2.9)$$

where $f_1, \ldots, f_H$ are prespecified functions, and the parameters (a_0, a_h and weights $w_h, w_{hj}, h = 1, \ldots, H$) are estimated by minimizing some loss function. Gradient descent, rather than the traditional Newton-Raphson method, is used to minimize the loss function. The "backpropagation" algorithm, which uses the chain rule of differentiation to iteratively compute the gradients of the weights for each layer, is combined with "minibatch gradient descent" which updates the network's parameters by applying gradient descent to a subset of the training data. The batch size and learning rate of the mini-batch procedure are called its hyperparameters of the procedure, whereas H and J in (2.9) are called hyperparameters of the NN model. Tuning these parameters suitably can improve performance; see Chapter 11 of Hastie et al. (2009) for details and examples. For large H, the network is called "deep."

Although Aoyama et al. (1990), Feng et al. (2003), Zhang et al. (2017) and others have found NNs of the type (2.9) useful and flexible to handle the complex nonlinearities in QSAR/QSTR models, difficulties in fitting these models and the tendency to overfit because of the large number of weights and parameters have been noted by Mosier and Jurs (2002), Baskin et al. (2009), Yee and Wei (2012) and others. There has been much recent progress, however, to address these difficulties in artificial intelligence using convolutional neural networks, with remarkable success in computer vision, speech recognition, natural language processing and drug discovery, but a comprehensive theory is still lacking.

Bagging and random forest. While AdaBoost and gradient boosting are sequential ensemble learning procedures, bagging is a parallel ensemble method, introduced by Breiman (1996), and applies the base learner to each bootstrap sample, which is drawn with replacement from the original dataset, therefore coming up with B classification or regression trees after B bootstrap samples are drawn; Supplement 2 in Section 2.7 provides the background for classification and regression trees (CART). We first explain bagging in the context of general regression problems, for which one applies regression to training sample $\mathbf{Z} = \{(\mathbf{x}_i, \mathbf{y}_i), 1 \leq i \leq n\}$ to derive a prediction $\hat{f}(\mathbf{x})$ of response at covariates $\mathbf{x}$. For each bootstrap sample $\mathbf{Z}_b^*$, $b = 1, \ldots, B$, fitting the regression model leads to the prediction $\hat{f}_b^*(\mathbf{x})$ and the "bagged" prediction is $\hat{f}_{\text{bag}}(\mathbf{x}) = B^{-1} \sum_{b=1}^{B} \hat{f}_b^*(\mathbf{x})$. In the case of regression trees, each bootstrap tree may involve features different from the original and may have a different number of terminal nodes. The bagged prediction is the average prediction (at $\mathbf{x}$) of the B trees.

For a classification tree that calculates a classifier $\hat{G}(\mathbf{x})$ at covariate $\mathbf{x}$ from the training sample $\mathbf{Z}$ in which y_i is a K-class response, we can regard $\hat{f}(\mathbf{x})$ as a vector-valued function with value 1 for the predicted class at $\mathbf{x}$ and value 0 for the remaining $K - 1$ classes. Then $\hat{f}_{\text{bag}}(\mathbf{x})$ is a K-dimensional vector whose kth component is the proportion of bootstrap trees predicting class k at $\mathbf{x}$. Moreover, the bagged classifier selects the class with the highest proportion, i.e., $\hat{G}_{\text{bag}}(\mathbf{x}) = \arg\max_{1 \leq k \leq K} \hat{f}_{\text{bag}}(\mathbf{x})$, which corresponds to the class with the "majority vote" by the B bootstrap trees. Supplement 2 in Section 2.7 provides the background for the majority voting characterization of Bayes classifiers.

Random forests, introduced by Breiman (2001), also use bootstrap resampling but modify the original bagging algorithm for selecting features (e.g., molecular descriptors in QSTR modeling) of the tree models. Because of the correlation of the trees from the B bootstrap samples, strong features (predictors of response in regression trees) tend to be selected by most of the trees. Random forests modify the bagging procedure by random selection of m features from a given set of M features at each node for determining the split in each tree, and the (unpruned) tree grows to maximum size when the tree learner stops further splitting. Concerning the selection of m, $m = \sqrt{M}$ is recommended for classification problems with M features and $m = M/3$ is recommended for regression problems with M predictors; see Hastie et al. (2009, p.592).

The idea of choosing a random subset of available decisions when splitting a node of a tree dated back to Amit and Geman (1997) for a single tree. In addition, Ho (1995, 1998) introduced the "random subspace method" for selecting a subset of features to use to grow each tree in a forest, and Dietterich (1998) introduced randomized node optimization for the decision at each node in constructing decision forests. Besides bagging, these are the precursors of random forests introduced in Breiman's seminal paper, which also describes the following method for measuring the importance of the features by making use of out-of-bag (OOB) estimates:

> Suppose there are M input variables (components of x). After each tree is constructed, the values of the mth variable in the out-of-bag examples are randomly permuted and the out-of-bag data is run down the corresponding tree. The classification given for each x_i that is out of bag is saved. This is repeated for $m = 1, \ldots, M$. At the end of the run, the plurality of out-of-bag class votes for x_i with the mth variable noised up is compared with the true class label of x_i to (estimate) the misclassification rate.

The OOB estimates are described in Appendix II of Breiman's paper. Hastie et al. (2009) explain the OOB error estimates in their Section 15.3.1 as follows: "For each observation $z_i = (x_i, y_i)$, construct its random forest prediction by averaging only those bootstrap trees in which z_i did not appear. (This) OOB error estimate is almost identical to that obtained by (leave-one-out) cross-validation (when the number of bootstrap trees is large). Hence unlike many other nonlinear estimates, random forest can be fit in one sequence, with cross-validation being performed along the way. Once the OOB error stabilizes (with the number of bootstrap trees, the training can be terminated", as illustrated in their Figure 15.4. Their Section 15.3.2 explains how "randomly permuting" the OOB sample values for the mth variable helps measure the importance of that variable, saying: "When the bth bootstrap tree is grown, the OOB samples are passed down the tree, and the prediction accuracy is recorded. Then the values for the mth variable are randomly permuted in the OOB samples, and the accuracy is again computed. The decrease in accuracy as a result of this permuting is averaged over all trees, and is used as a measure of the importance of the mth variable in the random forest." They note that "the randomization effectively voids the effect of a variable," much like how it works in linear regression shown in their Exercise 15.7:

Suppose we fit a linear regression model to n observations with response y_i and predictors $x_{i1}, \ldots, x_{iM}$; all variables are standardized to have mean 0 and standard deviation 1. Let RSS be the mean squared residual on the training data and $\hat{\beta}$ the vector of estimated regression coefficients. Denote by RSS* the mean squared residual on the training data using the same $\hat{\beta}$, but with the n values for the mth variable randomly permuted before the predictions are calculated. Show that $E_P(\text{RSS}^* - \text{RSS}) = 2\hat{\beta}_j^2$, where E_P denotes expectation with respect to the permutation distribution. Argue that this is approximately true when the evaluations are done using an independent test set.

Hastie et al. (2009) also describe open-source software implementation of random forest. It should be noted that in 2001 (at the dawn of big data era) Breiman's paper anticipated the "large M relative to n" issues that we have described above in connection with high-dimensional linear regression. In particular, the paper notes that "important recent problems, i.e., medical diagnosis and document retrieval, often have the property that there are many input variables, often in the hundreds or thousands, with each one containing only a small amount of information," hence the importance of selecting a manageable number of features (input variables). The paper also discusses the "dual role of correlation and strength" played by random forests in variable selection and Breiman's view that the sequential ensemble method AdaBoost "is emulating a random forest" in the later stages of its iterative scheme. Svetnik et al. (2003) give an overview of random forests and their application to QSAR modeling. Polishchuk et al. (2009) applied random forest approach to QSAR analysis of aquatic toxicity of chemical compounds tested on *Tetrahymena pyriformis*; Liaw and Svetnik (2015) demonstrated the utility of random forest and stochastic gradient boosting in predicting biological toxic activities from chemical structures.

2.1.4 Model validation

QSAR/QSTR models need to be validated for generalizability of the models' predicted toxicological response based on the molecular descriptors of the compound. Their validation should take into account both scientific validity (e.g., unambiguous algorithm, interpretable mechanism, domain applicability) and statistical measures of goodness-of-fit and predicttiveness (Gramatica, 2007; Roy and Mitra, 2011). Using models fitted by multiple linear regression and PLS regression as examples, Veerasamy et al. (2011) emphasize the importance of validation and outline strategies for both internal and external validation. Roy and Mitra (2011), Yousefinejad and Hemmateenejad (2015) and Gramatica and Sangion (2016) describe the metrics and terminologies used for statistical validation of QSAR/QSTR models. It is generally believed that the QSAR/QSTR models that have been appropriately validated externally can be considered practically reliable for both scientific and regulatory purpose (Tong et al., 2004; Roy and Mitra, 2011).

Internal validation. Internal validation of QSAR/QSTR models refers to a cross-validation process in which data from each compound contribute to both the training set and the test set, as in K-fold, or leave-K-out (LKO), cross-validation in which the model is constructed using data from $c - K$ compounds and validated using data from K compounds. To illustrate, consider leave-one-out (LOO) cross-validation. Let y_i be the toxicological response for the ith compound and $\hat{y}_i$ be the predicted value of y_i using the compound's molecular descriptors $\mathbf{x}_i = (x_{i1}, \ldots, x_{ip})$ and model parameters estimated using data from the remaining $c - i$ compounds. The process repeats c times until the predicted value $\hat{y}_i$ is estimated for each of the c compounds in the data set. The predictive coefficient of determination for the test set is given

$$Q^2_{\text{LOO}} = 1 - \frac{\sum_{i=1}^{c} \left(y_i - \hat{y}_i\right)^2}{\sum_{i=1}^{c} \left(y_i - \bar{y}^{(-i)}\right)^2} \tag{2.10}$$

where $\bar{y}^{(-i)} = \frac{1}{n} \sum_{j \neq i} y_j$ is the sample mean of y_j's for the c compounds without the ith one in the training set. A higher value of Q^2_{LOO} suggests a better model for prediction of toxicological response.

External validation. Unlike internal validation where data for every compound contribute to both the training and test sets, external validation requires data from each compound to be used only in the training set or test set for model validation, as in the holdout method that partitions the entire data set randomly into two subsets s_0 for training and s_1 for validation; the random partition uses the range of toxicological responses or that of molecular descriptors (Roy and Mitra, 2011). The predictive coefficient of determination for the test set is

$$Q^2_{\text{Ext}} = 1 - \frac{\sum_{i \in s_1} \left(y_i - \hat{y}_i\right)}{\sum_{i \in s_1} \left(y_i - \bar{y}_0\right)} \tag{2.11}$$

where $\bar{y}_0 = \frac{1}{|s_0|} \sum_{i \in s_0} y_i$ and $|s_0|$ denotes the number of compounds in the training set, for which (2.10) is an internal validation analog by using cross-validation. Schüürmann et al. (2008) show that using $\bar{y}_0$ in (2.11) over-estimates the prediction capability that is triggered by the difference between the training and test set activity means, and hence propose to use $\bar{y}_1 = \frac{1}{|s_1|} \sum_{i \in s_1} y_i$ instead of $\bar{y}_0$.

Validation of classification models. Validation of classification models basically involves evaluation of misclassification rates that can be estimated according to the scheme of dividing the original data into training

TABLE 2.1 Number of compounds with true and predicted classes.

Predicted	True state		
	Toxic	Non-Toxic	Total
Toxic	n_{11}	n_{01}	$n_{.1}$
Non-Toxic	n_{10}	n_{00}	$n_{.0}$
Total	$n_{1.}$	$n_{0.}$	n

and test sets. For example, consider external validation of a classification problem in which a compound is classified as either toxic or non-toxic. Let $n_{1.}$ and $n_{0.}$ denote the number of compounds that are actually toxic and non-toxic, respectively, and n_{11} and n_{00} the number of compounds that are correctly classified as toxic and non-toxic using a classification model; see Table 2.1. The sensitivity of the predictive model is $n_{11}/n_{1.}$ and its specificity is $n_{00}/n_{0.}$. The predictive accuracy is $\rho = (n_{01} + n_{10})/n$ and the misclassification rate is $1 - \rho$. Commonly used measures for external validation of classification models are (a) the harmonic mean of sensitivity and predictive positive value (defined as $n_{11}/n_{.1}$), (b) the kappa coefficient

$$\kappa = 1 - \frac{1 - \rho}{1 - p_e} \qquad (2.12)$$

of Cohen (1960), where $p_e = n_{1.}n_{.1}/n^2 + n_{0.}n_{.0}/n^2$ is the expected chance of agreement between the predicted and true states, and (c) Matthews' correlation coefficient $(n_{11}n_{00} - n_{01}n_{10})/\sqrt{n_{1.}n_{0.}n_{.1}n_{.0}}$; see Gorodkin (2004) who also gives its generalization to multi-class classification.

2.2 Pharmacokinetic-pharmacodynamic models

Whereas QSAR/QSTR models are concerned with the relationship between chemical structures measured by molecular descriptors and safety outcomes through AOPs, pharmacokinetic-pharmacodynamic (PK-PD) models are used to quantify responses of the human body to a drug through a concentration-response profile. PK-PD models are based on the assumptions that the magnitude of response (in particular, toxic response in the safety context) depends on drug concentration at the effect site.

The first phase in PK-PD modeling consists of a PK model that describes the time course of drug concentration in plasma or blood, as a proxy of concentration at the effect site, after administration during which the processes of drug absorption, distribution, metabolism, and elimination (ADME) are investigated. The premise for PK modeling is that the human body consists of multiple compartments and drug movement between compartments can be described by mathematical models. For example, drug concentration $C(t)$ in blood plasma at time t in a one-compartment model can be written as a function of the amount of drug in plasma at time t, denoted by $A(t)$, the volume V of the compartment, fractional rate k_a of absorption and k_e of elimination (Davidian, 2009):

$$C(t) = \frac{A(t)}{V} = \frac{k_a D F}{V(k_a - k_e)} \left[\exp(-k_e t) - \exp(-k_a t) \right], \qquad (2.13)$$

in which D denotes the amount of drug at time $t = 0$ at an absorption site and F denotes the bioavailability of the system. The elimination rate k_e is often expressed by $k_e = Cl/V$, where Cl represents clearance in terms of the volume of blood being "cleared" of the drug per unit time. The PK parameter vector $\theta = (k_a, V, Cl)$ is estimated at both the population and individual levels by using mixed effects models; see Bartroff et al. (2013), Bonate (2011) and Davidian (2009).

The second phase in PK-PD modeling consists of a PD model that describes the relationship between drug concentration at the effect site and therapeutic effects, which can be either efficacy effects or adverse effects or both. Bonate (2011) describes linear, log-linear, *Emax*, and sigmoidal PD models, the most popular of which is the *Emax* model

$$E(t) = E_0 + \frac{E_{\max} - E_0}{1 + C_{50}/C(t)}, \qquad (2.14)$$

where $E(t)$ denotes the response (toxic effect) at concentration $C(t)$ of time t, E_0 the response at zero (baseline) concentration, $E_{\max}$ the maximum response, and C_{50} the concentration generating 50% of $E_{\max}$. The PD parameter vector is $\lambda = (E_0, E_{\max}, C_{50})$. Putting PK and PD models together, one can design dosing regimens for concentrations that target desired therapeutic effects.

We next consider fitting PK-PD models. Let Y_{ij}^{PK} be the PK response variable for subject i at time t_{ij} and $\boldsymbol{Y}_i^{PK} = \{Y_{ij}^{PK} : j = 1, \ldots, n_i\}$, $i = 1, \ldots, N$. Let Z_{ik} be the kth covariate (e.g., dose received) for subject i and $\boldsymbol{Z}_i = \{Z_{ik} : k = 1, \ldots, K\}$. Let R_{il} be the lth covariate for the ith subject that does not change during the entire observation time, e.g., age in years, gender, and let $\boldsymbol{R}_i = \{R_{il} : l = 1, \ldots, L\}$ be "between-subject" covariates that are relevant only to how individual subjects differ but are not required to describe the response versus time relationship at the subject level. Letting $\boldsymbol{X}_i = (\boldsymbol{Z}_i, \boldsymbol{R}_i)$, the subject-specific PK models have the form

$$Y_{ij}^{PK} = m(t_{ij}, \boldsymbol{Z}_i, \boldsymbol{\theta}_i) + \epsilon_{ij}^{PK}, \qquad (2.15)$$

where $E(\epsilon_{ij}^{PK} | \boldsymbol{Z}_i, \boldsymbol{\theta}_i) = 0$ and $\boldsymbol{\theta}_i$ is the subject-specific PK parameter vector modeled by

$$\boldsymbol{\theta}_i = d(\boldsymbol{R}_i, \boldsymbol{\beta}, \boldsymbol{b}_i), \qquad (2.16)$$

a mixed effects model in which d is an r-dimensional function describing the relationship between θ_i and R_i, with parameter β associated with the fixed effects and with random effects b_i across subjects; see Davidian (2009) who also provides details of fitting PD models of the form similar to (2.16):

$$Y_{ij}^{PD} = \mu\left(m(t_{ij}, \boldsymbol{Z}_i, \boldsymbol{\theta}_i), \boldsymbol{\lambda}_i\right) + \epsilon_{ij}^{PD}. \qquad (2.17)$$

2.3 Analysis of preclinical safety data

Preclinical databases play an increasingly important role in safety evaluation. Statistical/machine learning approaches have been applied to these databases, e.g., Ring and Eskofier (2015) who use the US National Toxicology Program (NTP) database to identify patterns for the incidence of liver tumors, Festing (2014) who compares sub-acute toxicity effects among nine published studies, Vesterinen et al. (2014) who carry out meta-analysis of data from multiple animal studies, and Hothorn (2014) who reviews some commonly used statistical methods in toxicological studies and provides details on related software packages.

2.3.1 Carcinogenicity

Carcinogenicity studies represent one of the key components in toxicology assessment for exposure to agents with respect to tumor formation. In these studies, animals are given doses that are well above human exposure level, in order to observe the carcinogenicity effect within a short period of time in a relative small number of animals (e.g., 50-60 rats or mice) that are randomly allocated to several groups including a control group and treatment groups at multiple dose levels of a compound. Scheduled interim sacrifices take place during the experiment and at the end of the study when all surviving animals are sacrificed and subjected to necropsy. There are several statistical issues in the analysis of these experimental data. First, animals may die before tumors are formed and/or observed, and the cause of death may be difficult to ascertain. Second, animals living longer usually have a higher probability of developing tumors than those dying earlier. Third, tumors may or may not be lethal. In addition, tumor onset time is usually unknown and premature death from non-tumor cause prevents later development of tumors; see FDA (2001) and Hothorn (2014) for more discussion. Tumors can be classified as *incidental*, *fatal*, and *mortality independent*. Tumors that do not directly or indirectly cause the death of animals but are merely observed at autopsy are called *incidental*. Tumors that are directly or indirectly responsible for the death of animals are said to be *fatal* or *lethal*. Tumors (such as skin tumors) that are detected at times other than when the animal dies are called *mortality independent*.

TABLE 2.2 Count data for incidental tumors by time interval.

Time Interval	Outcome	Dose group 1	$\cdots$	I	Total
1	With tumors	y_{11}	$\cdots$	y_{I1}	$y._1$
	Without tumors	$n_{11} - y_{11}$	$\cdots$	$n_{I1} - y_{I1}$	$n._1 - y._1$
	Total deaths	n_{11}	$\cdots$	n_{I1}	$n._1$
$\vdots$	$\vdots$	$\vdots$	$\vdots$	$\vdots$	$\vdots$
j	With tumors	y_{1j}	$\cdots$	y_{Ij}	$y._j$
	Without tumors	$n_{1j} - y_{1j}$	$\cdots$	$n_{Ij} - y_{Ij}$	$n._j - y._j$
	Total deaths	n_{1j}	$\cdots$	n_{Ij}	$n._j$
$\vdots$	$\vdots$	$\vdots$	$\vdots$	$\vdots$	$\vdots$
J	With tumors	y_{1J}	$\cdots$	y_{IJ}	$y._J$
	Without tumors	$n_{1J} - y_{1J}$	$\cdots$	$n_{IJ} - y_{IJ}$	$n._J - y._J$
	Total deaths	n_{1J}	$\cdots$	n_{IJ}	$n._J$

Peto (1974) and Peto et al. (1979) have proposed the following method for the analysis of incidental tumors. Let n_{ij} be the number of animals in group i that die during time interval j from causes unrelated to the presence of tumor of interest, and y_{ij} be the number of animals with observed tumors in the incidental category, $i = 1,\ldots,I$ and $j = 1,\ldots,J$. Let $n._j = \sum_{i=1}^I n_{ij}$ and $y._j = \sum_{i=1}^I y_{ij}$; see Table 2.2. Let $p_{ij} = y_{ij}/n_{ij}$ be the proportion of animals with tumors in the ith group of the jth interval. Then under the null hypothesis of no treatment effect across multiple treatment groups, the expected number of tumors for the ith group of the jth interval is $E_{ij} = p_{ij}y._j$. Let $D_{ij} = y_{ij} - E_{ij}$. The covariance of D_{i_1j} and D_{i_2j} is given by

$$\text{Cov}\,(D_{i_1j}, D_{i_2j}) = \kappa_j p_{i_1j}(\delta_{i_1i_2} - p_{i_2j}) = V_{i_1,i_2;j}, \qquad (2.18)$$

where $\kappa_j = y._j(n._j - y._j)/((n._j - 1))$, and $\delta_{i_1i_2} = 1$ if $i_1 = i_2$ and 0 otherwise. Let $n_i. = \sum_{j=1}^J = n_{ij}$, $E_i. = \sum_{j=1}^J = E_{ij}$, $V_{i_1,i_2} = \sum_{j=1}^J V_{i_1,i_2;j}$ and d_i be the dose level of the ith group. Under the null hypothesis, the test statistic

$$Z_P = \frac{\sum_{i=1}^I d_i(n_i. - E_i.)}{\sqrt{\sum_{i_1=1}^I \sum_{i_2=1}^I d_{i_1} d_{d_2} V_{i_1,i_2}}} \qquad (2.19)$$

follows approximately a standard normal distribution.

For fatal tumors that cause the death of animals, a similar method can be used if the time interval is divided into J subintervals according to each time of tumor death. For the analysis of data with unknown cause of death, the Cochran-Armitage test (Cochran, 1954; Armitage, 1955) is often used to test for a linear trend in the proportions of animals with tumors across dose levels. Let n_i be the number of deaths in the ith treatment group at dose level d_i, and let y_i be the number of animals with observed tumors in the ith group. Let $y = \sum_{i=1}^{I} y_i$, $n = \sum_{i=1}^{I} n_i$, and $p_i = n_i/n$. Then under the null hypothesis, the expected number of animals with tumors in the ith group is given by $E_i = yp_i$. Let

$$ U = \sum_{i=1}^{I} d_i(y_i - E_i), \ \bar{d} = \frac{1}{n} \sum_{i=1}^{I} n_i d_i, \text{ and } V = \frac{y(n-y)}{n(n-1)} \sum_{i=1}^{I} n_i(d_i - \bar{d})^2. $$

$$ (2.20) $$

Under the null hypothesis, V is a consistent estimate of the variance of U, and the Cochran-Armitage test statistic $Z_{CA} = U/\sqrt{V}$ is approximately standard normal. An implicit assumption of the Cochran-Armitage test is equal risk of developing tumors across the dose groups over the study duration. To adjust for the differences in tumor rates among dose groups, Bailer and Portier (1988) propose a poly-k test that replaces n_i in the Cochran-Armitage test statistic by the number n_i^* of animals at risk for the ith dose group defined by

$$ n_i^* = \sum_{j=1}^{n_i} \omega_{ij}, \text{ where } \omega_{ij} = \begin{cases} 1 \text{ if a death with tumor occurs,} \\ (t_{ij}/t_{\max})^k \text{ otherwise,} \end{cases} \quad (2.21) $$

in which t_{ij} is the time when a tumor-free animal i dies, $t_{\max}$ is the time of terminal sacrifice, and k is suggested to be 3 or 6 (for a polynomial of order 3 or 6). Instead of fixing k in advance, Moon et al. (2003) propose to estimate k by equating the empirical lifetime tumor incidence rate (obtained from the data by using a fractional weighting scheme) to a separately estimated cumulative lifetime tumor incidence rate. They also propose a bootstrap-based age-adjusted improvement of the poly-k test.

2.3.2   Reproductive and developmental toxicity

Reproductive and developmental toxicity refers to toxic effects of a compound on the reproductive and developmental functions of animals and/or humans. FDA guidance on reproductive and developmental toxicology (FDA, 2011c) categorizes the toxicity into two broad classes, namely the class of reproductive (parental) toxicity which includes fertility of male and female, parturition and lactation, and the class of developmental (embryonic or fetal) toxicity which consists of mortality, dysmorphogenesis, developmental alterations and functional impairment. Consequently, the endpoints for reproductive toxicity include body weight and weight gain, fertility index, gestation length, and sperm count, while the endpoints for developmental toxicity consist of malformation, fetal weight and length, number of fetuses, survival rate; see Parker and Hood (2006) and Tyl and Marr (2006) for further details. Hothorn (2014) points out several special features in the statistical analysis of developmental toxicity data. First, correlated binary data (e.g., fetal death, malformation) can arise within a litter. Second, the dose-response relationship may include multiple endpoints, some of which are continuous (e.g., birth weight) while others are discrete. Third, experimental units such as birth rate cannot be randomized; instead, the experimental design should randomly assign pregnant females to different dose groups. In addition, confounding variables may also affect the outcome, e.g., a larger litter size may reduce the birth weight.

Correlated binary and trivariate outcomes within litters. Consider the analysis of a binary toxicity endpoint, such as the malformation or death of fetuses in a litter. Let Y_{ijk} be the binary outcome (e.g., death or malformation) for the kth fetus in the jth litter and ith dose group consisting of n_{ij} fetuses, $i = 1, \ldots, I$, $j = 1, \ldots, n_i$, and $k = 1, \ldots, n_{ij}$. Let $Y_{ij} = \sum_{k=1}^{n_{ij}} y_{ijk}$ be the total number of toxic responses and $p_{ij} = Y_{ij}/n_{ij}$ be the corresponding proportion of response in the jth litter and the ith dose group. Then, Y_{ij} follows a binomial distribution: $Y_{ij} \sim Bin(n_{ij}, p_{ij})$. Williams (1975) uses a random effects approach that assumes p_{ij} to vary among litters within the ith dose group according to a beta distribution $Beta(a_i, b_i)$. The resultant distribution of Y_{ij} is a beta-binomial distribution with density function

$$P\{Y_{ij} = y_{ij}\} = \binom{n_{ij}}{y_{ij}} \frac{B(a_i + y_{ij}, b_i + n_{ij} - y_{ij})}{B(a_i, b_i)}, \tag{2.22}$$

where $a_i > 0$, $b_i > 0$, $B(c_1, c_2) = \Gamma(c_1)\Gamma(c_2)/\Gamma(c_1+c_2)$ and $\Gamma(\cdot)$ is the gamma function. Let $\mu_i = a_i/(a_i + b_i)$ be the mean of the beta distribution. Then the mean and variance of Y_{ij} are

$$E(Y_{ij}) = n_{ij}\mu_i, \quad \text{Var}(Y_{ij}) = n_{ij}\mu_i(1 - \mu_i)\left[1 + (n_{ij} - 1)\phi_i\right], \tag{2.23}$$

where $\phi_i = 1/(a_i + b_i + 1) = \text{Cov}(y_{ijk_1}, y_{ijk_2})$ is the intra-litter correlation coefficient; see Catalano and Ryan (1994) and Chen (2005) who also uses logistic regression to model the increasing toxicity over doses. Chen et al. (1991) extend the beta-binomial distribution for Y_{ij} to a Dirichlet-trinomial distribution for (X_{ij}, Y_{ij}, Z_{ij}), where X_{ij}, Y_{ij}, and Z_{ij} denote respectively the number of deaths, malformations, and normal births. The probabilities p_{ij}, q_{ij} and r_{ij} of these events for the jth litter and the ith dose group (so that $p_{ij} + q_{ij} + r_{ij} = 1$) are assumed to follow a Dirichlet distribution with density function

$$g(p, q, r) = \frac{\Gamma(a_i + b_i + c_i)}{\Gamma(a_i)\Gamma(b_i)\Gamma(c_i)} p^{a_i - 1} q^{b_i - 1} r^{c_i - 1}. \tag{2.24}$$

Then the distribution of (X_{ij}, Y_{ij}, Z_{ij}), conditional on $X_{ij} + Y_{ij} + Z_{ij} = n_{ij}$, is a Dirichlet-trinomial distribution

$$f(x_{ij}, y_{ij}, z_{ij}) = \frac{n_{ij}! \Gamma(a_i + b_i + c_i) \Gamma(a_i + x_{ij}) \Gamma(b_i + y_{ij}) \Gamma(c_i + z_{ij})}{x_{ij}! y_{ij}! z_{ij}! \Gamma(a_i + b_i + c_i + n_{ij}) \Gamma(a_i) \Gamma(b_i) \Gamma(c_i)}. \quad (2.25)$$

Ryan and Molenberghs (1999) use a multivariate exponential family for multivariate binary outcomes which arise when each fetus in a litter is assessed for presence of multiple outcomes, e.g., death/resoprtion, malformation, low birth weight. The proposed model allows the response rates to depend not only on the dose level but also on the cluster size.

Characterizing the relationship between toxic response and dose levels. Under the beta-binomial distribution (2.22) for the number of toxic responses within a litter, the probability of toxic response at dose d_i is given by $P(d_i) = \mu_i = a_i/(a_i + b_i)$. The following models have been used to fit $P(d_i)$ directly:

- probit model: $P(d_i) = \Phi(\beta_0 + \beta_1 d_i)$,

- logit model: $P(d_i) = [1 + \exp(-\beta_0 + \beta_1 d_i)]^{-1}$,

- extreme value model: $P(d_i) = 1 - \exp[-\exp(-\beta_0 - \beta_1 d_i)]$,

- Weibull model: $P(d_i) = 1 - \exp(-\beta_0 - \beta_1 d_i^\omega)$,

where $\omega > 0$ brings more flexibility in the shape of the dose-response curve, which Hunt and Li (2006) propose to model nonparametrically by using regression splines.

2.4 Predictive cardiotoxicity

Cardiotoxicity refers to toxic effects on the heart that cause electrophysiological perturbation (e.g., QT interval prolongation, arrhythmias, polymorphic ventricular tachycardia) and/or structural changes (e.g., ischemia, cardiomyopathies) that may eventually lead to heart failure and/or sudden death (Braña et al., 2013; Yeh et al., 2014; López-Fernández and Thavendiranathan, 2017), and is one of the leading causes for drug attrition during preclinical and clinical development (Ferri et al., 2013), accounting for approximately 20% to 45% of drug withdrawal from market due to safety reasons (Ferri et al., 2013; Onakpoya et al., 2016). The FDA, together with Cardiac Safety Research Consortium and Health and Environmental Science Institute, held a Think Tank meeting on July 23, 2013, which concluded with a new paradigm for assessing cardiac safety during drug development. This paradigm, called the Comprehensive in vitro Proarrythmia Assay (CiPA), basically includes three components: (a) characterization of drug electrophysiological effects on multiple human cardiac ionic channels in heterologous expression systems, (b) application of *in silico* models to reconstruct human cellular ventricular action potential and early after-depolarization and repolarization instability, and (c) confirmation of the electrophysiological effects using human stem cell-derived cardiomyocytes (hSC-CMs); see Ferri et al. (2013) and Sun (2016). The FDA also initiated the CiPA project for validating hSC-CM technology for better predictive assessment of drug-induced cardiac toxicity (Turner et al., 2017). The CiPA paradigm, together with careful evaluation of drug effects on electrophysiological conduction in phase I studies (e.g., QT/QTc intervals), is expected to provide better prediction of drug cardiotoxicity potential.

2.4.1 Comprehensive in vitro Proarrythmia Assay (CiPA)

Proarrhythmic risk is mostly evaluated by using nonclinical *in vitro* human models based on pathophysiological mechanisms of Torsades de Pointes (TdP) proarrhythmias (Ferri et al., 2013). Two regulatory guidelines, i.e., ICH S7B and ICH E14, provide recommendations for studies of drug effects on the electrophysiological system of the heart. The ICH S7B (ICH, 2005b) recommends an *in vitro* assay to assess whether a compound and its metabolites block the potassium channel encoded by the human *ether-à-go-go* related gene (hERG), while the ICH E14 guideline (ICH, 2005a) describes the design, conduct, analysis, and interpretation of specific clinical studies called the "Thorough QT studies" (TQT) that are designed to assess the potential of a drug to delay cardiac repolarization as measured by corrected QT (QTc) interval prolongation on the surface of the electrocardiograph. The TQT is used to evaluate whether the drug has a threshold effect on QTc prolongation that is determined by the upper bound of the 95% confidence interval for the maximum time-matched mean effect on QTc of 10 milliseconds. Vicente et al. (2016) point out that after the implementation of ICH S7B and ICH E14 guidelines, no new marketed drugs have been identified to be associated with an unacceptable risk of polymorphic ventricular tachycardia. On the other hand, undue focus on hERG and QTc has resulted in drugs being inappropriately dropped from further development, because not all drugs that block the hERG potassium channel or prolong QTc interval cause TdP (Stockbridge et al., 2013). Vicente et al. (2016) give examples of marketed drugs that block hERG potassium channel and prolong QTc interval but have minimal risk of TdP because they also block additional inward currents. They comment that the hERG-QTc prolongation screening assays might be too sensitive for detection of drugs with TdP potential and hence lack the specificity of prediction for the screening of drugs that may actually not cause TdP.

Ion channels and QTc prolongation. Advances of cardiac electrophysiology have clarified the mechanism of the ion currents that play an important role in QTc prolongation and development of TdP. It is now understood that there are multiple ion channel currents, in addition to hERG, driving various phases of cardiac action and blocking hERG channel and leading to EAD (early after-depolarization) and then TdP (Gintant et al., 2016). Moreover, nonclinical studies have shown that EADs associated with drug-induced hERG potassium channel blockade can be suppressed by blocking late sodium or L-type calcium currents such that the repolarization reserve of the myocyte is compromised, which explains why some QTc prolonging drugs that block inward currents, in addition to hERG, have minimum TdP risk (Vicente et al., 2016). Recent clinical studies have demonstrated that blocking late sodium current can reduce drug-induced QTc prolongation caused by hERG potassium channel blockade and mitigate recurrent TdP caused by the long QT syndrome. CiPA aims at incorporating this mechanistic understanding into cardiac safety evaluation of new drugs (FDA, 2017b). The Ion Channel Working Group (ICWG), under the auspices of the Safety Pharmacology Society of the CiPA initiative, has chosen the following seven ion channels for drug effect evaluation (Vicente et al., 2016; FDA, 2017b):

- hERG channels that mediate I_{K_r},

- L-type Ca^{2+} channels that mediate I_{Ca},

- $Na_v1.5$ channels that mediate peak and late I_{Na},

- $K_v4.3$ channels that mediate I_{to},

- KCNQ1 and KCNE1 channels that mediate I_{Ks},

- $K_{ir}2.1$ channels that mediate I_{K1}.

In silico models. These models should use measures that are mechanistically based, experimentally verifiable, and directly related to the changes in cellular electrical activities that are known to be associated with TdP and its triggers (Colatsky et al., 2016). After careful evaluation of several candidate models, an expert group of modelers under the CiPA initiative eventually selected the O'Hara-Rudy (ORd) model (O'Hara et al., 2011) as a leading *in silico* model for further development for regulatory applicaitons. The model provides a mathematical description of undiseased human ventricular myocyte electronphysiology and Ca^{2+} cycling, and its open-source codes are available in `http://rudylab.wustl.edu`, in which all constants and initial conditions for state variables and scaling factors are pre-defined. Several improvements of the ORd model have recently been made to incorporate time, voltage, state and temperature-dependent dynamic drug interactions with the hERG channel (Di Veroli et al., 2014; Li et al., 2016, 2017). With respect to the proarrhythmic risk measure to qualify or quantify torsadegenesis of a drug, several candidates, such as action potential duration (APD), the appearance of EAD, balance between inward and outward currents, have been considered. Two mechanistically based measures, namely the percent change of integral of inward currents (late sodium and L-type calcium) and the percent change of the integral of inward currents minus outward currents, are recommended because of their ability to separate the twelve CiPA training drugs into their low, medium, and high TdP risk categories at concentrations around Cmax and even at $25\times$ Cmax (Li et al., 2017), where Cmax is the maximum serum concentration that a drug achieves in a specified compartment or test area of the body after the drug has been administered.

Stem-cell derived cardiomyocyte assays. As another key component in the CiPA initiative, *in vitro* assays on human stem-cell derived cardiomyocytes (hSC-CM) not only provide further confirmation of drug effects identified by *in silico* models of ionic current studies, but can also identify potential gaps in cellular electrophysiologic effects that are not detected by the *in silico* ionic current reconstructions but may have TdP risk (Colatsky et al., 2016). The rationale underlying hSC-CM assays is the myocytes' ability to recapitulate the integrated critical drug effects that influence electrophysiology in human myocytes and reported as drug-induced repolarization abnormalities. Currently there are two major experimental approaches, namely, high throughput microelectrode arrays (to reveal prolongation of field potential duration of stem-cell cardiomyocytes) and voltage-sensing optical (to capture the changes in repolarization shape); see Colatsky et al. (2016), Millard et al. (2017), Renganathan et al. (2017), Walker et al. (2017) and Roquemore et al. (2017) for further details and recent developments.

2.4.2 Phase I ECG studies

Another key component of the CiPA initiative involves ECG assessment in the first-in-human (FiH) clinical studies, with single dose or multiple ascending doses (exposure-response modeling), to determine if there are unexpected ion channel effects, e.g., human-specific metabolites or protein binding, in comparison with the preclinical ion channel data (Colatsky et al., 2016). As briefly discussed in Section 2.4.1, drugs that block the hERG potassium channel may also block other channels that mitigate TdP risk. The CiPA Phase I ECG Working Group aims at identifying new ECG biomarkers, in addition to QTc and QTS, which can differentiate drugs blocking only hERG channels from those blocking multi-ion channels and which are sensitive enough to detect ion channel effects in phase I exposure-response studies that usually have relatively small sample sizes (Colatsky et al., 2016). Through the analysis of two FDA sponsored clinical trials, the CiPA ECG Working Group has identified heart rate corrected J-T_{peak} (J-T_{peak}c) as the best biomarker for differentiating QT prolonging drugs with selective hERG blockade, from QT prolonging drugs with hERG and late sodium or calcium current blockade; see Johannesen et al. (2014), Johannesen et al. (2016), and Vicente et al. (2016). Johannesen et al. (2016) have also developed an automated algorithm for assessment of J-T_{peak}c and $T_{peak} - T_{end}$ intervals that can be applied in clinical studies to determine if there are unexpected ion channel effects in humans compared to preclinical evidence, and the open-source code is available at https://github.com/fda/ecglib. Despite such progress, much work is still needed in the design of exposure-response ECG studies with relatively small sample sizes and in the performance evaluation of using J-T_{peak}c interval for TdP risk assessment (Colatsky et al., 2016).

2.4.3   Concentration-QTc (C-QTc) modeling

After the implementation of ICH E14, it has been observed that drugs blocking the hERG potassium channel exhibit a nearly linear relationship between drug concentration and QTc prolongation, and that the QTc interval prolongation at the maximum drug concentration can be predicted by using concentration-response models. Evidence from various studies has supported the replacement of TQT by C-QTc modeling in FiH trials to provide definitive assessment of potential drug-induced QTc interval prolongation during clinical development of new drugs (Florian et al., 2012; Darpo et al., 2014; Zhang et al., 2015; Darpo et al., 2015; Nelson et al., 2015; Garnett et al., 2016); see also ICH E14 Guideline (Questions & Answers) Revision 3 issued in December 2015 (ICH, 2015).

A linear random effects model and some refinements. Consider a placebo-controlled C-QTc study in which n subjects are randomly assigned to a placebo group with n_0 subjects or to a treatment (new test drug) group with n_1 subjects so that $n = n_0 + n_1$. Suppose that ECGs are taken from each subject at baseline $t = 0$ and at predefined time points $t = 1, \ldots, T$ after drug administration, and the QTc interval at time t is obtained by using some heart rate correction method; see Vandenberk et al. (2016) for details. Let $\Delta\mathbf{QTc}(t) = \mathbf{QTc}(t) - \mathbf{QTc}(0)$ be the baseline-adjusted QTc interval at time t, $t = 1, \ldots, T$. A linear random effects model is commonly used to describe the C-QTc relationship:

$$\Delta\mathbf{QTc}_{ij}(t) = \alpha_{ij} + \beta_{ij}C_j(t) + \epsilon_{ij}, \qquad (2.26)$$

where $\alpha_{ij} \sim N(\alpha_i, \sigma_\alpha^2)$ denotes the random intercept, $\beta_{ij} \sim N(\beta, \sigma_\beta^2)I(i = 1) + 0I(i = 0)$ the random slope, $C_j(t)$ the plasma concentration in raw scale or log transformed scale of test drug at time t, $\epsilon_{ij} \sim N(0, \sigma^2)$, $i = 0$ (control group) or 1 (treatment group) and $j = 1, \ldots, n_i$; see Tsong et al. (2008). Under this model, $\Delta \text{QTc}_j(t)$ of subject j reaches the maximum at $C_{j,\max} = \max_{1 \le t \le T} C_j(t)$. Assuming in addition that $C_{j,\max} \sim N(\mu_c, \sigma_c^2)$, the difference in $\Delta \text{QTc}_j(t)$ between treatment ($i = 1$) and placebo ($i = 0$), denoted by $D\Delta \text{QTc}_j(t)$, satisfies

$$E\left(\max_{1 \le t \le T} D\Delta \text{QTc}_j(t)\right) = (\alpha_1 - \alpha_0) + \beta\mu_c. \tag{2.27}$$

Therefore, the regulatory concern of drug threshold effect (defined by a 10 millisecond threshold) can be formulated by testing the null hypothesis

$$H_0 : (\alpha_1 - \alpha_0) + \beta\mu_c \ge 10. \tag{2.28}$$

Note that under the linear random effects model,

$$E\left[(\alpha_{1j} - \alpha_{0j}) + \beta_{1j}C_{j,\max}\right] = (\alpha_1 - \alpha_0) + \beta\mu_c,$$
$$\text{Var}\left[(\alpha_{1j} - \alpha_{0j}) + \beta_{1j}C_{j,\max}\right] = 2\sigma_\alpha^2 + \sigma_\beta^2\sigma_c^2.$$

Letting z_q denote the qth quantile of the standard normal distribution, an approximate $100(1 - \gamma)\%$ confidence interval for $(\alpha_1 - \alpha_0) + \beta\mu_c$ is

$$\frac{1}{n_i} \sum_{j=1}^{n_1} \max_{1 \le t \le T} D\Delta \text{QTc}_j(t) \pm z_{1-\gamma/2} \sqrt{\left(2\sigma_\alpha^2 + \sigma_\beta^2\sigma_c^2\right)/n_1}. \tag{2.29}$$

To avoid confounding, one can use a cross-over design in which every subject is given the treatment drug and placebo in sequence. Assuming no sequence and carry-over effects, the difference in baseline-adjusted QTc interval between treatment and placebo for the jth subject at time t, denoted by $D\Delta \text{QTc}_j(t)$, can be related to concentration $C_j(t)$ by

$$D\Delta \text{QTc}_j(t) = \alpha_j + \beta_j C_j(t) + \epsilon_j, \tag{2.30}$$

where $\alpha_j \sim N(\alpha, \sigma_\alpha^2)$ represents the random intercept, $\beta_j \sim N(\beta, \sigma_\beta^2)$ the random slope, $C_j(t)$ the drug concentration at time t, and $\epsilon_j \sim N(0, \sigma^2)$ the random error for subject j. Under the linear random effects model (2.30) and $C_{j,\max} \sim N(\mu_c, \sigma_c^2)$, for which $D\Delta \text{QTc}_j(t)$ reaches its maximum at $C_{j,\max}$, the following analog of (2.27) also holds for the sequence design:

$$E\left(\max_{1 \le t \le T} D\Delta \text{QTc}(t)\right) = \alpha + \beta\mu_c, \tag{2.31}$$

The regulatory concern of drug threshold effect can be similarly formulated by testing the null hypothesis $H_0 : \alpha + \beta\mu_c \ge 10$, and an approximate $100(1 - \gamma)\%$ confidence interval for $\alpha + \beta\mu_c$ is (2.29).

Tsong et al. (2008) have pointed out that violation of model assumptions, e.g., linearity of the C-QTc relationship, may lead to severe bias in testing and estimation. Sébastien et al. (2016) propose to use a model averaging approach in which different candidate models (linear, exponential, Emax) are fitted to C-QTc data and the final estimate of drug effect on QTc is obtained by a weighted average of the estimates generated from the candidate models. They show that the model averaging approach is robust with respect to the control of type I error and also less sensitive to model misspecification than the commonly used linear model.

2.5 Toxicogenomics in predictive toxicology

Toxicogenomics (TGx) is an interdisciplinary science that incorporates multiomics (including genomics, transcriptomics, proteomics, metabolomics and epigenomics) into toxicology to study the adverse effects of exposure to biopharmaceutical products on human health (National Research Council, 2007; Waters, 2016). TGx provides insights into drug-gene interactions and the response of biological pathways to toxicant-specific alterations in gene, protein, and metabolite expressions (National Research Council, 2007). It thereby plays a critical role in predictive toxicology in (a) facilitating more efficient screening of compounds with respect to both toxicity and efficacy, (b) elucidating genetic susceptibility at every level of genomic profiling, (c) identifying safety biomarkers for personalized therapy and regulatory decision making, and (d) enhancing the ability to extrapolate more accurately from experimental animals to humans with respect to risk assessment and prediction (National Research Council, 2007; Zhang et al., 2014; Nandedkar and Waykole, 2016).

2.5.1 TGx science and technology

The development and applications of TGx rely on the combined evolving core technologies of genomics, transcriptomics, proteomics, and metabolomics. Genomics is the study of individual genomes containing a complete set of DNA within a single cell of an organism and genomic technologies refer to those that facilitate more efficient, large-scale studies of individual genomes, e.g., high-throughput gene sequencing using microarrays for detection of DNA sequence variation between individual genomes (often referred to as single nucleotide polymorphisms or simply SNPs), and DNA methylation assays for epigenomic studies. Transcriptomics is the study of the complete set of RNA transcripts produced by the genome for identification of differentially expressed genes in distinct cell populations or tissues. Currently relying on microarray technologies, transcriptomics is an emerging and continually evolving field in safety biomarker discovery and risk assessment (Gupta, 2014). Proteomics is the study of collections of proteins (proteomes) in a living organism. Because proteins carry out most functions encoded by genes, analysis of proteomes provides insights into abnormalities in protein production and/or function that might be associated with drug exposure. The most commonly used technologies for proteomics are 2-dimensional gel electrophoresis and mass spectrometry for protein separation and characterization. Although genomics, transcriptomics, and proteomics provide information on structural and/or functional alterations at gene and/or protein level, they do not inform about the dynamic metabolic status of a living organism. Metabolomics provides the information on dynamic biological states through the analysis of metabolites during the metabolic processes in cells or living organisms. The importance of such analysis is that drug-induced pathophysiological changes in cellular functionality and structure can be reflected in altered compositions of a drug and its metabolites in body fluids (e.g., blood, urine, cerebrospinal fluid), which are readily available from human subjects. Metabolomic analysis relies primarily on nuclear magnetic resonance (NMR) and mass spectrometry to detect differences in metabolic profiles that correspond to various modes of toxicity (Nandedkar and Waykole, 2016; Oziolor et al., 2017).

2.5.2 TGx biomarkers

The concept of safety biomarkers has evolved from conventional biological indicators of toxic exposure to TGx biomarkers which are defined by gene-expression, protein and/or metabolic profiles and which serve as susceptibility indicators of adverse outcomes. Amur et al. (2015) have pointed out that the most commonly used biomarkers in drug development belong to one of the following four categories:

(a) *Response biomarkers*: They measure the biological responses of a patient to treatment and consist of pharmacodynamic-based biomarkers, safety biomarkers and efficacy-response biomarkers. Safety biomarkers can be used to monitor adverse effects on the biological system of humans. Amur et al. (2015) present response biomarkers that are qualified through the Biomarker Qualification Program at FDA and EMA; examples include β2-microglobulin for detection of nephrotoxicity and cardiac troponins T and I for detection of heart muscle damage. TGx biomarkers mostly belong to this category.

(b) *Prognostic biomarkers*: They provide information on the natural course of a disease and hence inform the anticipated status of the disease in the absence of therapeutic intervention or under standard care. Prognostic biomarkers identify patients who are likely at high risk of adverse disease-related outcomes or accelerated deterioration of their health status. Examples of prognostic biomarkers are BRCA1 with high expression implying worse prognosis in untreated breast cancer patients (Mehta et al., 2010), local atherosclerotic plaques for secondary manifestations of atherosclerotic disease (de Kleijn et al., 2010), and S100A12 for major adverse cardiovascular events in patients with heart failure (He et al., 2015).

(c) *Predictive biomarkers*: They identify a subset of patients who respond to a particular treatment and hence are used to enrich the cohort of individuals who are likely to benefit from the therapy. Unlike prognostic biomarkers, predictive biomarkers are related to treatment and hence help forecast favorable or unfavorable response of a patient to one or more therapies. Examples are EGFR mutation in non-small cell lung cancer (Ballman, 2015), metabolite markers for personalised intervention regimes for patients with type 2 diabetes (Andersen et al., 2014), and PD-1/PD-L1 expression for treatment of multiple cancers including malignant melanoma, non-small cell lung cancer, renal cell carcinoma, classical Hodgkin lymphoma, and recurrent or metastatic head and neck squamous cell carcinoma (Vareki et al., 2017).

(d) *Diagnostic biomarkers*: They are used to distinguish patients with a particular disease from those who do not have the disease. Examples of diagnostic biomarkers are prostate-specific antigen (PSA, a protein produced by cells of the prostate gland) for prostate cancer (Velonas et al., 2013) and an integrated biomarker system comprising 5 genes, 40 metabolites, and 6 clinical manifestations for early diagnosis of type 2 diabetic nephropathy (Huang et al., 2013).

TGx biomarkers play an increasingly important role in early prediction of toxicities in specific forms or to specific organs, such as hepatotoxicity, nephrotoxicity, cardiotoxicity, carcinogenicity, immunotoxicity, reproductive and developmental toxicity. Uehara et al. (2015) review available toxicogenomic biomarkers for etiological and outcome-based hepatotoxicity, nephrotoxicity, and carcinogenicity. Because of the complexity and variety of mechanisms that are responsible for organ-specific toxicities, one would expect a wide range of biomarkers for each of the specific organ toxicities. For example, genomic biomarkers have been identified for various types of hepatotoxicity, enabling prediction of the likelihood of occurrence of hepatotoxicity upon certain amount of exposure (dosage + time); see Boverhof and Gollapudi (2011), Uehara et al. (2013), Uehara et al. (2015), Campion et al. (2013) and Thomas and Waters (2016) for further details. Although some TGx biomarkers have been recommended by regulatory agencies for incorporation into drug discovery and development, many of them still have one or more of the following weaknesses to help actual drug approval: (a) lack of accurate phenotypic anchoring of TGx profiles to confirmed outcomes and conventional toxicity endpoints, (b) limited sensitivity and/or specificity in predicting clinical toxicities, (c) lack of optimal analytical assessment, (d) difficulty in analyzing high-dimensional TGx data, (e) incomplete knowledge in adverse outcome pathways and network, (f) lack of consensus in result interpretation of TGx data (Qin et al., 2016; Nandedkar and Waykole, 2016).

2.6 Regulatory framework in predictive toxicology

In laying out the strategic plan for advancing regulatory science, the FDA has identified eight priority areas among which modernizing toxicology to enhance product safety tops the list (FDA, 2011a). The agency's report stipulates implementation strategies to improve prediction of product safety by focusing on preclinical data and collaborative research in the areas of modeling human adverse outcomes, biomarkers, endpoints used in nonclinical and clinical evaluation, and computational and *in silico* models.

2.6.1 Regulatory guidelines

In addition to the guidelines on late stage clinical safety described in Chapter 1, there are documents issued by ICH covering a broad range of areas in preclinical safety studies from genotoxicity, immunotoxicity, reproductive toxicity, carcinotoxicity to general nonclinical safety studies (http://www.ich.org/products/guidelines/safety/article/safety-guidelines.html). Particularly noteworthy is the recently finalized nonclinical testing strategy for assessing cardiotoxicity through QT/QTc interval prolongation. While adopting ICH guidelines, the FDA produces its own guidelines for sponsors' preclinical toxicology and clinical pharmacology studies to be included in submissions to the agency. For example, the guidance for safety testing of drug metabolites by the FDA (FDA, 2016), developed on the basis of multiple ICH guidelines, provides general considerations and more specific instructions on safety assessment of disproportionate drug metabolites between animal species and humans with respect to general toxicity, genotoxicity, developmental toxicity, and carcinogenicity. The FDA also provides guidelines on nonclinical toxicological studies in some therapies, disease areas or specific safety concerns, e.g., nonclinical safety evaluation of reformulated drug products, endocrine-related drugs, enzyme replacement therapies, therapeutic radiopharmaceutics, and drugs for osteoporosis. For a complete list of FDA guidelines in pharmacology and toxicology, see https://www.fda.gov/drugs/guidancecomplianceregulatoryinformation/guidances/.

2.6.2   Safety biomarker qualification

Safety biomarkers are a critical component in predictive toxicology. The discovery, development, qualification, regulatory acceptance and utilization of safety biomarkers represent important steps toward accurate and precise prediction of adverse effects of drugs on humans. Biomarkers including safety biomarkers must be qualified before being used in a particular context of preclinical and/or clinical research. The FDA defines a qualification as "a conclusion that within the stated context of use, a biomarker can be relied upon to have a specific interpretation and application in drug development and regulatory review" (FDA, 2014c). The regulatory agency has established a biomarker qualification program in which a three-stage approach (initiation, consultation and advice, and review and decision) is provided to guide biomarker qualification process. Recently the FDA and EMA have collaborated with academic and industrial researchers to identify and qualify safety biomarkers for detection of drug-induced renal toxicity using preclinical animal models, and have endorsed a number of safety biomarkers that are more sensitive and specific than traditional tests (Amur et al., 2015).

2.6.3   In silico models in predictive toxicology

One of the objectives of the FDA's Critical Path Initiative is to improve product safety through prediction of drug-induced toxicity in early development stages. The FDA has used computational methods and *in silico* models in the prediction of human risk using chemical structure-activity relationship (SAR). Along this line, the FDA has developed methods and tools for the analysis and integration of complex omics (genomics, transcriptomics, proteomics, and metabolomics) datasets (Benz, 2007; Valerio, 2011; Hong et al., 2016). In the FDA guideline on the evaluation of genotoxic and carcinogenic impurities in drug substances and products (FDA, 2008a; Valerio and Cross, 2012), the use of *in silico* predictive models based on SAR and QSAR approaches is recommended for structural alerts and for assessing whether potential genotoxicity is below the qualification threshold. In particularly, *in silico* models have been used for prediction of drug-induced liver injuries (Chen et al., 2013), drug-induced phospholipidosis and P450 inhibition (Valerio, 2011), adverse drug-drug interactions (Zhang et al., 2009) and mutagenic potential of drug impurities (Valerio and Cross, 2012). In its strategic plan for advancing regulatory science, the FDA elaborates priority areas in which modernizing toxicology to enhance product safety tops the list (FDA, 2011a). The strategic plan specifically describes the development and use of computational methods and *in silico* models (a) to improve the SAR models in the prediction of human risk and integrate this analysis into the review process, (b) to link to chemical structures and substructures to product safety, disease targets, and toxicity mechanisms, and (c) to integrate PK, PD, mechanistic safety data to predict clinical risk-benefit and confirm post-marketing safety.

2.7 Supplements and problems

1. *Exercise.* There are many toxicity endpoints that can be measured along the AOPs. Give at least one example of toxicity measurement at the molecular, cellular, and organ levels respectively for (a) hepato-toxicity, (b) nephrotoxicity, (c) cardiotoxicity, (d) neurotoxicity, and (e) hematotoxicity.

2. *Statistical methods for QSAR/QSTR.* We supplement here the list of methods in Section 2.1.3 and provide details on classification and regression trees.

   Gaussian process regression (GPR). Consider the training set $D = \{(\mathbf{x}_i, y_i) : i = 1, \ldots, n\}$, where $\mathbf{x}_i$ is a vector of dimension d and y_i the target response. In GPR, each target response y_i is related to $\mathbf{x}_i$ through a basis function $f(\mathbf{x}_i)$ such that

   $$y_i = f(\mathbf{x}_i) + \epsilon_i, \qquad i = 1, \ldots, n \tag{2.32}$$

   where ϵ_i denotes the noise and a Gaussian process (GP) defines a prior distribution on the functions f so that inference takes place directly in function space. A GP is a set of random variables such that any finite number of them have a multivariate Gaussian distribution and is therefore determined by its mean function $E[f(\mathbf{x}_i)] = m(\mathbf{x}_i)$ and covariance function $\mathrm{Cov}(f(\mathbf{x}_i), f(\mathbf{x}_j)) = E[f(\mathbf{x}_i) - m(\mathbf{x}_i)][f(\mathbf{x}_j) - m(\mathbf{x}_j)] = k(\mathbf{x}_i, \mathbf{x}_j)$. To predict $f(\mathbf{x}^*)$ for a new compound characterized by $\mathbf{x}^*$, one can use the Bayes rule (Rasmussen and Williams, 2006; Schwaighofer et al., 2007), which gives a normal distribution for the predicted response with mean

   $$\bar{f}(\mathbf{x}^*) = \sum_{i=1}^{n} \alpha_i k(\mathbf{x}_i, \mathbf{x}^*) \tag{2.33}$$

   and variance

   $$\sigma(\mathbf{x}^*) = k(\mathbf{x}^*, \mathbf{x}^*) - \sum_{i=1}^{n} \sum_{j=1}^{n} k(\mathbf{x}_i, \mathbf{x}^*) k(\mathbf{x}_j, \mathbf{x}^*) L_{ij} \tag{2.34}$$

   where $\alpha = (\alpha_1, \ldots, \alpha_n)^T$ is a solution of the linear system $(\mathbf{K} + \sigma^2 \mathbf{I}) \alpha = \mathbf{y}$, $\mathbf{y} = (y_1, \ldots, y_n)^T$, $\mathbf{K} = \{k(\mathbf{x}_i, \mathbf{x}_j) : 1 \leq i, j, \leq n\}$, and

L_{ij} are the elements of the matrix $\mathbf{L} = (\mathbf{K} + \sigma^2 \mathbf{I})^{-1}$. GPR has been applied by Burden (2001) to analyze the effects of benzodiazepine on muscarinic receptors and the toxicity effect of substituted benzenes to the ciliate, by Obrezanova et al. (2007) to build regression models of absorption, distribution, metabolism, and excretion, and by Jin et al. (2014) to three-dimensional QSTR modeling and prediction of acute toxicity of organic contaminants on algae.

k-nearest neighbor methods for classification and regression. Let $\mathbf{x}_i = (x_{i1}, \ldots, x_{ip})$ represent a vector of p-dimensional molecular descriptors and y_i be toxicological response with categorical values so that the training set consists of $\{(\mathbf{x}_i, \mathbf{y}_i), i = 1, \ldots, n\}$. For a new compound with molecular descriptors $\mathbf{x}^* = (x_1^*, \ldots, x_p^*)$, its distance $d(\mathbf{x}^*, \mathbf{x}_i)$ to $\mathbf{x}_i$ is determined by using one of the following commonly used distance measures

$$
d_i = \begin{cases}
\sqrt{\sum_{j=1}^p (x_{ij} - x_j^*)^2} & \text{Euclidean distance,} \\
\sum_{j=1}^p |x_{ij} - x_j^*| & L_1\text{-distance,} \\
\left[\sum_{j=1}^p |x_{ij} - x_j^*|^q \right]^{1/q} & \text{Minkowski distance } (1 < q < 2), \\
\sum_{j=1}^p I(x_{ij} \neq x_j^*)/p & \text{Hamming distance,}
\end{cases}
\tag{2.35}
$$

in which the Hamming distance is used for categorical descriptors and the other distance measures are used for numerical descriptors. The k-nearest neighbors (k-NN) of $\mathbf{x}^*$ are defined by the k smallest distances $d_{(1)} \leq d_{(2)} \leq \ldots \leq d_{(k)}$ and the k-NN method defines $k_j = \sum_{i=1}^k I(y_{(i)} = j)$ for response class j, where $y_{(i)}$ is the class indicator corresponding to the compound in the training set with the ith smallest distance, and assigns the new compound with descriptors $\mathbf{x}^*$ to class m if $k_m \geq \max_j k_j$. For $j_1 \neq j_2$, both attain $\max_j k_j$, this would result in assigning a compound to more than one class, and one can break the ties by choosing the class with the smallest d_j.

An enhancement of the preceding method is weighted k-NN approach which uses weights w_i ($1 \leq i \leq k$) and defines k_j by $k_j' = \sum_{i=1}^k w_i I(y_{(i)} = j)$. Different choices of w_i have been proposed including $w_i = (d_{(k)} - d_i) / (d_{(k)} - d_{(1)})$ and $w_i = \exp(-d_i)/\sum_{\nu=1}^k \exp(-d_\nu)$; see Webb (2003). Using weights that sum to 1 enables one to extend to kNN regression problems, which estimates the toxicological response of a new compound by averaging the responses of all the compounds in the k-NN, i.e., $y = \sum_{i=1}^k w_i y_i$ (Altman, 1992).

It should be pointed out that the molecular descriptors $\mathbf{x}_i$ in the training set may be measured at different scales, e.g., some with wide ranges and others with relatively narrow windows, or as a mixture of numerical and categorical variables. For numerical descriptors at various scales, a standardization of the descriptor variables at raw scales should be taken to ensure that each unit of the calculated distance d_i contributes approximately the same in identifying the k-NN. Some commonly used standardization methods include

$$x_{ij}^* = \begin{cases} (x_{ij} - \bar{x}_j)/\hat{\sigma}_j, & \text{Auto-scaling,} \\ x_{ij}/(\max_i x_{ij}), & \text{Maximum scaling} \\ (x_{ij} - \min_i x_{ij})/(\max_i x_{ij} - \min_i x_{ij}), & \text{Range scaling} \end{cases}$$

where $\bar{x}_j = \frac{1}{n}\sum_{i=1}^n x_{ij}$, $\hat{\sigma}_j = \frac{1}{n-1}\sum_{i=1}^n (x_{ij} - \bar{x}_j)^2$, and $\max_i$ and $\min_i$ are taken over the n compounds for each of the p molecular descriptors. With respect to the size of the neighborhood, one can choose a small k (e.g., $k = 1$) initially and increase the neighborhood size and then determine the optimal k based on classification errors in validation. Some other choices of optimal k include a local linear discriminant analysis of Hastie and Tibshirani (1996), statistical confidence-based neighborhood selection of Wang et al. (2006), a Bayesian optimal choice of Ghosh (2006) and stochastic k-neighborhood selection using neighborhood component analysis of Tarlow et al. (2013).

Because of its simplicity and easy implementation, k-NN approach has been extensively used in QSAR/QSTR modeling for classification and regression of predictive toxicological response of new compounds. For example, Liu et al. (2012) used adaptive nearest neighbors for predicting toxicological effects of structurally diverse compounds with applications to human maximum recommended daily dose; Gadaleta et al. (2014) employed the k-NN approach to predicting sub-chronic oral toxicity in rats, which provided valuable toxicity assessment of compounds in subsequent development; Chavan et al. (2016) illustrated the utility of k-NN classification models based on 172 molecular structures for the prediction of the hERG (human ether-a-go-go related gene) toxicity that is related to QT interval prolongation; specifically, they applied the developed k-NN models to FDA withdrawn substances and found that the models are able to differentiate mechanisms underlying QT interval prolongation (i.e., hERG-derived and non-hERG derived QT prolongations); Zhang et al. (2016) applied five different machine learning algorithms including k-NN to classify compounds, based on 13 molecular descriptors combining, five fingerprints and molecular descriptors combining fingerprints at four IC50 (half maximal inhibitory concentration) thresholds, as either hERG blockers or non-hERG blockers.

Bayesian classification, discriminant analysis, classification and regression trees. Suppose $(\mathbf{X}, Y)$ takes values in $\mathbb{N}^M \times \{1, \dots, K\}$, where Y is the class label of $\mathbf{X}$. A classifier is a function $C : \mathbb{N}^M \to \{1, \dots, K\}$

that classifies x to the class $C(\mathbf{x})$. Let $\pi(k)$ be the prior probability of class k and let $(\mathbf{X}_i, Y_i)$, $1 \leq i \leq n$, be a training sample which has the same distribution as $(\mathbf{X}, Y)$ and from which a classifier C_n is developed. The misclassification probability of the classifier is $P\{C_n(\mathbf{X}) \neq Y\}$, where $(\mathbf{X}, Y)$ is a future realization independent of the training sample. With the 0-1 loss function (that has loss 1 for misclassification and loss 0 for correct classification), the Bayes classifier minimizes the posterior risk, or equivalently, $C_n^{\text{Bayes}}(\mathbf{x})$ chooses class k that maximizes the posterior probability $\pi_n(Y = k | \mathbf{X} = \mathbf{x})$. Hence the Bayes classifier is a majority voting rule.

Discriminant analysis (DA) is often used for determination of discriminant scores based on toxicological responses and a set of molecular descriptors of compounds in the training set. The scores are further used for classifying untested compounds with known molecular structures. Linear DA (LDA) tries to find a hyperplane that achieves greatest separation between classes. The hyperplane is defined by a linear discriminant function L that is a linear combination of molecular descriptors $L = \sum_{j=1}^{p} \omega_j x_j$, where ω_j is the weight corresponding to descriptor x_j. The discriminant function L is obtained by optimizing the set of weights $\omega = \{\omega_j : j = 1, \ldots, p\}$ that maximize the ratio of between-class to within-class variances. Quadratic DA is similar to LDA, except that the covariance matrices may differ between classes and therefore must be estimated for each class; see Hastie et al. (2009, Sections 4.3, 12.5, 12.6 and 12.7) for details and refinements of LDA. Partial least squares DA is essentially partial least squares regression (Hastie et al., 2009, Section 3.5.2) with binary response variables that are correlated with molecular descriptors through latent variables that are determined by using classification parameters (Ståhle and Wold, 1987; Ghorbanzadeh et al., 2016).

CART (classification and regression tree) is a statistical/machine learning method for constructing prediction models through recursive partitioning of training data sets in order to obtain subsets that are as homogeneous as possible in a given target class. Classification trees (CT) are designed for response variables that take on a finite number of unordered values, and regression trees (RT) are for response variables that take continuous or ordered discrete values (Hastie et al., 2009). Consider a classification problem in which a training data set contains n compounds with the ith compound having a toxicological response variable y_i that takes on values $1, 2, \ldots, K$, and p molecular descriptors $\mathbf{x}_i = (x_{i1}, \ldots, x_{ip})$, $i = 1, \ldots, n$. A CT solution is to recursively partition the $\mathbf{x} = (\mathbf{x}_1, \ldots, \mathbf{x}_n)$ space in the training data set into M disjoint sets $R_1, \ldots, R_M$, such that the predicted value of y_i is k if $\mathbf{x}_i$ belongs to R_m, for $k = 1, \ldots, K$ and $m = 1, \ldots, M$. The partition is based on *splitting rules*, also called *impurity functions*, that help achieve the maximum homogeneity within subsets after each splitting. For subset R_m with n_i compounds, let

$$\hat{p}_{mk} = \frac{1}{n_i} \sum_{\mathbf{x}_i \in R_m} I(y_i = k) \tag{2.36}$$

be the estimated probability of class k compounds in subset R_m. The splitting rule of CT is often determined by the *Gini impurity measure* G or *entropy index* E:

$$G = \sum_{k=1}^{K} \hat{p}_{mk}(1 - \hat{p}_{mk}), \quad E = -\sum_{k=1}^{K} \hat{p}_{mk} \log(\hat{p}_{mk}), \tag{2.37}$$

which becomes small if the $\hat{p}_{mk}$'s are close to 0 or 1.

Next consider a regression tree (RT) in which the toxicological response y_i is continuous and which is used to predict the response of a new compound with molecular descriptors $\mathbf{x}$, using a predictor of the form

$$f(\mathbf{x}) = \sum_{m=1}^{M} c_m I(\mathbf{x} \in R_m). \tag{2.38}$$

Hastie et al. (2009, Section 9.2.2) describe the basic ideas for constructing $\hat{f}$ based on a training sample $\{(\mathbf{x}_i, y_i), 1 \leq i \leq n\}$. The splitting rule for RT proceeds as follows. Starting with all of the data, consider a splitting variable j and split point s, and define the pair of half-places

$$R_1(j, s) = \{\mathbf{x} | x_j \leq s\} \text{ and } R_2(j, s) = \{\mathbf{x} | x_j \leq s\}.$$

The greedy algorithm finds the splitting variable j and split point s that solve

$$\min_{j,s} \left[\min_{c_1} \sum_{\mathbf{x}_i \in R_1(j,s)} (y_i - c_1)^2 + \min_{c_2} \sum_{\mathbf{x}_i \in R_2(j,s)} (y_i - c_2)^2 \right]. \tag{2.39}$$

For any choice j and s, the inner minimization is solved by

$$\hat{c}_1 = \frac{1}{|R_1(j,s)|} \sum_{i:\mathbf{x}_i \in R_1(j,s)} y_i \text{ and } \hat{c}_2 = \frac{1}{|R_2(j,s)|} \sum_{i:\mathbf{x}_i \in R_2(j,s)} y_i.$$

For each splitting variable, the determination of the split point s can be done very quickly. Having found the best split, we partition the data into the two resulting regions and repeat the splitting process on each of the two regions. Then this process is repeated on all of the resulting regions; see Hastie et al. (2009) who also ask: "How large shoould we grow the tree? Clearly a very large tree might overfit the data, while a small tree might not capture the important structure." Hastie et al. (2009, pp. 308, 310–317) discuss these and other issues, not only for RTs, but also for CTs.

Support vector machine (SVM). This is a supervised learning method for pattern recognition and has gained much popularity in many applied fields due to its flexibility in modeling nonlinear relationships and robust performance (Abe, 2010). For classification problems, it is an alternative to discriminant analysis and to its variants including logistic regression for classification, classification trees, and neural network. In the biomedical field, SVMs have been used to develop prediction models for disease prognosis in a clinical setting, e.g., Cleophas et al. (2013), and compound classification and toxicity prediction in predictive toxicology, e.g., Furey et al. (2000); Yap et al. (2004); Ferrari et al. (2009); Zhang et al. (2016) and Koutsoukas et al. (2016).

Consider a simple binary classification problem in which a compound can be classified as either toxic or non-toxic with respect to some measurable toxicological response based on two molecular descriptors x_1 and x_2. For linearly separable data as in Figure 2.3, apparently there are many different ways to define a hyperplane that separates the two clusters of compounds, e.g., the two dashed lines representing such linear hyperplanes. An SVM approach tries to find a hyperplane with the maximum margin that is defined as the sum of distances from the hyperplane to the closest sample sets of both classes. These data points are called support vectors. The rationale of this choice is that an optimal hyperplane will not change much if the observations that are far away from the hyperplane are removed, but will change significantly if any of the support vectors are removed. Thus, the support vectors are critical observations in the data set for determining the classification rules.

Now consider a binary classification with a data set of n observed training pairs $(\mathbf{x}_i, y_i)$, $\mathbf{x}_i \in \mathbb{R}^d$ and $y_i \in \{-1, 1\}$, $i = 1, \ldots, n$. For any separation hyperplane $\mathbf{w}\mathbf{x} + a = 0$, where $\mathbf{w}$ denotes the weight vector, two parallel hyperplanes can be derived, one passing through the support vectors on toxic side $\mathbf{w}\mathbf{x} + a = -1$ and another on non-toxic side $\mathbf{w}\mathbf{x} + a = 1$ (Figure 2.3). Therefore, the margin D can be computed during learning from the distance between the two hyperplanes, i.e., $D = 2/\|\mathbf{w}\|$ and maximizing the margin is equivalent to minimizing

$$f(\mathbf{w}) = \frac{\|\mathbf{w}\|}{2} \qquad (2.40)$$

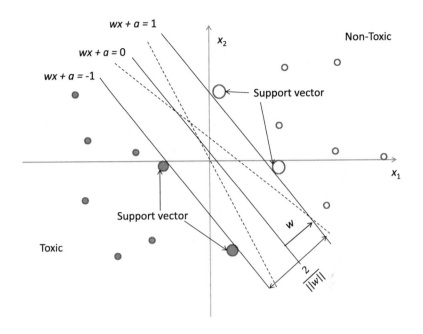

FIGURE 2.3 Illustration of support vector machine with linear separation.

subject to

$$\begin{cases} \mathbf{wx}_i + a \geq 1, & \text{if } y_i = 1 \\ \mathbf{wx}_i + a \leq -1, & \text{if } y_i = -1 \end{cases} \qquad (2.41)$$

for $i = 1, \ldots, n$. Or equivalently

$$\begin{cases} \min_{\mathbf{w}} \|\mathbf{w}\|^2 \\ y_i \left(\mathbf{wx}_i + a \right) \geq 1, \quad i = 1, \ldots, n \end{cases} \qquad (2.42)$$

which is a quadratic optimization problem subject to linear constraints with a unique minimum.

Now consider a linearly inseparable case in which there exist some margin violations or misclassifications as shown in Figure 2.4. Let $\xi_i \geq 0$ be a slack variable measuring the error of instance $\mathbf{x}_i$ (margin violated and misclassified observations). Then the "soft" margin

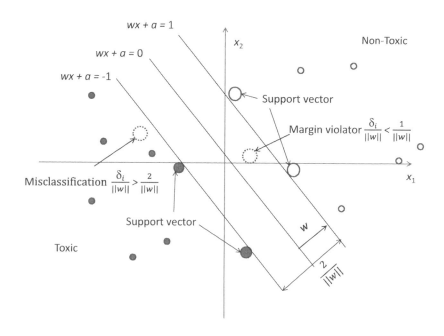

FIGURE 2.4 Illustration of support vector machine with margin violation and misclassification.

solution for optimization becomes

$$\begin{cases} \min\limits_{\mathbf{w},; \, \xi_i \geq 0} ||\mathbf{w}||^2 + C \sum\limits_{i=1}^{n} \xi_i \\ y_i \left(\mathbf{w}\mathbf{x}_i + a \right) \geq 1 - \xi_i, \quad i = 1, \ldots, n \end{cases} \qquad (2.43)$$

where C is a regularization parameter defined by user. A small C implies a large margin, making the constraint to be easily ignored, while a large C implies a narrow margin and hence makes the constraint more influential (Cortes and Vapnik, 1995).

For non-linear classification, one can formulate a non-linear function $\psi(\mathbf{x}_i)$ of $\mathbf{x}_i$ and replace $\mathbf{x}_i$ by $\psi(\mathbf{x}_i)$ in (2.42) or (2.43); see Abe (2010), Ferrari et al. (2009) and Hastie et al. (2009, Section 12.3) for implementation details.

3. *Exercise.* Consider a dataset for incidental tumors that include the number n_i of animals and the number y_i of animals with tumors at

dose i for $i = 1, \ldots, I$ with increasing doses. Let $n = \sum_{i=1}^{I} n_i$ and $y = \sum_{i=1}^{I} y_i$. Conditional on the margins n and y, derive an exact test for testing the null hypothesis of equal probabilities of tumor occurrence across the I dose levels against an increasing probability of tumor occurrence over dose.

TABLE 2.3 Developmental toxicity data for DEHP.

Dose	Dams	Live fetuses	(111)	(110)	(101)	(100)	(011)	(010)	(001)	(000)
							Malformation			
0.000	30	330	0	0	0	0	0	5	4	321
0.025	26	288	0	0	0	3	0	1	1	283
0.050	26	277	0	5	2	8	2	13	8	239
0.100	24	137	3	0	5	16	6	12	11	84
0.150	25	50	8	7	8	4	1	9	7	6

4. *Exercise.* Ryan and Molenberghs (1999) describe five developmental toxicity studies investigating the effects in mice of five different chemicals, one of which is di(2-ethylhexyl)-phthalate (DEHP), a chemical compound used as a plasticizer. In the DEHP developmental toxicity study, there are five dose groups including a control with zero dose, and 24-30 dams in each dose group. Recorded for each offspring are malformation types that were classified as being "external," "visceral," and "skeletal" (denoted by y_1, y_2, and y_3, respectively). Some animals were found to have multiple malformation types. Table 2.3 summarizes the recorded malformation data for DEHP where the column (111) represents the number of fetuses with all three malformations, i.e., $(111) = (y_1 = 1, y_2 = 1, y_3 = 1)$, the column labeled (110) the number of fetuses with external and visceral malformation but no skeletal malformation, i.e., $(110) = (y_1 = 1, y_2 = 1, y_3 = 0)$, and so on. One of the study objectives was to determine whether the probability of malformation for each type and the number of malformations for all types increase with dose.

   (a) Derive a likelihood function that can be used to answer the above questions,

   (b) Use either SAS or R codes to obtain the maximum likelihood estimates of the parameters,

   (c) Draw conclusions based on results obtained in (b).

3

Benefit-Risk Assessment of Medical Products

Safety evaluation in biopharmaceutical product development has three primary objectives. First is the identification of signals that are likely or possibly associated with the candidate drug or vaccine. Second is the development of a comprehensive risk management plan to assure that any potential adverse outcomes to patients are minimized and dealt with in an appropriate manner. Third is the assessment of the benefit-risk trade-off, which is the main focus of this chapter. A favorable benefit-risk (B-R) profile has always been the regulatory standard for approval of new drug and vaccine products. However, there are shortcomings with traditional methodologies for B-R analysis, compounded by limitations in the available data. In the Innovative Medicines Initiative (IMI) PROTECT (Pharmacaepidemiological Research on Outcomes of Therapeutics by a European Consortium), Mt-Isa et al. (2014) have identified 49 methodologies categorized as frameworks, metrics, estimation techniques, and utility survey techniques for the assessment of benefit and risk of medicines. The set is further down to recommend 13 of the 49 methodologies. There is now growing interest in approaching the B-R questions with better approaches; see Jiang and He (2016).

The challenges in undertaking a comprehensive benefit-risk analysis have been well-recognized; see Guo et al. (2010). A thorough evaluation involves multiple sources of evidence and different disciplines, from clinical medicine to statistics and policy. Available clinical trial data are usually quite limited and need to be supplemented by other sources of epidemiological data, and the evaluations need to continue into the post-marketing setting. Judgment has played an important role and there are numerous examples of subjective judgment in interpreting clinical outcomes to reach the conclusions of an evaluation. Because of the critical nature of benefit-risk analysis in the decision process concerning safety, regulatory agencies, the pharmaceutical industry, and the academic community have undertaken several initiatives to review the available methodologies and make recommendations on best practices. In particular, the European Medicines Agency (EMA) established a working group with the goal of providing recommendations on ways to improve the methodology, consistency, transparency, and communication of the evaluations. This effort resulted in a reflections paper (EMA, 2009) and a recommendations paper (Phillips, 2011). The IMI-PROTECT team reviewed and developed a set of tools and methods for real life case studies (Hughes et al., 2014). Hammad and Pinto (2016) recently described some key changes in guidelines for benefit-risk analysis and the implications for drug development programs and requirements on the data and analysis, to address the scientific and operational challenges of benefit-risk assessments. Many regulatory agencies have started implementing measures to provide consistency and transparency, as in the EMA Benefit-Risk Methodology Project (Phillips, 2011) and FDA's guidelines for benefit-risk assessment (FDA, 2013b, 2017a). In June 2016, an International Conference on Harmonization (ICH) expert working group finalized revision of the guidance for Benefit and Risk Conclusions. The revisions provide greater specificity regarding how to structure and report the benefit-risk assessment.

In the first three sections of this chapter, we give examples in which B-R assessments play an important role in the FDA's decisions on whether to withdraw certain medical products from the market, and then describe some critical ingredients for a comprehensive B-R evaluation, and in particular the guidance of regulatory agencies and drug manufacturers' consortia. We next proceed to introduce the multi-criteria statistical decision theory underlying B-R trade-offs in the stakeholders' decisions in Section 3.4, and provide additional statistical methods for B-R analysis in Sections 3.5 and 3.6. Supplements and problems are given in Section 3.7.

3.1 Some examples of B-R assessments in regulatory decisions

3.1.1 Tysabri

Tysabri was the first monocolonal antibody that was approved by the FDA in 2004 for the treatment of multiple sclerosis. Shortly after approval, Tysabri was removed from the market after two patients taking the drug developed progressive multifocal leukoencephalopathy (PML), a rare (about 1 in 1000 patients during an 18-month follow-up period) untreatable and frequently fatal brain infection (Ransohoff, 2007). About a year later after Tysabri's withdrawal from the market, an FDA advisory committee met to decide whether the product could be re-introduced with a restricted distribution program, and eventually concluded that the drug was so effective in comparison with other available treatments that patients considered the risk worth taking. Upon reassessment of the benefit-risk of the product and an improved risk management program proposed by the manufacturer, FDA announced in 2006 the remarketing of Tysabri with the statement that "Tysabri is indicated for use as monotherapy...for patients who have not responded adequately to, or cannot tolerate, other treatments for MS." The remarketing, however, required careful monitoring and limited distribution through registered providers (Kachuck, 2011).

3.1.2 Lorcaserin

Lorcaserin is a selective serotonin receptor agonist that regulates appetite and reduces food intake. Before the first New Drug Application (NDA) for the indication of weight loss, the manufacturer evaluated Lorcaserin in two phase II and three phase III studies. According to the FDA guidance document for weight-management products (FDA, 2015b), a drug is considered effective if, after 1 year of application, either of the following is achieved: (a) the difference in mean weight loss between the active-product and placebo-treated groups is at least 5% and the difference is statistically significant, or (b) the proportion of subjects who lose $\geq 5\%$ of baseline body weight is at least 35% in the active-product group and is at least twice that in the placebo-treated group, and the difference between the group proportions is statistically significant. For (a), none of the three Lorcaserin phase III studies achieved a 5% mean weight loss difference. On the other hand, two of the three phase III trials achieved (b), and it was noted that the percentage of weight loss was based only on completers, and there was a high drop-out rate in Lorcaserin patients (34–45%). On the risk side, the incidence rates of serious adverse events were similar for Lorcaserin and placebo subjects, but an increased risk of mammary fibroadenomas and adenocarcinomas in female rats administered with very high doses of Lorcaserin had been reported. Based on those data, a September 2010 FDA advisory committee voted 9 to 5 to recommend rejection of the new drug application for Lorcaserin because of mediocre weight loss and high risk for adenocarcinoma in rats. The manufacturer then conducted additional clinical studies and readjudicated the animal carcinogenicity data to address these concerns. Upon reviewing the additional information, the advisory committee agreed that Lorcaserin's benefit outweighed its potential risk when used long-term in overweight and obese patients and that the clinical relevance of Lorcaserin-induced adenocarcinoma was inconclusive. The committee voted 18 to 4 in favor of approving Lorcaserin, and subsequently the FDA approved Lorcaserin for chronic weight management (Morrato and Allison, 2012; Miller, 2013).

3.1.3 Crizotinib

Lung cancer is the leading cause of cancer deaths in both men and women in the United States. In the past decade, FDA approved multiple products for the treatment of advanced non-small cell lung cancer (NSCLC). Traditionally, the approval of new NSCLC treatments has been based on the improvement of overall survival (OS) or progression-free survival (PFS). However, if surrogate endpoints such as overall response rate (ORR) can reasonably predict clinical benefits, they can be used for accelerated approval. On the risk side, harms can be either fatal or non-fatal adverse events. Crizotinib received FDA's accelerated approval in 2013 with a single-arm study and ORR as the primary endpoint. Specifically, the approval decision was based on the target disease with unmet medical need, statistically significant and clinically meaningful benefit over control with respect to ORR and PFS, and risk that was lower than the control risk. In their analysis of the benefit-risk data from 20 NSCLC drugs that were submitted to the FDA for NDA, Raju et al. (2016) used crizotinib as an example to illustrate the importance of benefit-risk assessment and decision analysis.

3.2 Ingredients for comprehensive B-R evaluation

3.2.1 Planning process

B-R evaluations should use a structured and well-defined planning process. The Benefit Risk Action Team (BRAT) formed by PhRMA (Pharmaceutical Research as Manufacturers of America) has developed a framework (the BRAT framework) for such planning and to help decision makers select, organize, and communicate the evidence underlying B-R decisions. FDA has also published guidance for a structured approach (FDA, 2013b) that provides evidence of benefit (or beneficial outcomes) and risk (or harmful outcomes), severity of conditions and current treatment options, risk management measures to mitigate risk, and implications and explanations for decision making. Moreover, EMA has adopted the PrOACT-URL decision-making framework developed by the IMI-PROTECT Benefit-Risk group. The PrOACT-URL framework is a generic decision-making guide with 8 steps: Problems, Objectives, Alternatives, Consequences, Trade-offs, Uncertainty, Risk tolerances, and Linked decisions; see Table 3.1.

3.2.2 Qualitative and quantitative evaluations

Evaluating treatment options on the basis of benefit-risk trade-offs involves subjective judgment regardless of whether it is termed a qualitative or quantitative evaluation. In a qualitative framework the favorable and unfavorable effects need to be clearly identified and summarized us-

TABLE 3.1 Summary of PrOACT-URL components.

Components	Further explanation
Problem	Determine the nature of the problem and its context.
Objective	Establish objectives that indicate the overall purposes to be achieved and criteria for favorable and unfavorable effects.
Alternatives	Identify the options to be evaluated against the criteria.
Consequences	Describe how the alternatives perform for each of the criteria, i.e., the magnitude of all effects, and their desirability or severity, and the incidence of all effects.
Trade-off	Assess the balance between favorable and unfavorable effects.
Uncertainty	Report the uncertainty associated with the favorable and unfavorable effects, and consider how the balance between favorable and unfavorable effects is affected by uncertainty.
Risk tolerance	Judge the relative importance of the decision maker's risk attitude for this product.
Linked decisions	Consider the consistency of this decision with similar past decisions, and assess whether taking this decision could impact future decisions.

ing a common scale, and an overall assessment is made using clinical judgment. In a quantitative framework the effects are integrated using either specified weights as in Gail et al. (1999), or a rank ordering system as in Chuang-Stein et al. (1991) and Claggett et al. (2014). The resulting score does not have the same interpretation of a truly objective quantity such as mortality, blood pressure, or body weight. For this reason, quantitative findings are sometimes interpreted with skepticism (Phillips et al., 2013) and the need for rigor in clarity and communication is amplified.

3.2.3 Benefit-risk formulations

The B-R formulation of Gail et al. (1999) provides insights into the data needed and interpretation of the analysis for a treatment developed to prevent exacerbations of chronic obstructive pulmonary disease (COPD). Their model uses a metric defined by a weighted average of the treatment differences over K toxic or disease outcomes:

$$S = \sum_{k=1}^{K} w_k (P_{0k} - P_{1k}), \tag{3.1}$$

where P_{0k} and P_{1k} are the proportions of patients responding to the control and candidate treatment regimens, respectively, and the weights w_k are chosen to reflect the relative importance of the outcomes. Positive values $P_{0k} - P_{1k}$ are considered favorable and negative values unfavorable. The score S provides an integrated overall indicator such that $S > 0$ can be considered associated with a favorable benefit-risk profile, and $S < 0$ an unfavorable profile. This is the essence of a quantitative benefit-risk evaluation framework, which has been a source of unease concerning quantitative benefit-risk evaluations. Decision makers are concerned — rightly — that such score as (3.1) is inadequate to replace the collective clinical and regulatory judgments inherent in their decisions. However, when used properly and in the proper decision context, quantitative methods can facilitate decisions by providing relevant data and appropriate summaries and guide the decision process in the presence of these data. Moreover, they can be very helpful for planning purposes at the initial stage of a clinical development program. The aforementioned model of Gail et al. (1999) uses the proportions of patients responding to treatment and control, but other forms of outcome variables (e.g., normalized effect sizes) can also be applied so that the evidence across different types of toxic or disease outcomes can be integrated. It is also important to determine weights which reflect the patients' propensity to accept or avoid risk and which incorporate the frequency and severity of adverse events that patients may experience with the therapy. Various perspectives from different groups of stakeholders need to be considered in quantitative B-R evaluation. Adoption of and adherence to a common set of principles can result in widespread acceptance of the benefit-risk decisions. A multidisciplinary approach is recommended, helping statistical and data scientists learn fast and work well with scientists from other disciplines.

3.3   Benefit-risk methods using clinical trials data

Weighted categories of patients. Chuang-Stein et al. (1991) describe methods that incorporate patient-level data from randomized clinical trials in the overall evaluation of benefits and risks of a treatment. Each patient in a trial is assigned to one of five categories defined according to the subject's response to efficacy and the presence and severity of side effects: (a) efficacy, no serious side effects; (b) efficacy, serious side effects; (c) no efficacy, no serious side effects; (d) no efficacy, serious side effects; (e) side effects leading to patient's withdrawal from the study. Three measures are used to evaluate the categories simultaneously by using weights W_1, W_2, W_3, W_4, W_5 to reflect the relative importance of the categories for the patient. The simplest of the three measures uses the linear score

$$m = W_1 + W_2 - W_3 - W_4 - W_5. \tag{3.2}$$

A positive value of m indicates a favorable score and a negative value of m is unfavorable. The scores for each treatment can be compared statistically and graphical displays can also be included for visualization. Two ratio measures are also proposed that relate more to a benefit/risk ratio score. Chuang-Stein et al. (1991) use the hypertension example discussed in the previous section to illustrate the application of these measures. The two trials compare a test drug + HCTZ (hydrochlorothiazide) with a standard + HCTZ for treating hypertension. The results are consistent across both trials and show that the test drug is efficacious but is also associated with more side effects.

Categorical weights for individual patients. Chuang-Stein (1994) derive a score for each patient by reducing the observed benefit response by the patient's risk score. The safety endpoints are divided into J classes, and into L_j levels of severity for the jth class. Weights w_{jk} are assigned to level $k = 1, \ldots, L_j$ and class $j = 1, \ldots, J$. A risk score $r_i = \sum_{j=1}^{J} \sum_{k=1}^{L_j} w_{jk} I_{ijk}$ is computed for patient i, where $I_{ijk} = 1$ if patient i has experienced side effect j at severity level k, and $I_{ijk} = 0$ otherwise. The weights w_{jk} are monotonically related to the severity level k of the side effect. The efficacy score e_i for patient i is reduced by r_i for the risk-adjusted benefit score

$$e_i^* = e_i - fr_i, \tag{3.3}$$

where f is penalty per unit of risk and depends on the severity of the underlying disease being treated. In particular, because pediatric vaccines are administered to otherwise healthy infants, the value of f would be relatively large. Chuang-Stein (1994) provides an example using data from two randomized clinical trials of an investigational medicine for patients with exertional angina. In this example, ten classes of safety endpoints are divided into 4 grades and the weights are developed in collaboration with a cardiovascular physician.

Ranked categories for patients' outcomes. Claggett et al. (2014) compare treatments in the setting of a randomized clinical trial when each subject in the trial has time-to-event outcome variables, using data from the Beta-Blocker Evaluation of Survival Trial that include mortality and morbidity outcomes. Although the patient's overall survival time is the primary outcome variable, other important endpoints are also collected, such as hospitalization due to heart failure. Their analysis compares treatments on a benefit-risk scale using categorical responses for the patients. They simplify their outcome variables by using a categorical system consisting of clinically meaningful categories that are usually defined as a key part of the study protocol. Their analysis shows that defining ranked categories is simpler than defining preference weights across a set of multiple endpoints. This ranking approach circumvents the need for weights and can incorporate event time and censoring by using ordered categorical responses; see Cai et al. (2011).

3.4 Multi-criteria statistical decision theory

3.4.1 Multi-criteria decision analysis

Multi-Criteria Decision Analysis (MCDA) is a methodology for making decisions that involve multiple alternatives and multiple conflicting criteria, for which the competing alternatives would involve trade-offs of positive/negative effects across the multiple criteria under consideration. An example from financial economics is to form a portfolio of risky assets so that the portfolio return for a future period has a high mean and low variance; this is known as the mean-variance portfolio optimization problem. Essentially, MCDA is an optimization tool that is described by Keeney and Raiffa (1993) as "an extension of decision theory that covers any decision with multiple objectives." Supplement 1 in Section 3.7 illustrates this with the mean-variance portfolio optimization problem.

To develop a quantitative framework for B-R assessment, Mussen et al. (2007) propose to use the principles and formulation of MCDA to (a) account for multiple benefits and risk criteria, (b) incorporate judgments on the evidence and potential uncertainties, and (c) make trade-offs of benefits against risks. The MCDA methodology consists of a seven-step process (Table 3.2) that needs to be initiated early in clinical development process since it defines the essential data needed for a comprehensive B-R analysis to gain regulatory approval. MCDA brings complete transparency into the analysis and is integrated with the clinical development program; see the comprehensive review of MCDA for medical products by Phillips et al. (2013) who also consider application of MCDA to a drug for rheumatology, for which a one-day workshop was convened to develop the B-R model for the evaluation. During that workshop, referred to as a decision conference, the participants used an effects tree that clearly delineated favorable and unfavorable variables, assigned value weights to the effects, and applied an overall preference score for each alternative under consideration. There were three alternatives including a placebo control and two doses (low and high) of the candidate drug for regulatory approval against the background of methotrexate.

For Step 5 in Table 3.2, MCDA uses a method known as "swing weighting". A plausible range for the lower and upper limits is identified for

TABLE 3.2 A seven-step process for MCDA in benefit-risk assessment.

1.	Establish the decision context
2.	Identify the options to be appraised
3.	Identify objectives and criteria
I	Identify criteria for assessing the consequences for each option
II	Organize the criteria using high-level and lower-level objectives
4.	Assess the expected performance of each option against the criteria ("scoring")
I	Describe the consequences of each option
II	Score the options on the criteria
III	Check the consistency of the scores on each criterion
5.	Assign weights for the criteria to reflect their relative importance to the decision
6.	Calculate weighted scores at each level in the hierarchy and calculate overall weighted scores
7.	Examine the result and conduct sensitivity analysis

each variable, and the swing weights express the relevance of each variable based on a difference between the low and high limits. The highest weight is assigned to the criterion that yields the most important change in patient outcomes. Using the low(L) and high(H) weights $v_k^{(L)}$ and $v_k^{(H)}$ for criterion k, the MCDA socre for a given alternative in Table 3.2 is

$$S = \sum_{k=1}^{K} w_k (x_k - v_k^{(L)})/(v_k^{(H)} - v_k^{(L)}), \qquad (3.4)$$

where x_k is the criterion value and w_k is the weight assigned to criterion k. Such score S_j is computed for each alternative j ($j = 1, ..., M$) under consideration and the one with the highest score is preferred. For the rheumatology application of Phillips et al. (2013), the scores show a preference of both doses over the placebo control, and a preference of the low dose over the high dose. Application of the MCDA methodology to B-R assessment has been considered a major advance in the evaluation of medicinal products. It improves (3.1) by using swing weighting to map the criteria to a common scale and provides transparency and clear documentation of the values of the parameters used in the assessment. Uncertainty in the scoring is addressed using sensitivity analysis. Sensitivity analysis can be used to assess the robustness of the conclusions of the assessment.

3.4.2 Stochastic multi-criteria acceptability analysis and statistical decision theory

Stochastic multi-criteria acceptability analysis (SMAA) has been developed to address the limitations of MCDA in handling uncertainty in the weights and in the estimated values of the criteria. It is a family of methods that explicitly model the sources and amount of uncertainty in multi-criteria decisions. Tervonen and Lahdelma (2007) apply SMAA to the benefit-risk analysis for drugs. In MCDA the benefit-risk criteria are based only on point estimates of the favorable and unfavorable effects and on assigned weights for the criteria to reflect their relative importance to the decision, and uncertainty in these estimates and weights is handled by sensitivity analysis. SMAA incorporates two types of uncertainty that need to be incorporated in the analysis: (a) sampling variability in the estimated effect sizes, and (b) the weights used to scale the relative importance of the different criteria, for which SMAA methods are based on finding regions in the weight space to rank the criteria and make extensive use of Monte Carlo simulation to incorporate uncertainties in these regions and effect size estimates. As in MCDA, SMAA also considers benefit-risk decisions among M alternatives based on K criteria. Each of the alternatives has criterion values $x^j = (x_1^j, \ldots, x_K^j)$ for $j = 1, \ldots, M$, where x_k^j is the performance measure of alternative j for criterion k and is treated as a random variable that has a distribution quantifying uncertainty and which can be a continuous measurement, or categorical variable, or time to an event or another outcome variable from a clinical trial. Similarly, the weights are assumed to be random variables in the feasibility region $w_k > 0$ and $\sum w_k = 1$. A complete lack of preference can be specified by a uniform distribution for the weight vector **w**, but a patient with a mild disease may have a preference for fewer symptomatic adverse events over efficacy, whereas a patient at a severe disease stage may consider efficacy to be more important. The preference for any point in the K-dimensional space can be represented by

$$S_j(x^j, w) = \sum_{k=1}^{K} w_k u(x_k^j), \qquad (3.5)$$

where $u(x_k^j) = (x_k^j - v_k^{(L)})/(v_k^{(H)} - v_k^{(L)})$ is the utility function of the criterion x_k^j using the low and high swing weights $v_k^{(L)}$ and $v_k^{(H)}$ for criterion k as in (3.4) for MCDA. The SMAA formulation in (3.5) incorporates uncertainty by assuming the criteria and the weights to be random variables. A method called "inverse weight space analysis" (Lahdelma and Salminen, 2010, p.290) can be used to assign particular ranks to the M treatment options. While the weight space is given by $\Omega = \{\mathbf{w} \in \mathbb{R}^K : w_k \geq 0 \text{ and } \sum w_k = 1\}$, the inverse weight space is defined as the set of weights for which r is the rank of treatment j, $1 \leq r \leq M$.

Monte Carlo simulation is performed using data generated from the assumed distribution for the criterion effects x_k^j and for the weights w_k. The preference score $S_j(x^j, w)$ is computed for each realization and each alternative. Then the rank acceptability index, denoted by b_j^r, is the proportion of all possible values of the weight vector for which alternative j has rank r. Tervonen and Lahdelma (2007) provide computational implementation details of this and other SMAA methods.

As an alternative to weighting in MCDA and inverse weighting for SMAA, Wang et al. (2016) introduce the "stochastic multi-criteria discriminatory method" (SMDM), which assumes the weight vector w to be random, using a uniform distribution for w if no information is available or a distribution reflecting partial information such as ranking of the criteria. For two treatment options A and B, let $\Delta(w) = S_A(x^A, w) - S_B(x^B, w)$ denote the difference in scores for the values of the K-dimensional vectors x^A and x^B and the weight vector w. Thus, a value of $\Delta(w) > 0$ indicates a preference for A and $\Delta(w) < 0$ a preference for B. However, to include the variance of $\Delta(w)$ as part of the decision metric, SMDM uses a more stringent cutoff than 0, favoring A if $\Delta(w) \geq \text{cutoff}(w)$ and B if $-\Delta(w) \geq \text{cutoff}(w)$, with cutoff(w) determined by the following "discriminatory probabilities":

$$d_A = P\{\Delta \geq \text{cutoff}(w)\}, d_B = P\{-\Delta \geq \text{cutoff}(w)\}. \tag{3.6}$$

Clearly, if the discriminatory cutoff is 0, then $d_A + d_B = 1$. On the other hand, if cutoff(w) is too high, then d_A and d_B can be both low, meaning that a clear preference cannot be determined. A useful visual display is provided by plots of d_A and d_B against the value of the cutoff. Wang et al. (2016) recommend using Monte Carlo simulation to determine d_A and d_B and apply SMDM to the data of a clinical trial comparing a standard to a test drug for hypertension reported by Chuang-Stein et al. (1991); see Section 3.3. The patient data are grouped into five categories ordered from the best outcome (efficacy without serious side effects and labeled category 1) to the worst outcome (side effects leading to patient's withdrawal from the study, labeled category 5). Wang et al. (2016) show how to simulate the weight distribution according to the ranking.

Multi-criteria statistical decision theory. Similar to MCDA, SMAA methods originated from decision optimization applications that are broader than health care; see Tervonen and Figueira (2008), Lahdelma and Salminen (2010), and Tervonen et al. (2011). Supplements 1 and 2 of Section 3.7 illustrate this point for the mean-variance portfolio optimization problem. Supplement 1 assumes the means and covariances of the returns $r_i(i = 1, ..., p)$ of p risky assets over a single future time period to be known so that the portfolio has return $\mu = \sum_{i=1}^p w_i \mathbb{E}(r_i)$ and variance $\sigma^2 = \sum_{1 \leq i,j \leq p} w_i w_j \text{Cov}(r_i, r_j)$, in which the w_i denote the portfolio weights such that $\sum_{i=1}^p w_i = 1$, with $w_i \geq 0$ if short selling is not allowed but with some w_i taking positive and other w_i taking negative values for long-short portfolios. The portfolio optimization problem is to choose the weights such that μ is maximized according to the mean criterion and σ is minimized according to the variance (representing "risk") criterion. The solution to this multi-criteria decision problem is the "efficient frontier" in the (σ, μ) plane, which was first discovered by Markowitz (1952) who won the Nobel Prize in Economics for this seminal work and also showed how to compute the efficient (i.e., minimum-variance) portfolio for a target level μ_* of mean return. In practice, however, $\mathbb{E}(r_i)$ and $\text{Cov}(r_i, r_j)$ are usually unknown, and substituting them by their estimated values based on historical data can lead to portfolios that may perform much worse than the case of known means and covariances; this is known as the "Markowitz enigma". Lai et al. (2011) address this problem by using statistical decision theory, which treats the unknown parameters as states (with prior distributions quantifying their uncertainty), to reformulate the portfolio optimization problem in terms of SMAA. They use an empirical Bayes approach to solve this SMAA problem and bootstrap methods to implement the solution; details are given in Supplement 2.

3.5   Quality-adjusted benefit-risk assessments

3.5.1   Q-TWiST

Q-TWiST (Quality-adjusted Time Without Symptoms of disease and Toxicity of treatment) is a health index in the classification of benefit-risk methods described by Mt-Isa et al. (2014). It relies on individual patient-level data and is considered most relevant to healthcare providers and regulatory agencies. Q-TWiST builds on the Quality-Adjusted Life Year (QALY) measure which is a well-established metric used by health economists for conducting cost-effectiveness analyses. Weinstein et al. (2009) gave an overview on the foundations and origins of the QALY and its use in economic evaluations. The incremental cost-effectiveness ratio is defined as $\Delta C / \Delta Q$, where ΔC and ΔQ are the incremental changes in cost and QALYs, respectively, in comparing a novel test program to a standard control. Guo et al. (2010) used Q-TWiST to compare therapies, incorporating duration and quality of life (QOL), in the comparison. Patients were assumed to move progressively through a sequence of clinical health states but cannot backtrack. The method partitions the area under the Kaplan-Meier survival curve and calculates the average duration a patient spends in each health state. In this way, the Q-TWiST is a quality-adjusted version of TWiST by converting time into QALYs. It penalizes the QALYs gained due to the efficacy of the drug by the QALYs lost due to the impact of adverse drug experiences. Essentially the method tracks the progression of patients through the series of health states each of which has a specific QOL. The method is particularly well suited for cancer therapies and many applications have been reported that use the Q-TWiST; see Gelber et al. (1996) who also provide a graphical tool that partitions the survival plot showing the time with toxicity, time in TWiST, time after relapse, and overall survival. For cancer outcomes, the method measures the time with toxicity (TOX), disease-free survival (DFS), and the overall survival (OS). The original TWiST was defined as TWiST = DFS − TOX and the period after a relapse until death is REL = OS − DFS. TWiST has utility score $\mu = 1$, and incorporating the utility scores μ_{TOX} and μ_{REL} for TOX and REL leads to the definition of Q-TWiST as

$$Q\text{-}TWiST = \mu_{\text{TOX}} \times \text{TOX} + \text{TWiST} + \mu_{\text{REL}} \times \text{REL}. \qquad (3.7)$$

Gelber et al. (1995) recommend estimating the Q-TWiST for specified values of μ_{TOX} and μ_{REL} since the times that patients spend in each health state are available from the clinical trial data. A major complication, however, arises in the presence of censoring. Censoring occurs if patients are not followed until the final health state of death because they are either still alive at the end of the study or lost to follow-up. This is not a problem when $\mu_{\text{TOX}} = \mu_{\text{REL}} = 1$ and the analysis is strictly based on time. However, when μ_{TOX} and/or μ_{REL} is < 1, the censoring is informative and the Kaplan-Meier estimate of the mean is biased. Zhao and Tsiatis (2001) have developed a modified log-rank test that is suitable for testing the equality of survival functions of quality-adjusted lifetime, including the Q-TWiST, which is the topic of the next two subsections.

3.5.2 Quality-adjusted survival analysis

As pointed out by Zhao and Tsiatis (1997), quality-adjusted survival analysis arises in treatment evaluation of chronic diseases, such as cancer or AIDS, for which "extending overall survival time may not be the only goal of a new therapy, since patients might have to endure longer time of toxicity from the drug and life after disease recurrence might be painful." The quality adjusted lifetime (QAL) is defined by $U = \sum_{j=1}^{k} q_j S_j$, where $q_1, \ldots, q_k$ are the utility coefficients assigned to each of the k health states, and $S_1, \ldots, S_k$ are times spent in each state. In a typical application, a patient undergoing treatment would first go through a period S_1 that is subject only to toxicity, then at time $S_1 + S_2$ may have a relapse, and finally at time $S_1 + S_2 + S_3$ would die. Because patients typically enter a survival trial over a period of time and the study is terminated before all the information for every patient is observed (Bartroff et al., 2013, Chapter 6), this also "results in varying amounts of follow-up and censored or incomplete quality-adjusted survival time." Zhao and Tsiatis (1997) first considered an asymptotically unbiased, normally distributed estimator of the quality-adjusted survival distribution. Subsequently, they developed a more efficient estimator by using inverse probability weighting, proposed by Robins and Rotnitzky (1992), to (a) define the set of influence functions for all regular asymptotically linear estimators for the distribution of QAL, (b) construct a class of estimators that have these influence functions, (c) use the Cauchy-Schwarz inequality to find the form of the most efficient estimator and obtain the efficiency bound, and (d) derive an estimator that is much easier to construct than the most efficient estimator and is more efficient than their earlier estimator introduced in 1997; details are described below.

Assume that there are $K + 1$ states of health denoted by $s \in S = \{1, ..., K, 0\}$. It is assumed that state 0 is absorbing and corresponds to death or disease (for example, cancer relapse). For n individuals under study, the ith individual's health over time is described by a discrete-state continuous-time stochastic process $\{V_i(t), t \geq 0\}$, where $V_i(t)$ takes values in the state space S. Let T_i denote the time taken by the ith subject to move into the absorbing state 0; T_i can be considered as the overall survival time. Let $V_i^H(t) = \{V_i(u) : u \leq t\}$ be the ith subject's health history up to time t and Q denote a utility function which maps the state space S to the interval $[0, 1]$; it maps the absorbing state to 0. The functional form of Q can vary for individuals according to their own assessment of quality of life for the different health states; the assessment may also vary over time to reflect the patient's change of perception. With this notation, the ith individual's QAL, denoted by U_i, is $U_i = \int_0^{T_i} Q_i(t, V_i(t)) \, dt$. In most studies, the entire health history for all individuals is not observed because of various types of censoring. To accommodate this, suppose the ith subject has a potential time to censoring C_i with survival function $K(u)$, which is the same for all individuals, and assume that censoring is independent of the health history. In a well-controlled clinical trial in which patients' follow-up is complete during the course of the study, censoring occurs only when a patient is still alive at the end of the study; this is called administrative censoring. For such situations, independent censoring may be reasonably assumed. Because of the presence of censoring, QAL can only be defined within the time frame of observation as it is not possible to estimate nonparametrically the distribution of QAL beyond some time point. Zhao and Tsiatis (1999) choose a value L such that $K(L) > 0$ and redefine QAL as $U_i = \int_0^L Q_i(t, V_i(t)) \, dt$.

The health status data for a sample of n individuals that include the possibility of censoring can be described as $\{X_i = \min(T_i, C_i), \delta_i = I(T_i \leq C_i), V_i^H(X_i), i = 1, ..., n\}$. To estimate the QAL-adjusted survival distribution $S(x) = P(U > x), x \geq 0$, from such a sample, Zhao and Tsiatis (1997) use the idea of inverse probability weighting proposed by Robins and Rotnitzky (1992) to construct a weighted estimator:

$$\hat{S}_{\text{wt}}(x) = n^{-1} \sum_{i=1}^{n} \frac{\delta_i I(U_i > x)}{\hat{K}(T_i)},$$

with

$$\hat{K}(T_i) = \prod_{u \leq T_i} \left\{ 1 - \frac{dN^c(u)}{Y(u)} \right\},$$

where $N^c(u) = \sum N_i^c(u) = \sum I(X_i \leq u, \delta_i = 0)$ and $Y(u) = \sum Y_i(u) = \sum I(X_i \geq u)$. Thus, $\hat{K}(T_i)$ is the Kaplan-Meier estimator of $K(T_i)$, recalling that K is the common survival function of the C_i. Statistical properties of this estimator can be derived by exploiting the martingale theory for counting processes (Bartroff et al., 2013, Section 6.6), which Zhao and Tsiatis (1999) use to derive the approximation

$$n^{1/2}\{\hat{S}_{wt}(x) - S(x)\} \approx n^{-1/2} \sum_{i=1}^{n} \{B_i - S(x)\}$$
$$- n^{-1/2} \sum_{i=1}^{n} \int_0^\infty \{B_i - G(B, u)\} \frac{dM_i^c(u)}{K(u)},$$

where $B_i = I(U_i > x)$, $S_T(u) = P(T > u)$, $G(Z, u) = E\{Z_i I(T_i \geq u)\}/S_T(u)$ for any i.i.d. random variables Z_i, and $M_i^c(u) = N_i^c(u) - \int_0^u \lambda^c(t) Y_i(t)\, dt$ is the martingale process, in which $\lambda^c(u)$ is the common hazard function for the censoring variables C_i. The approximation is used to show that $\hat{S}_{\text{wt}}(x)$ is consistent and asymptotically normal, and that the asymptotic variance is

$$S(x)\{1 - S(x)\} + \int_0^\infty \frac{S_T(u)}{K(u)} G(B, u)\{1 - G(B, u)\}\lambda^c(u)\, du,$$

which Zhao and Tsiatis (1999) argue to be inefficient because $\hat{S}_{\text{wt}}(x)$ does not use the health status information that is accrued for each individual over the course of the study. Noting that the influence function for complete data is $B_i - S(x)$, they consider the class of influence functions

$$B_i - S(x) - \int_0^\infty [B_i - G(B, u)] \frac{dM_i^c(u)}{K(u)}$$
$$+ C \int_0^\infty [e(V_i^H(u)) - G(e, u)] \frac{dM_i^c(u)}{K(u)},$$

where $e(V_i^H(u))$ is any function of the ith subject's health history up to time u and C is the regression coefficient of the first stochastic integral on the second one. They give consistent estimates $\hat{C}$, $\hat{G}(B, u)$ and $\hat{G}(e, u)$ and use the Cauchy-Schwarz inequality to show that the most efficient choice of $e(V_i^H(u))$ is $E(B_i|V_i^H(u))$, thereby deriving the semiparametric efficiency bound for estimating the quality-adjust survival function. They point out, however, that $E(B_i|V_i^H(u))$ is very difficult to estimate and suggest using $e_i^*(V_i(u)) = \int_0^u Q_i(t, V_i(t)) \, dt$ instead. This yields their estimator to improve $\hat{S}_{\text{wt}}(x)$:

$$\hat{S}_{\text{imp}}(x) = \frac{1}{n} \sum_{i=1}^n \frac{\delta_i^*(x) I(U_i > x)}{\hat{K}(T_i^*(x))}$$

$$+ \frac{\hat{C}}{n} \sum_{i=1}^n \int_0^\infty \left[e_i^*\left(V_i^H(u)\right) - \hat{G}(e^*, u) \right] \frac{dN_i^c(u)}{\hat{K}(u)}, \qquad (3.8)$$

in which $T_i^* = \min\{T_i, s_i^*(x)\}$ and $\delta_i^*(x) = I(T_i^*(x) \le C_i)$, where $s_i^* = \inf\left\{s : \int_0^s Q_i(t, V_i(t)) \, dt \ge x\right\}$ and "all functions of the survival time, such as $\hat{K}(u)$ and $N^c(u)$, should be indexed by x" although such indexing is omitted "for ease of notation." They show that $\hat{S}_{\text{imp}}(x)$ "is easy to compute and is substantially more efficient than previously proposed estimators."

3.5.3 Testing QAL differences of treatment from control

Zhao and Tsiatis (2001) study the hypothesis testing problem to compare QAL from independent treatment and control groups. They say:

> The log-rank test is the most commonly used test for comparing the survival distribution among two treatments in clinical trials. In the special case where the utility coefficient is one for all health states except death, an individual's quality-adjusted lifetime is the same as their survival time. However, except for this special case, the log-rank test applied to censored QAL data would be biased. This is due to the induced informative censoring... Specifically, an individual who has a high utility coefficient accumulates QAL faster compared with an individual who has a poor quality of life. Hence, when censoring is present, even though the censoring is independent of the survival time, a large censored QAL often indicates a large uncensored QAL and vice versa. ... We propose here a test statistic for comparing the distribution of quality-adjusted lifetime that becomes the standard log-rank test when quality-adjusted lifetime equals survival time but is unbiased otherwise.

They use inverse probability weighting as in the preceding subsection to tackle informative censoring. Let Z_i (=1 or 0) be the treatment indicator for the ith individual, taking the value 1 for the treatment group, and n_1 (or n_0) denote the number of subjects in the treatment (or control) group. Let $K(t) = P(C_i > t)$ as in the preceding subsection, and define

$K(t, z) = P(C_i > t | Z_i = z)$ for $z = 0, 1$, $w(t) = K(t, 1)K(t, 0)/K(t)$,

$$\psi_i = \int_0^\infty w(u) \left[Z_i - \frac{E\{Z_i I(V_i \geq u)\}}{E\{I(V_i \geq u)\}} \right] dM_i^V(u), \qquad (3.9)$$

where V_i is the QAL defined in the preceding subsection. The martingale $M_i^V(u)$ is based on the counting processes for the QAL and can be written as $M_i^V(u) = I(V_i \leq u) - \int_0^u \lambda^V(t)I(V_i \geq t)dt$, where $\lambda^V(t)$ is the hazard function for V_i, which under H_0 is independent of Z_i. Since $K(u)$ and $K(u, z)$ are typically unknown, Zhao and Tsiatis (2001) propose to substitute them in (3.9) by their Kaplan-Meier estimates, assuming that "the probability of observing complete data is bounded away from zero," as in the use of L such that $K(L) > 0$ in the integral $\int_0^L$ defining V_i in the preceding subsection. With these substitutions, replacing $dM_i^V(u)$ by $dN_i^V(u)$ in ψ_i under the null hypothesis yields the test statistic

$$\frac{1}{\sqrt{n}} \sum_{i=1}^n \frac{\delta_i}{\hat{K}(T_i, Z_i)} \frac{\hat{K}(V_i, 1)\hat{K}(V_i, 0)}{\hat{K}(V_i)}$$

$$\times \left[Z_i - \frac{\sum_{j=1}^n \frac{\delta_j}{\hat{K}(T_j, Z_j)} Z_j I(V_j \geq V_i)}{\sum_{j=1}^n \frac{\delta_j}{\hat{K}(T_j, Z_j)} I(V_j \geq V_i)} \right], \qquad (3.10)$$

which they show to be asymptotically normal and derive a consistent estimate of the asymptotic variance in their Appendix 2 and Eq. (2). They also illustrate their method with a breast cancer study in which patients entering the study first experience toxicity and then a period of good health until their disease relapses, for which QAL "is defined to be the time spent between the end of toxicity and the start of disease relapse," which is equivalent to setting the utility function to 1 (for the healthy period) or 0 (otherwise).

For traditional survival endpoints (without quality adjustments), the logrank statistic is asymptotically efficient for proportional hazards alternatives, but other test statistics can have considerably higher power at alternatives where hazard ratios can be time-varying. Murray and Tsiatis (1999) and Chen and Tsiatis (2001) have followed up on the aforementioned work by Zhao and Tsiatis (1999). Their basic idea is the restricted mean survival time (RMST) curve of a survival endpoint T: $\text{RMST}(t) = E\left(\min(T, t)\right)$, which is the area under the survival curve of T up to time t. Thus $\text{RMST}(t)$ can be estimated by the area of the corresponding Kaplan-Meier curve up to time t. This idea can likewise be applied to the QAL V in lieu of T, and can also be extended to the difference between the RMST curves of the treatment and control groups; see Zhao et al. (2016) for details.

3.6 Additional statistical methods

3.6.1 Number needed to treat (NNT)

NNT (number needed to treat) is defined as the number of patients who need to be treated for preventing a disease endpoint to occur. The measure, originally proposed by Laupacis et al. (1988), is used for trials with binary endpoints so that the results can be summarized by the proportions of patients in each of two groups who experience the outcome of interest. When the outcome is the occurence of an adverse event, such as death or disease, the absolute risk reduction (ARR) is defined by ARR= $P_0 - P_1$ for the proportions of patients in the active and control groups experiencing the outcome. When the outcome is a favorable outcome, such as an improvement or cure in the disease, then ARR= $P_1 - P_0$; see Cook and Sackett (1995) who use NNT to measure the benefit of an active treatment over a control. In either case NNT = 1/ARR. Moreover, for benefit-risk analysis, ARR is preferred to relative measures of treatment effect such as relative risk, relative risk reduction, and odds ratio, as it is especially relevant to evaluating and integrating effects across favorable and unfavorable outcomes with possible different background incidence rates. Note that when the treatment effect is near 0, ARR is small, then the NNT can be very large, which can cause complications with confidence interval estimates of NNT; see Altman (1998). An alternative to NNT is NNH, which is the proportion of patients who experience an adverse drug reaction.

3.6.2 Incremental net benefits

The incremental net benefit (INB) is an incremental change in a patient's health benefit minus by an incremental change in patient's risk. It was originally proposed to evaluate the cost-effectiveness of a pharmaceutical product and was later used to assess the net gain in health by patients using the product (Willan, 2004; Garrison et al., 2007; Lynd et al., 2010). Because it allows comparison of changes in treatment benefits reduced by the changes in treatment risks over treatment groups, it incorporates time and utility in benefit-risk assessments. To illustrate, consider a randomized trial comparing two groups. Let p_{ij} denote the probability of experiencing the jth beneficial outcome in the ith treatment group, and q_{ik} the probability of experiencing the kth harmful outcome in the ith treatment group, with $i = 1, 2$, $j = 1, \ldots, J$ and $k = 1, \ldots, K$. For example, p_{ij} is the probability of survival (or the probability of having a myocardial infarction if the benefit is a reduction in myocardial infarction incidence) and q_{ik} is the probability of dying if the harm is death (or the probability of experiencing a hypersensitivity episode if the harm is hypersensitivity).

Let $\Delta p_j = p_{2j} - p_{1j}$ be the difference in probabilities of having beneficial outcome j and $\Delta q_k = q_{2k} - q_{1k}$ the difference in probabilities of experiencing harmful outcome k. Najafzadeh et al. (2015) introduce weights ϕ_j and ψ_k and a factor γ to quantify the trade-off between benefit and risk in the definition

$$\text{INB} = \sum_{j=1}^{J} \phi_j T_j \Delta p_j - \gamma \sum_{k=1}^{K} \psi_k \tau_k \Delta q_k, \tag{3.11}$$

where T_j (τ_k) represents the duration of impact of the jth beneficial (kth harmful) outcome; the choice $\gamma = 1$ implies that benefits and risks are equally important to the decision maker, whereas $\gamma > 1$ places more weight on harmful than beneficial effects. They also define

$$\text{MAR}_{jk} = \frac{\phi_j / \Delta p_j}{\psi_k / \Delta q_k} \tag{3.12}$$

as a measure of the increase in risk of a harmful event k that an individual is willing to accept in exchange for an increase in the benefit of outcome j. Letting u_j (or ν_k) denote the utility associated with outcome j (or k) after treatment and u_0 be the baseline utility of patients before treatment, they define the quality-adjusted life-years INB as

$$\text{INB}_{\text{QALY}} = \sum_{j=1}^{J} (u_0 - \nu_j) T_j \Delta p_j - \gamma \sum_{k=1}^{K} (u_0 - \nu_k) \tau_k \Delta q_k, \tag{3.13}$$

where $(u_0 - \nu_j) T_j$ can be thought of as the QALY gained when experiencing a beneficial event and $(u_0 - \nu_k) \tau_k$ as the QALY lost when having a harmful event.

3.6.3   Uncertainty adjustments and Bayesian methods

Weights have played an important role in the aforementioned quantitative B-R evaluations. Flexible weights should be used to reflect patient preference, severity of outcome, cost, and other major considerations that can enhance the robustness and acceptance of the B-R assessments. As noted in Section 3.4.2, SMAA has the appealing ability to account for sampling variability and missing data. To address the issue of uncertainty adjustments in B-R analysis, Zhao et al. (2014) and Waddingham et al. (2016) have provided case studies that demonstrate the potential for Bayesian analysis to output a posterior distribution of the overall benefit-risk balance through simulations. In particular, Zhao et al. (2014) introduce a Bayesian model for a global benefit-risk score which assigns patients ranks 1 to 5 based on efficacy and side effects; details are given in Supplement 4 (which also summarizes how they apply the Bayesian model to longitudinal data from a clinical trial of a pain medicine) and Supplement 5 of Section 3.7 reviews the Bayesian sensitivity analysis of Waddingham et al. (2016). For the related problem of cost-effectiveness, Stinnett and Mullahy (1998) have used the Bayesian approach in their net health benefit analysis and cost-effectiveness acceptability curve.

A workshop was convened by the Institute of Medicine (IOM) in 2014 for characterizing the uncertainty in assessing benefits and risks of pharmaceutical products (Caruso et al., 2014). IOM subsequently recommended the development of systematic and structured approaches, in addition to improvements in transparency and communication to reduce uncertainty, understanding the heterogeneous patient populations and health care systems, clinical factors, and economic and cultural factors, development of disease and treatment models to integrate the available epidemiological and clinical trial data such as the model of Gail et al. (1999) concerning the benefits and harms of Tamoxifin in treating breast cancer. Effective evaluation of benefits and risks should consider data sources outside a single clinical study or even a clinical program of several studies, and include supplemental data on the treatment effects of a drug and its comparators, structured literature reviews and meta-analyses of existing studies, and real-world observational database studies. Epidemiological studies of baseline risks for both beneficial and harmful outcomes and separate studies of patient preferences can provide important information and data. The benefit-risk profile of a drug should be updated as new information becomes available. A risk management plan and post-marketing safety studies should be in place at the onset to mitigate the unforeseen risks that may arise, taking precaution for rare but severe adverse events that only become evident when a sufficiently large number of patients have taken the drug.

3.6.4 Endpoint selection and other considerations

The key components of a B-R analysis are the endpoints selected for the analysis, the weights used for integrating the criteria values, and the uncertainties discussed in the preceding subsection. Ma et al. (2016) have discussed how these components relate to one another and the complexity they contribute to the overall evaluation. Benefit endpoint selection is relatively easy because the phase III protocol has to define the primary and secondary endpoints, but the safety endpoints are much harder to prespecify as adverse effects may be identified only during the course of clinical trials or in postmarketing studies. The benefits and risk outcomes in a benefit-risk analysis carry differing levels of importance. The derivation of weights for the benefit and risk endpoints can in principle be based on the trade-off between them; see Guo et al. (2010) who use NNT or NNH to address the relative weights to be assigned. Weighting for multiple outcomes used in MCDA is more challenging, particularly with respect to uncertainty adjustments. There are uncertainties in the evidence for the multiple endpoints that define the benefits and the risks, and there is also uncertainty in the relative importance characterized by weights or ranks of the benefits and risks.

Benefit-risk analysis (BRA) involves a complex and multifaceted set of data, methods and judgement on the part of all stakeholders, as pointed out by Jiang and He (2016, page 171): "Although numerous approaches and frameworks have been proposed in recent years, there is no single approach or framework that can be applied and utilized in every setting and a combination of methods may be needed for each BRA." Structured BRA is a multidisciplinary effort involving teams of experts in clinical science, safety assessment, decision science, epidemiology, economics, and statistics. Below is a list of statistical considerations for BRA:

(a) Sound statistical analyses are the foundational basis for the evidence used for qualitative value assessments of the available data, and quantitative benefit-risk analysis should incorporate statistical principles and widely accepted frameworks such as BRAT or PRoACT.

(b) Clear and complete effects tabulation should include a clear delineation of favorable and unfavorable effects.

(c) The impact of uncertainty as represented in the model assumptions and sampling variability, implemented by Monte Carlo simulation and presented by graphical displays, should be incorporated in BRA, which cannot be adequately addressed using hypothesis-driven study designs and P-value summaries.

(d) Statistical decision theory under uncertainty can provide basic techniques and expert judgement to identify the most important benefits and risks and to assign weights based on their importance.

(e) Simple methods that are clearly understood by clinicians and graphical displays showing the integration of both benefits and risks can effectively communicate the results.

(f) Supplementing randomized clinical trials data with appropriate epidemiological, health outcomes and observational data is often helpful and necessary for a comprehensive benefit-risk analysis.

3.7 Supplements and problems

1. *Multi-objective optimization and efficient frontier in mean-variance portfolio optimization.* Let $\mathbf{f} : \mathbb{R}^n \to \mathbb{R}^m$ be a vector-valued function of

n decision variables such that $f_i(\mathbf{x})$ represents the ith objective function in a multi-objective optimization problem. There may also be inequality and equality constraints on the decision variables so that the optimization problem can be represented by maximization of $\mathbf{f}(\mathbf{x})$ over $\mathbf{x} \in S$, where S is the constrained set and $\mathbf{x} \in S$ dominates $\mathbf{x}' \in S$ if $f_i(\mathbf{x}) \geq f_i(\mathbf{x}')$ for every $i = 1, ..., m$, with strict inequality for some i. A vector of decision variables is said to be *Pareto optimal* if there does not exist $\mathbf{x} \in S$ that dominates it. The set of Pareto optimal elements of S is called the *Pareto boundary*. If $\mathbf{x}$ is a random variable, then the f_i are certain expected functionals of $\mathbf{x}$; see Guo et al. (2017, pp.49-50), who also relate Markowitz's mean-variance portfolio optimization problem, a two-objective stochastic optimization problem, with $f_1(\mathbf{w}) = E(\mathbf{w}^T\mathbf{r})$ and $f_2(\mathbf{w}) = -\mathrm{Var}(\mathbf{w}^T\mathbf{r})$. The mean-variance portfolio optimization theory, introduced by Markowitz (1952) to incorporate the impact of risk into investment decisions, is a single-period theory on the choice of portfolio weights providing the optimal tradeoff between the mean μ (measure of profit) and the standard deviation σ (measure of risk) of return for a future period. Markowitz first approached the problem by considering the geometry of optimal portfolio as follows. The set of points in the (σ, μ) plane that corresponds to returns of portfolios of a given set of p stocks is called a *feasible region*; it is convex to the left in the sense that given any two points in the region, the line segment joining them does not cross the region's left boundary. The left boundary of the feasible region is called the *minimum-variance set*: for a given value μ of the mean return, the feasible point with smallest σ lies on this left boundary, corresponding to the *minimum-variance portfolio*. For a given value σ of volatility, investors prefer the portfolio with largest mean return, achieved at an upper left boundary point of the feasible region; the upper portion of the minimum-variance set is called the *efficient frontier*. Given the mean vector μ and the covariance matrix Σ of the stock returns in the future period for which the portfolio is to be constructed, Markowitz also solved for the optimal portfolio weight vector $\mathbf{w}$ that minimizes the variance $\mathbf{w}^T\Sigma\mathbf{w}$ of the portfolio return under the constraints that the weights sum to 1 and the mean return $\mathbf{w}^T\mu$ of the portfolio attains some target level μ_*.

2. *Incorporating parameter uncertainty to resolve the Markowitz enigma.* Whereas the problem of minimizing $\mathrm{Var}(\mathbf{w}^T\mathbf{r}_{n+1})$ subject to a given level μ_* of the mean return $E(\mathbf{w}^T\mathbf{r}_{n+1})$ is meaningful in Markowitz's framework, in which both $E(\mathbf{r}_{n+1})$ and $\mathrm{Cov}(\mathbf{r}_{n+1})$ are known, the surrogate problem of minimizing $\mathbf{w}^T\hat{\Sigma}\mathbf{w}$ under the constraint $\mathbf{w}^T\hat{\mu} = \mu_*$ ignores the fact the sample estimates $\hat{\mu}$ and $\hat{\Sigma}$ have inherent errors (risks) themselves. Lai et al. (2011) consider the more fundamental

problem

$$\max\{E(\mathbf{w}^T\mathbf{r}_{n+1}) - \lambda\mathrm{Var}(\mathbf{w}^T\mathbf{r}_{n+1})\} \qquad (3.14)$$

when μ and Σ are unknown and treated as state variables whose uncertainties are specified by their posterior distributions given the observations $\mathbf{r}_1, ..., \mathbf{r}_n$ in a Bayesian framework. The random vector w in (3.14) consists of weights that depend on $\mathbf{r}_1, \ldots, \mathbf{r}_n$. If the prior distribution puts all its mass at (μ_0, Σ_0), then the minimization (3.14) reduces to Markowitz's portfolio optimization problem that assumes μ_0 and Σ_0 are given. The Lagrange multiplier λ in (3.14) can be regarded as the investor's risk-aversion index when variance is used to measure risk. Lai et al. (2011) solve (3.14) by rewriting it as the following maximization problem over η:

$$\max_{\eta}\{E[\mathbf{w}^T(\eta)\mathbf{r}_{n+1}] - \lambda\mathrm{Var}[\mathbf{w}^T(\eta)\mathbf{r}_{n+1}]\}, \qquad (3.15)$$

where $\mathbf{w}(\eta)$ is the solution of the stochastic optimization problem

$$\mathbf{w}(\eta) = \arg\min_{\mathbf{w}}\{\lambda E[(\mathbf{w}^T\mathbf{r}_{n+1})^2] - \eta E(\mathbf{w}^T\mathbf{r}_{n+1})\}. \qquad (3.16)$$

Let μ_n and $\mathbf{V}_n$ be the posterior mean and second moment matrix given the set $\mathcal{R}$ of current and past returns $\mathbf{r}_1, ..., \mathbf{r}_n$. Since w is based on $\mathcal{R}_n$, it follows from $E(\mathbf{r}_{n+1}|\mathcal{R}_n) = \mu_n$ and $E(\mathbf{r}_{n+1}\mathbf{r}_{n+1}^T|\mathcal{R}_n) = \mathbf{V}_n$ that $E(\mathbf{w}^T\mathbf{r}_{n+1}) = E(\mathbf{w}^T\mu_n)$, $E[(\mathbf{w}^T\mathbf{r}_{n+1})^2] = E(\mathbf{w}^T\mathbf{V}_n\mathbf{w})$. When short selling is allowed without limits, $\mathbf{w}(\eta)$ in (3.16) is given explicitly by

$$\begin{aligned}\mathbf{w}(\eta) = \arg\min_{\mathbf{w}:\mathbf{w}^T\mathbf{1}=1}\{\lambda\mathbf{w}^T\mathbf{V}_n\mathbf{w} - \eta\mathbf{w}^T\mu_n\} \\ = \frac{1}{C_n}\mathbf{V}_n^{-1}\mathbf{1} + \frac{\eta}{2\lambda}\mathbf{V}_n^{-1}\left(\mathbf{V}_n^{-1} - \frac{A_n}{C_n}\mathbf{1}\right),\end{aligned} \qquad (3.17)$$

where $A_n = \mu_n^T\mathbf{V}_n^{-1}\mathbf{1} = \mathbf{1}^T\mathbf{V}_n^{-1}\mu_n$, $B_n = \mu_n^T\mathbf{V}_n^{-1}\mu_n$, $C_n = \mathbf{1}^T\mathbf{V}_n^{-1}\mathbf{1}$. When there are limits on short selling, they become inequality constraints on w in (3.16) and quadratic programming can be used to compute $\mathbf{w}(\eta)$.

The Bayesian approach requires full specification of the prior distribution of (μ, Σ) besides the distribution of $\mathbf{r}_{n+1}$ given (μ, Σ), even though (3.15) and (3.16) only involve $E[(\mathbf{w}^T\mathbf{r}_{n+1})^2]$ and $E(\mathbf{w}^T\mathbf{r}_{n+1})$. Lai et al. (2011) use the bootstrap method to estimate $E_{\mu,\Sigma}[(\mathbf{w}^T\mathbf{r}_{n+1})^2]$ and $E_{\mu,\Sigma}(\mathbf{w}^T\mathbf{r}_{n+1})$, which is tantamount to a nonparametric empirical Bayes (NPEB) approach without explicitly specifying the prior distribution of (μ, Σ) and the distribution of $\mathbf{r}_{n+1}$ given (μ, Σ). The discussion so far has assumed i.i.d. returns $\mathbf{r}_1, ..., \mathbf{r}_{n+1}$. More importantly, the NPEB approach can be extended to incorporate time series effects of the stock returns; see Lai et al. (2011) for details and for their choice of λ to optimize a widely used performance measure called "information ratio" along the NPEB efficient frontier.

3. *Desirability of outcome ranking and Win Ratio.* Although almost all clinical study protocols have separate hypotheses and statistical analysis plans for efficacy and for safety, Evans and Follmann (2016) argue that clinical trials should use the totality of evidence in a pragmatic way that allows more direct benefit-risk determination. Whereas the traditional practice is to construct separate summary measures of efficacy and safety before an integrated analysis at the population level, Evans and Follmann (2016) argue for the use of intra-patient analysis that combines efficacy and safety outcomes at the patient level to yield a composite benefit-risk outcome so that inter-group comparison can be made using these composite endpoints for patients in each treatment group; an example of this is the Q-TWiST method described in Section 3.5.1. They also describe a method, called DOOR (desirability of outcome ranking), to rank all trial participants. Other methods that involve ranking patient histories based on the multiple outcomes include the Win Ratio (Pocock et al., 2011) and the global benefit-risk score (Chuang-Stein et al., 1991). These integrated statistical methods for benefit-risk analysis are useful for policy decisions regarding the approvability and clinical utility to patients, although separate analyses of efficacy and safety remain the mainstay for understanding the clinical and biological mechanisms of candidate drugs and vaccines.

4. *Bayesian framework for longitudinal benefit-risk assessment.* Using the five outcome categories of individual patients proposed by Chuang-Stein et al. (1991), Zhao et al. (2014) have developed a Bayesian framework for longitudinal benefit-risk assessment in a clinical trial setting. Suppose there are K scheduled visits in a two-arm randomized clinical trial. Let n_{ijk} denote the number of subjects in the ith treatment group falling into the jth category (as described in Section 3.3) at the kth visit, and $n_{i \cdot k} = \sum_{j=1}^{5} n_{ijk}$ be the number of subjects in the ith treatment group at the kth visit, with $i = 1$ for new treatment and 2 for the control, $j = 1, \ldots, 5$ and $k = 1, \ldots, K$. Let p_{ij} be the proportion of subjects falling into the jth category for the ith treatment group; note that $\sum_{j=1}^{5} p_{ij} = 1$. Let $\mathbf{p}_i = \{p_{ij} : j = 1, \ldots, 5\}$ and $\mathbf{n}_{i \cdot k} = \{n_{ijk} : j = 1, \ldots, 5\}$. Assuming independence of $\mathbf{p}_1$ and $\mathbf{p}_2$, Zhao et al. (2014) consider a common prior of $\mathbf{p}_i \sim D(\boldsymbol{\alpha})$, where $D(\boldsymbol{\alpha})$ is the Dirichlet distribution (Carlin and Louis, 2000) and $\boldsymbol{\alpha} = \{\alpha_j : j = 1, \ldots, 5\}$, yielding a prior mean $E(p_{ij}) = \alpha_j / \left(\sum_{h=1}^{5} \alpha_h \right)$. Noting that the posterior density of $\mathbf{p}_i$ given the longitudinally observed data $\mathbf{n}_{i \cdot k}, k = 1, \ldots, K$, is

$$ f(\mathbf{p}_i | \mathbf{n}_{i \cdot 1}, \ldots, \mathbf{n}_{i \cdot k}) \propto D(\boldsymbol{\alpha}) f(\mathbf{p}_i | \mathbf{n}_{i \cdot 1}, \ldots, \mathbf{n}_{i \cdot k-1}) f(n_{i \cdot k} | \mathbf{p}_i), \qquad (3.18) $$

Zhao et al. (2014) use Gibbs sampling to compute credible intervals of the benefit-risk measures besides the posterior mean and covariance matrix of $\mathbf{p}_i$.

5. *A hierarchical Bayesian model for structured benefit-risk analysis.* A hierarchical Bayesian approach to probabilistic sensitivity analysis has been proposed by Waddingham et al. (2016) who assume that $X_{ijk} \sim \text{Bin}(n_{ijk}, \pi_{ijk})$, where X_{ijk} is the number of patients having event k in arm $j \in \{1,2\}$ of trial i, n_{ijk} is the number of patients in arm j of trial i and π_{ijk} is the corresponding probability of event occurrence. They define $\mu_{i \cdot k} = [\text{logit}(\pi_{i1k}) + \text{logit}(\pi_{i2k})]/2$, the mean of the log odds of both arms for event k and trial i, and $\delta_{i \cdot k} = \text{logit}(\pi_{i1k}) - \text{logit}(\pi_{i2k})$, which is the log odds ratio between arm 1 and arm 2. Hence $\text{logit}(\pi_{i1k}) = \mu_{i \cdot k} + \delta_{i \cdot k}/2$ and $\text{logit}(\pi_{i2k}) = \mu_{i \cdot k} - \delta_{i \cdot k}/2$. The hierarchical Bayesian model assumes that $\mu_{i \cdot k} \sim N(0, 0.25)$ and $\delta_{i \cdot k} \sim N(d, \tau)$ with hyperpriors $d \sim \text{Uniform}(-1, 1)$ and $\tau \sim \text{Gamma}(a, b)$.

TABLE 3.3 Number (%) patients having the most common adverse events by treatment and grade.

	Trabectedin (N = 340)			Dacarbazine (N = 155)		
	All Grades	Grade 3	Grade 4	All Grades	Grade 3	Grade 4
Nausea	247 (73)	18 (5)	0	76 (49)	3 (2)	0
Fatigue	228 (67)	20 (6)	0	79 (51)	2 (1)	1 (1)
Neutropenia	165 (49)	70 (21)	56 (16)	45 (29)	17 (11)	15 (10)
Alanine aminotransferase increased	154 (45)	85 (25)	4 (1)	9 (6)	1 (1)	0
Vomiting	149 (44)	16 (5)	0	33 (21)	2 (1)	0
Anemia	134 (39)	49 (14)	0	45 (29)	17 (11)	1 (1)
Constipation	121 (36)	3 (1)	0	44 (28)	0	0
Aspartate aminotransferase increased	120 (35)	40 (12)	4 (1)	8 (5)	0	0
Decreased appetite	116 (34)	7 (2)	0	31 (20)	0	1 (1)
Diarrhea	115 (34)	6 (2)	0	35 (23)	0	0
Thrombocytopenia	101 (30)	27 (8)	31 (9)	56 (36)	15 (10)	13 (8)
Dyspnea	84 (25)	12 (4)	1 (< 1)	30 (19)	1 (1)	0
Peripheral edema	83 (24)	3 (1)	0	21 (14)	1 (1)	0
Headache	78 (23)	1 (< 1)	0	29 (19)	0	0
Blood alkaline phosphatase increased	69 (20)	5 (1)	0	11 (7)	0	0
Cough	61 (18)	1 (< 1)	0	32 (21)	0	0

6. *Exercise.* A randomized multi-center phase III clinical trial was conducted to compare the efficacy and safety of trabectedin with dacarbazine in patients with metastatic liposarcoma or leiomyosarcoma after failure of prior therapies. The trial enrolled a total of 518 patients with 2:1 randomization ratio that assigned 345 patients to trabectedin and 173 patients to dacarbazine. In the final analysis of progression-free survival and interim analysis of overall survival (64% censored), Demetri et al. (2015) report a 45% reduction in the risk of disease progression or death (hazard ratio = 0.55, $p < 0.001$) and a slightly better and statistically insignificant benefit in overall survival (hazard ratio = 0.87, $p = 0.37$) for patients receiving trabectedin over patients treated with dacarbazine. They also report the most common adverse

events (defined as $\geq 20\%$ frequency) and their severity grades in Table 3.3.

Suppose that (a) the reported adverse events in Table 3.3 are equally important, (b) grade 1 events are equally weighted with grade 2 events, (c) grade 4 events are given weights that are twice those for grade 3 events, and the weights for grade 1 or grade 2 events are half of those for grade 3 events, (d) death rates for the two groups are approximately equal, and (e) the less common adverse events ($< 20\%$ frequency) are negligible. Without access to individual patients' data and assuming that the benefit for patients treated with trabectedin is similar to that of patients treated with dacarbazine in terms of survival time, compute the MCDA score for each treatment group using the algorithm described in Section 3.4, and the risk-adjusted benefit for each group using the method described in Section 3.3. Discuss your conclusion on treatment preference.

4

Design and Analysis of Clinical Trials with Safety Endpoints

Safety evaluation is an important component of the design and analysis of clinical trials for the development of pharmaceutical, biological, and vaccine products. In early-phase clinical trials, the evaluation is mostly exploratory with a focus on serious adverse reactions to the product and is based on relatively small sample sizes and shorter study durations. In later phases of clinical development, the safety profile is characterized more fully because of larger numbers of patients and longer study durations of clinical trials. Some clinical trials may be designed with specific safety hypotheses concerning the equivalence or superiority of the candidate drug or vaccine to a control agent. Depending on the stage of clinical development, the objectives of the clinical trials may differ substantially. Although safety endpoints may or may not be of primary interest in these clinical trials, safety data are collected in various forms, including clinical adverse events, vital signs, laboratory test outcomes, and imaging results. This chapter presents study designs and data analysis methods that are commonly used to address pre-defined safety or toxicity issues in clinical trials. Section 4.1 begins with dose-escalation designs in phase I studies. Section 4.2 describes safety considerations in the design and analysis of phase II, phase III, and phase II/III clinical trials. In Section 4.3 we introduce clinical trial designs with both efficacy and safety endpoints. Section 4.4 presents the typical tabular formats for summarizing safety data from clinical trials. Statistical methods for their analysis are given in Section 4.5, and commonly used graphical displays of these data are described in Section 4.6. Section 4.7 concludes with supplements and problems.

4.1 Dose escalation in phase I clinical trials

Phase I trials are generally conducted on healthy volunteers (although patients with certain diseases may also be used in some disease areas such as cancer), with the objective of determining (a) the absorption, distribution, metabolism, and excretion through pharmacokinetics (PK) modeling, (b) the safety, minimum effective dose (MED) and maximum tolerated dose (MTD) through pharmacodynamics (PD) studies, and (c) bioavailability of a biopharmaceutical agent. As the first-in-human studies, phase I trials may encounter much uncertainty in the selection of design parameters, e.g., starting dose, dose increment scheme, dose escalation and/or de-escalation method, number of patients per dose level, specification of dose-limiting toxicity (DLT), target toxicity level, and recommended dose for phase II trials; see Ting (2006), Le Tourneau et al. (2009), Julious et al. (2010), and Cook et al. (2015). Dose- limiting toxicity (DLT) refers to the toxic effects which are considered unacceptable because of their severity and/or irreversibility, and which prevents further administration of the agent to subjects at that level. DLTs are generally defined in the study protocol which describes pre-specified toxic effects and severities using a standardized grading criteria. In particular, a DLT may refer to any Grade 3 or 4 adverse event using the Common Terminology Criteria for Adverse Event (CTCAE) that has been reviewed in Section 1.4.2. The CTCAE Grade 3 is considered a severe AE and Grade 4 a life-threatening or disabling AE; such events may include skin toxicity, diarrhea, vomiting, central nervous system (lung or renal) toxicity, elevation of liver transaminase or bilirubin lasting more than 1 week. DLTs are also used in determining the maximum tolerated dose (MTD) in cancer trials, in which the dose of a cytotoxic agent is set as high as possible for efficacy subject to the probability constraint of experiencing DLTs being no more than a pre-defined threshold value, say, 33%. Note that the MTD may also be defined as the highest dose at which the probability of experiencing the DLTs is no more than a pre-defined threshold value, say, 33% (Le Tourneau et al., 2009; Storer, 1989).

Before a phase I trial, preclinical *in vitro* and *in vivo* studies are conducted to evaluate toxicity and the pharmacologic actions of the drug, thereby coming up with estimates of a good starting dose for phase I trials with human subjects, as already noted in Section 2.3. Because of safety considerations for subjects in the trial, the drug is usually initiated at a low, safe dose and sequentially escalated to show toxicity at a level where some therapeutic response occurs. For relatively benign drugs, phase I trials involve healthy volunteers from whom intensive blood sampling is conducted over time. In particular, the pharmacologically-guided dose escalation (PGDE) design employs pharmacokinetics-pharmacodynamics (PK-PD) parameters such as AUC (area under the drug concentration in blood plasma versus time curve) and toxicity response to guide the dose escalation or de-escalation in the next cohort of subjects. The specific assumptions for the PGDE design are that the quantitative relationship between drug exposure, as measured by drug concentration over time, and toxicity effects is consistent across species, and that the dose-limiting toxicity correlates with, and thereby can reasonably be predicted by, drug concentration in plasma (Collins et al., 1990). In this design, doses are escalated with one patient per dose level and with 100% dose increment if the plasma concentration is below a pre-specified threshold. Drawbacks for the PGDE design include inaccurate prediction of toxicities by plasma concentration of drugs and time delay in estimating PK-PD parameters and computing the subsequent dose for the next subject (Modi, 2006; Holford, 2006; Le Tourneau et al., 2009).

For cytotoxic treatments of cancer, the MTD is determined in phase I clinical trials by sequentially testing increasing or decreasing doses on different groups of subjects until the highest dose with acceptable toxic effects is found. The methods to determine an MTD can be classified into two basic categories: rule-based designs and model-based designs. The rule-based designs assume no dose-toxicity curves and allow for dose escalation or de-escalation based on pre-defined rules and observed toxicities in the specified DLT period of prior dose levels, while the model-based designs assume pre-defined dose-toxicity curves that are modified or updated with accumulated toxicity data that in turn determine the next dose level.

4.1.1 Rule-based designs for cytotoxic treatments

One of the major features for the rule-based designs is that they do not rely on pre-specified parametric or nonparametric models or curves that describe the dose-toxicity relationship. Instead, the designs use simple rules to escalate or de-escalate by a fraction of preceding dose, depending on the presence or absence of DLT in the previous cohort of treated subjects. Among the commonly used rule-based designs in clinical practice are the traditional 3+3 design and the accelerated titration design. In the traditional 3+3 design, a cohort consisting of 3 subjects is treated sequentially at each dose level starting with an initial dose that is considered to be safe, based on prior information including extrapolation of *in vivo* toxicity data. The next cohort of 3 subjects will be treated at the next higher dose (escalation) if none of the 3 subjects in the previous cohort experiences DLT, or at the next lower dose level (de-escalation) if 2 or more of the 3 subjects experience DLT, or at the current dose level if 1 of the 3 subjects experiences DLT. Using toxicity data from this second cohort, the next dose is set at the next higher dose level if 1 of the 6 subjects experiences DLT, or at the lower dose level if 2 of the 6 subjects experience DLT. Moreover, if a dose is de-escalated to the previous dose level, then either enroll 3 more subjects or terminate the study and declare it the MTD if the dose is de-escalated to the initial dose or if 6 subjects had already been treated at the previous dose level. A modified Fibonacci sequence is often used for dose increments so that the dose incremental ratios become smaller with increasing dose (Ting, 2006; Dancey et al., 2006; Le Tourneau et al., 2009).

Although the traditional 3+3 design is easy to implement and has therefore been widely used in dose-finding studies, it has been shown to expose more subjects to sub-therapeutic doses if the initial dose is chosen substantially below the MTD and may also take relatively long to finish the phase I study. Calling the traditional 3+3 design (with 3 subjects in each cohort and 40% dose-step increment) Design 1, Simon et al. (1997) propose a family of *accelerated titration dose-escalation designs*, consisting of the following three generic designs in which decision rules for dose escalation or de-escalation are based on pre-defined dose-limiting toxicity and moderate toxicity:

- Design 2 uses single-subject cohorts in its accelerated phase, and changes to Design 1 when the first instance of the first-course DLT or the second instance of the first-course moderate toxicity is observed.

- Design 3 is the same as Design 2 but with 80% dose-step increments in the initial acceleration stage, which terminates if the first instance of the first-course DLT or the second instance of the first-course moderate toxicity is observed.

- Design 4 is similar to Design 3, except for the criterion of triggering the end of accelerated phase that is defined as the first instance of any-course DLT or the second instance of any-course moderate toxicity.

In Designs 2–4, the traditional 3+3 design is adopted upon termination of the rapid initial accelerated phase, and MTD is estimated with all toxicity data collected in the study by using a recommended model which also allows for estimation of cumulative toxicity and inter-subject variability; see Simon et al. (1997) for details.

4.1.2   CRM, EWOC and other model-based designs

Unlike the rule-based designs, model-based approaches use prespecified statistical models or dose-toxicity response curves to toxicity data collected from all enrolled subjects to estimate the dose at which the probability of dose-limiting toxicity reaches a prescribed level. The models can be conveniently formulated by using the Bayesian framework in which the posterior probability of toxic response is updated with data from subjects enrolled at each dose level.

Continual Reassessment Method. This method, usually referred to as CRM, was proposed by O'Quigley et al. (1990). It models the toxicity response through a dose-toxicity function, which is continually updated by using all the data collected so far and which is in turn used to determine for the next subject the dose level that is closest to attaining a prespecified target toxicity rate θ. Consider a dose-finding trial with K dose levels d_k, $k = 1, \ldots, K$, such that $d_1 < \ldots < d_K$. Letting Y_i denote the binary variable that indicates either occurrence ($Y_i = 1$) or non-occurrence ($Y_i = 0$) of toxicity for the ith subject treated at dose level $x_i \in \{d_1, ..., d_K\}$, define

$$E(Y_i|x_i) = P\{Y_i = 1|x_i, \beta\} = \psi(x_i, \beta) \tag{4.1}$$

as the working model with β being unknown parameter, where $\psi(d, \beta)$ is a strictly increasing function of d. The following choices of $\psi(d, \beta)$ have been suggested by O'Quigley et al. (1990), Goodman et al. (1995) and O'Quigley and Conaway (2010):

$$\psi(d, \beta) = \begin{cases} d^\beta, \\ [(\tanh d + 1)/2]^\beta, \\ \exp(a + \beta d)/[1 + \exp(a + \beta d)], \end{cases} \tag{4.2}$$

where a is a fixed constant; these are called empirical, hyperbolic, and logistic models, respectively. The parameter β in (4.2) is constrained to be positive to ensure that (4.1) increases with the dose level d. To remove this positivity constraint, Cheung (2011) reparameterizes (4.2) as

$$\psi(d, \beta) = \begin{cases} d^{\exp(\beta)}, \\ [(\tanh d + 1)/2]^{\exp(\beta)}, \\ \exp[a + d\exp(\beta)]/\{1 + \exp[(a + d\exp(\beta))]\}. \end{cases} \tag{4.3}$$

Let $Y_i = 1_{\{x_i=d_k\}}$ be the number of subjects who experience the toxicity among the n subjects. The likelihood function of β is given by

$$L_n(\beta) = \prod_{i=1}^{n} (\psi(x_i, \beta))^{Y_i} (1 - \psi(x_i, \beta))^{1-Y_i}. \tag{4.4}$$

The original formulation of CRM by O'Quigley et al. (1990) uses a Bayesian approach in which the parameter β is assumed to have a prior density function h. The posterior distribution of β given the observed data $D_n = \{(x_i, y_i) : 1 \le i \le n\}$ has density function

$$\pi(\beta|D_n) = \frac{L_n(\beta)h(\beta)}{\int L_n(\beta)h(\beta)d\beta}, \tag{4.5}$$

and the posterior probability of toxicity at dose d is

$$\tilde{\psi}(d) = \int \psi(d, \beta)\pi(\beta|D_n)d\beta. \tag{4.6}$$

The recommended dose for the $(n+1)$st subject is

$$x_{n+1} = \min_{d \in \{d_1, ..., d_k\}} \left|\tilde{\psi}(d) - \theta\right|, \tag{4.7}$$

where θ is the pre-specified target rate of toxicity (usual choice $25 - 30\%$).

Modified CRMs. Several modifications of the original CRM have been proposed by O'Quigley et al. (1990), Goodman et al. (1995) and Møller (1995), including (a) restricted dose escalation by pre-defined levels, (b) using cohorts of size 2-3 subjects (instead of 1 subject at each dose), and (c) splitting the CRM design into two stages, the first stage of which uses the traditional 3+3 design until a dose-limiting toxicity is observed, whereupon the design enters into the second stage that uses the CRM to estimate the dose-toxicity function as described above. In addition, Cheung and Chappell (2000) have developed a sequential CRM to allow for late-onset toxicities for determining dose levels based on time-to-event toxicities. This approach incorporates information from partially observed subjects by using a weight function that depends on the amount of time during which a subject is followed.

Escalation with Overdose Control. Noting that CRM may cause unnecessary exposure of subjects to high toxic doses, Babb et al. (1998) introduced this design, often referred to as EWOC, that imposes measures to prevent future subjects from being exposed to high toxic doses. Specifically, EWOC considers the probability of exceeding the MTD for each higher dose after each patient, prohibiting dose escalation if this probability exceeds some pre-specified value. Let γ denote the MTD, and d_1 and d_K respectively the minimum and maximum doses that are considered for the trial such that $\gamma \in [d_1, d_k]$. Denote by Y the indicator variable for the occurrence of DLT. The dose-toxicity relationship is modeled by

$$P\{Y = 1|x = d\} = F(\beta_0 + \beta_1 d), \tag{4.8}$$

in which F is a prespecified distribution function and β_0 and β_1 are unknown parameters, with $\beta_1 > 0$ to ensure that the probability of a DLT increases with the dose. Since the MTD γ is the dose level at which the probability of DLT is θ, it then follows that

$$\gamma = \frac{F^{-1}(\theta) - \beta_0}{\beta_1} = d_1 + \frac{F^{-1}(\theta) - F^{-1}(\theta_0)}{\beta_1}, \tag{4.9}$$

where θ_0 is the probability of DLT at the starting dose d_1. Letting Y_i be the toxicity response for the ith subject who is administered dose x_i, the likelihood function is given by

$$L_n(\beta_0, \beta_1) = \prod_{i=1}^{n} [F(\beta_0 + \beta_1 x_i)]^{Y_i} [1 - F(\beta_0 + \beta_1 x_i)]^{1-Y_i}. \tag{4.10}$$

Similar to CRM, EWOC also specifies the prior density $h(\beta_0, \beta_1)$ and applies Bayes theorem to obtain the posterior density $\pi(\beta_0, \beta_1|D_n)$ that replaces β in (4.5) by (β_0, β_1), from which the posterior distribution of the MTD γ can be obtained through the transformation of $T(\beta_0, \beta_1) = (\theta_0, \gamma)$.

The EWOC design can be described as follows. Let α be the pre-defined threshold for the posterior probability of a dose x exceeding the MTD, which is called feasibility bound. The first subject receives dose d_1 and the doses for subsequent subjects are determined sequentially such that the posterior probability (given D_{k-1}) that the selected dose x_k exceeds the MTD is equal to the feasibility bound α. Babb et al. (1998) also propose to use the following asymmetric loss function for dose x:

$$l_\alpha(x, \gamma) = \begin{cases} \alpha(\gamma - x), & \text{if } x \leq \gamma, \text{ i.e., } x \text{ is an underdose} \\ (1 - \alpha)(x - \gamma), & \text{if } x > \gamma, \text{ i.e., } x \text{ is an overdose.} \end{cases} \tag{4.11}$$

Tighiouart et al. (2014) have extended the EWOC method that assigns weights to account for the time it takes a subject to develop a DLT.

Threshold Designs. These designs, introduced by Ji et al. (2007), use thresholds on toxicity probabilities to determine whether to escalate, or de-escalate, or remain at the current dose. Ji et al. (2007) assume independent Beta distributions for the toxicity probabilities p_i at dose d_i, $i = 1, \ldots, k$, where k is the total number of candidate doses. Suppose that n_i subjects are treated at dose d_i and m_i of them experience DLT. Then the likelihood function is

$$L(p_1, ..., p_k) \propto \prod_{i=1}^{k} p_i^{m_i} (1 - p_i)^{n_i - m_i}. \tag{4.12}$$

Using independent beta priors $B(0.005, 0.005)$ to approximate vague priors for p_i, the posterior distribution of $(p_1, ..., p_k)$ is that of independent $B(0.005 + m_i, 0.005 + n_i - m_i)$ random variables whose means are close to the observed toxicity proportions at doses d_i. Partition the interval $(0, 1)$ as $(0, \theta - K_1\sigma_i) \cup [\theta - K_1\sigma_i, \theta + K_2\sigma_i] \cup (\theta + K_2\sigma_i, 1)$, where θ is the target toxicity probability associated with the MTD, σ_i is the posterior standard deviation of p_i and K_1 and K_2 are prescribed positive constants such as $0 < \theta - K_1\sigma_i < \theta - K_2\sigma_i < 1$. The three intervals represent respectively the low, acceptable, and high probability of toxicity of a dose relative to that of the MTD. Let E, S, and D denote respectively the action of dose escalation, staying in current dose, and dose de-escalation. For $a \in \{D, S, E\}$, define

$$q(a, i) = \begin{cases} P\{p_i - \theta > K_2\sigma_i | \mathcal{D}_{i-1}\}, & \text{if } a = D \\ P\{-K_1\sigma_i \leq p_i - \theta \leq K_2\sigma_i | \mathcal{D}_{i-1}\}, & \text{if } a = S \\ P\{p_i - \theta < -K_1\sigma_i | \mathcal{D}_{i-1}\}, & \text{if } a = E, \end{cases} \tag{4.13}$$

where $\mathcal{D}_{i-1}$ represents the data for the first $i - 1$ subjects. Ji et al. (2007) propose to choose $a_i = \arg\max_{a \in \{D, S, E\}} q(a, i)$ for the ith subject. Noting that escalation may not be safe if data suggest that the next higher dose is likely to be highly toxic, they define the indicator variable $\mathcal{T}_i = I\left(P\{p_i > \theta | \mathcal{D}_{i-1}\} > \xi\right)$, where $\xi \in (0,1)$ is a cutoff value, e.g., $\xi = 0.95$, beyond which dose escalation is not allowed. The threshold dose assignment rule is given by $\arg\max_{a \in \{D,S,E\}} q(a,i)(1 - \mathcal{T}_i)$.

Liu and Yuan (2015) and Yuan et al. (2016) propose an alternative threshold design in which the thresholds are determined by Neyman-Pearson tests of three simple hypotheses $H_0 : p_j = \theta, H_1 : p_j = \theta_1$ and $H_2 : p_j = \theta_2$, where θ is the target toxicity probability associated with the MTD as before, $\theta_1(< \theta)$ is the highest toxicity probability that is deemed sub-therapeutic so that dose escalation should be made, and $\theta_2(> \theta)$ is the lowest toxicity probability that is deemed overly toxic so that dose de-escalation is required. Let $\hat{p}_j = m_j/n_j$ be the observed toxicity rate at the current dose level $x_i = d_j$. Liu and Yuan propose to

- escalate to level d_{j+1} if $\hat{p}_j \leq \lambda_{1j}$,

- de-escalate to level d_{j-1} if $\hat{p}_j > \lambda_{2j}$,

- stay at level d_j, if $\lambda_{1j} < \hat{p}_j \leq \lambda_{2j}$,

until the maximum sample size n is reached. Let $\mathcal{R}$ (retainment), $\mathcal{E}$ (escalation) and $\mathcal{D}$ (de-escalation) denote the correct decision for H_0, H_1 and H_2, respectively. With specified probability (prevalence) $P(H_j)$ for the occurrence of H_j, $j = 0, 1, 2$, the probability of making an incorrect decision (or decision error rate) at each dose assignment step is given by

$$P(H_0)P(\bar{\mathcal{R}}|H_0) + P(H_1)P(\bar{\mathcal{E}}|H_1) + P(H_2)P(\bar{\mathcal{D}}|H_2)$$
$$= P(H_0)\left[\mathbf{Bin}(n_j\lambda_{1j}; n_j, \theta) + 1 - \mathbf{Bin}(n_j\lambda_{2j}; n_j, \theta)\right]$$
$$+ P(H_1)\left[1 - \mathbf{Bin}(n_j\lambda_{1j}; n_j, \theta_1)\right] + P(H_2)\mathbf{Bin}(n_j\lambda_{2j}; n_j, \theta_2), \quad (4.14)$$

where $\bar{R}$ denotes the complement of R and $\mathbf{Bin}(\cdot; n, p)$ denotes the Binomial (n, p) distribution function. In the case $P(H_0) = P(H_1) = P(H_2) = 1/3$, (4.14) is minimized by

$$\lambda_{1j} = \log\left(\frac{1-\theta_1}{1-\theta}\right) \Big/ \log\left(\frac{\theta(1-\theta_1)}{\theta_1(1-\theta)}\right),$$
$$\lambda_{2j} = \log\left(\frac{1-\theta}{1-\theta_2}\right) \Big/ \log\left(\frac{\theta_2(1-\theta)}{\theta(1-\theta_2)}\right),$$

which are independent of n_j and does not vary with j. Liu and Yuan (2015) recommend the choice $\theta_1 = 0.6\theta$ and $\theta_2 = 1.4\theta$ as the default values.

4.1.3   Individual versus collective ethics and approximate dynamic programming

Bartroff and Lai (2010, 2011) point out that if the objective of a phase I cancer trial is just to estimate the MTD γ, then one should consider

Bayesian sequential designs that are optimal, in some sense, for this estimation problem; see Whitehead and Brunier (1995) and Haines et al. (2003) who use the theory of optimal design of experiments to construct Bayesian c- and D-optimal designs and further impose a relaxed Bayesian feasibility constraint on the design to avoid highly toxic doses. They also point out, however, that CRM or EWOC treats the next patient at the dose x that minimizes $E_\Pi[\ell(\gamma, x)]$ for $\ell(\gamma, x)$ given by $(\gamma - x)^2$ or by $\alpha(\gamma - x)I(x \leq \gamma) + (1 - \alpha)(x - \gamma)I(x > \gamma)$, where Π is the current posterior distribution. This is tantamount to dosing the next patient at the best guess of γ, where "best" means "closest" according to some measure of distance from γ. On the other hand, a Bayesian c- and D-optimal design aims at generating doses that provide most information for estimating the dose-toxicity curve to benefit future patients. To resolve this dilemma between treatment of patients in the trial and efficient experimental design for post-trial parameter estimation, Bartroff and Lai (2010) consider the finite-horizon optimization problem of choosing the dose levels $x_1, x_2, \ldots, x_n$ sequentially to minimize the global cost function

$$E_{\Pi_0}\left[\sum_{i=1}^n h(\gamma, x_i) + g(\hat{\gamma}_n, \gamma)\right], \qquad (4.15)$$

in which Π_0 denotes the prior distribution of θ, $h(\gamma, x_i)$ represents the loss for the ith patient in the trial, $\hat{\gamma}_n$ is the terminal estimate of the MTD (of benefit to future patients) and g represents a terminal loss function. They show how approximate dynamic programming can be used to compute the optimizing doses x_i which depend on $n - i$, where the horizon n is the sample size of the trial, and which therefore are not of the form $x_i = f(\Pi_{i-1})$ considered above. In terms of "individual" and "collective" ethics, note that (4.15) measures the individual effect of the dose x_k on the kth patient through $h(\gamma, x_k)$, and its collective effect on future patients through $\sum_{i>k} h(\gamma, x_i) + g(\hat{\gamma}_n, \gamma)$. By using a discounted infinite-horizon version of (4.15), Bartroff and Lai (2011) provide solutions that have form $x_i = f(\Pi_{i-1})$ for some functional f that only depends on Π_{i-1}. Specifically, take a discount factor $0 < \delta < 1$ and replace (4.15) by $E_{\Pi_0}[\sum_{i=1}^\infty h(\gamma, x_i)\delta^{i-1}]$ as the definition of global risk.

The main complexity of the infinite-horizon problem is that the dose x for the next patient involves also consideration for future patients who will receive optimal doses themselves; these future doses depend on the future posterior distribution. Bartroff and Lai (2011) reduce the complexity by considering two (instead of infinitely many) future patients, and choose the next dose x to minimize $E_\Pi\ell(\gamma, x; \Pi)$ when the current posterior distribution of β is Π, where β denotes the parameter vector of the dose-response relationship, e.g., $\beta = (\beta_0, \beta_1)$ in (4.8).

$$\ell(\gamma, d; \Pi) = h(\gamma, x) + \lambda E_\Pi\left\{E_\Pi[h(\gamma', x') \mid x_1 = d, y_1]\right\}. \qquad (4.16)$$

In (4.16), $\gamma' = F_{\beta'}^{-1}(\theta)$ with $\beta' \sim \Pi'$, and Π' and x' defined as follows. The first summand in (4.16) measures the toxicity effect of the dose x on the patient receiving it. The second summand considers the patient who follows and receives a myopic dose x' that minimizes the patient's posterior loss; the myopic dose is optimal because there are no more patients involved in (4.16). The effect of x on this second patient is through the posterior distribution Π' that updates Π after observing (x_1, Y_1), with $x_1 = d$. Since Y_1 is not yet observed, the expectation outside the curly brackets is taken over $Y_1 \sim \mathrm{Bern}(F_\beta(x))$, with $\beta \sim \Pi$.

A closely related approach is used in the "Bayesian decision-theoretic design" of Fan et al. (2012). They assume a "working Bayesian" model with beta priors $\mathrm{Beta}(a_i, b_i)$ for the toxicity rates p_i at increasing doses x_i belonging to a prescribed discrete set. Monotonicity in the prior means $\mu_i = a_i/(a_i + b_i)$ is achieved by fixing $c = a_i + b_i$ and choosing $a_i = r_i c$ with increasing r_i. From this conjugate family of Beta prior distributions, they also apply a "working" adjustment of the data via the "Pool Adjacent Violators" algorithm in isotonic regression to ensure that the adjusted sample toxicity rates also satisfy the monotonicity constraint. Analogous to the global cost function, they use a utility function that reflects an individual's benefit by participating in the trial and the gain for future patients in terms of the accuracy of the MTD estimate. They propose to initialize by assigning a cohort to the lowest dose and then to escalate the dose, one increment at a time, until the first toxicity occurs. Then they use a two-step-look-ahead rule similar to (4.16). They also allow for early termination "whenever the evidence for the current conclusion is considered sufficient," similar to a stopping criterion for CRM proposed by Heyd and Carlin (1999).

4.1.4 Extensions to combination therapies

Lee et al. (2017) have considered extending the approach in the preceding paragraph to a combination therapy involving two cytotoxic anticancer agents. They still use the Beta prior distribution $\mathrm{Beta}(a_j, b_j)$ for agent $j = 1, 2$, and introduce a partial order $\prec$ of the dose-agent combinations such that $p_{ij} \le p_{hk}$ whenever $(i, j) \prec (h, k)$. They show how the prior parameters can be elicited from clinicians and adjusted to satisfy the partial ordering as follows: The clinician provides his/her best estimate of $\mu_{ij} = a_{ij}/(a_{ij} + b_{ij})$ at each dose-agent combination, and is asked to adjust the estimate so that the order restriction $\mu_{ij} \le \mu_{hk}$ for $(i, j) \prec (h, k)$ is satisfied. A statistical default option that assumes independent toxicities of the agents is also provided. Extrapolation of a subject's response at a single dose-agent combination to worse (respectively, better) combinations (by the partial ordering) if the subject experiences (does not have) a DLT leads to the following updates of the parameters of the posterior Beta distribution. Suppose a cohort of n_{ij} patients were tested at (i, j), among whom t experienced DLTs. Then $a_{ij}^{\text{new}} = a_{ij}^{\text{old}} + t$ and $b_{ij}^{\text{new}} = b_{ij}^{\text{old}} + n_{ij} - t$, and

$$
(a_{h,k}^{\text{new}}, b_{h,k}^{\text{new}}) = \begin{cases} (a_{hk}^{\text{old}} + t, b_{hk}^{\text{old}}), & \text{for } (h,k) \succ (i,j) \\ (a_{hk}^{\text{old}}, b_{hk}^{\text{old}} + n_{ij} - t), & \text{for } (h,k) \prec (i,j) \\ (a_{hk}^{\text{old}}, b_{hk}^{\text{old}}), & \text{for all other}(h,k). \end{cases}
$$

These posterior means satisfy the order restrictions. Because of the complexity of the problem, Lee et al. (2017) only consider myopic rules and provide a partial extension of the single-agent case in the preceding paragraph. Other adaptive phase I designs for combination therapies have been proposed by Mandrekar et al. (2007), Yin and Yuan (2009), Yuan and Yin (2011), Braun and Wang (2010) and Wages et al. (2011).

4.1.5 Modifications for cytostatic cancer therapies

A cytostatic therapy works by stopping the cancer cells from multiplying. The usual clinical trial design for a cytotoxic agent aims at finding the MTD for the agent to shrink the tumor. In contrast, cytostatic agents may slow or stop the growth of tumors without shrinking existing tumors. Therefore, standard cytotoxic trial designs are unsuitable for cytostatic agents, as pointed out by Freidlin and Simon (2005): "In the early stages of development, reliable assays to identify the sensitive patients that express the target are often not available. This complicates evaluation of targeted agents as a result of the dilution of the treatment effect by the presence of the patients who do not benefit from the agent. Furthermore, some of these agents are thought to be cytostatic and are only expected to inhibit tumor growth without shrinking existing tumors. Traditionally, clinical development of cytotoxic agents involved a single arm phase II evaluation of the response rate. In most cases, this approach is no longer adequate for the development of cytostatic agents." Millar and Lynch (2003) and Korn et al. (2001) have pointed out the urgency of developing new designs to avoid rejecting a clinically useful cytostatic agent because it uses a standard cytotoxic trial design. Rosner et al. (2002) propose a randomized discontinuation design that initially treats all patients with the agent and then randomizes in a double-blind fashion to continuing therapy or placebo only for those patients whose disease is stable. They claim that by doing this, investigators can determine whether the slow tumor growth is due to the drug with naturally slow-growing tumors. In their evaluation of the randomized discontinuation design, Freidlin and Simon (2005) agree that the design "can be useful in some settings in the early development of targeted agents where a reliable assay to select patients expressing the target is not available." Stone et al. (2007), however, advocate randomized controlled (rather than single-arm) trials, and further suggest that the endpoint for testing the activity of cytostatic agents should be progression-free survival, instead of tumor response in cytotoxic trial designs. Xu et al. (2016) have proposed a two-stage Bayesian adaptive design for cytostatic agents via model adaptation, in which Stage I uses the standard Bayesian approach to search for the MTD and Stage 2 uses a Bayesian outcome-adaptive randomization scheme (randomizing according to the posterior probabilities of the effectiveness of the candidate doses) to search for the optimal dose under the constraint that it does not exceed the MTD.

4.2   Safety considerations for the design of phase II and III studies

The primary objective of a phase I trial is to find suitable dose levels that can be tolerated by patients and recommended for further investigation in a phase II study in which the intended therapeutic effects (efficacy) of the compound are investigated with the recommended dose(s). Phase II trials can sometimes be further categorized into phase IIA and phase IIB trials. Whereas a phase IIA trial evaluates clinical efficacy, pharmacokinetics and safety in selected populations of patients with the target disease or condition to be treated, a phase IIB trial fine-tunes further the target patient population and collects more efficacy and safety information for "Go/No Go" decision to phase III trials which are designed with sufficient statistical power to confirm clinical efficacy through randomized controlled designs and to establish the safety profile of the product.

Whereas the scope of toxic effects (e.g., DLT in general) in phase I studies is usually well defined, safety endpoints in phase II and III trials may or may not be as well defined. Even though safety evaluation is most likely stated as a primary (or a major secondary) objective in study protocols, safety endpoints are not commonly used as primary endpoints in designing phase II and III trials with statistical power to detect major safety concerns due to the following reasons. First, designing a trial to demonstrate the presence or absence of some serious safety events with statistical power usually results in a much larger sample size, as in the double-blind prospective trial using pharmacogenetic screening to reduce adverse drug reaction (Hughes et al., 2008) and the rotavirus efficacy and safety trial (Heyse et al., 2008). Second, unlike efficacy evaluation for which assessment standards are well established by regulatory authorities and drug developers, commonly accepted evidentiary standards for ascertaining safety are not available, as noted by Singh and Loke (2012). Third, randomized clinical trials are generally conducted in selected target patient populations with well-defined treatment regimens (e.g., daily dosage) in a relatively short period of time during which some chronic adverse events may not be observed.

In most cases, prior evidence of safety concerns, especially serious safety events, may not be strong enough to design phase III trials to investigate the serious safety issues. However, when prior information from various sources (e.g., preclinical studies, literature reports of similar agents) suggests serious side effects, a large statistically powered study may be needed to provide convincing evidence on the safety profile of the agent, as in the aforementioned rotavirus efficacy and safety trial (REST) which was suggested by a strong association of a similar vaccine product with intussusception, a rare yet serious adverse event during infancy (De-lage, 2000; Murphy, 2001; Murphy et al., 2003). This association caused the withdrawal of RotaShield® from the US market and triggered further scrutiny for the association with intussusception of other rotavirus vaccines under development. REST used a group sequential design, with a maximum sample size of 100,000 and a minimum of 60,000 infants with complete safety follow-up, to detect a 10-fold increase in relative risk of intussusception in vaccinees during the 42-day follow-up period after vaccination (Heyse et al., 2008), as described in the reminder of this section.

4.2.1 Conditioning on rare adverse events

Consider a randomized two-arm trial with $1 : r$ randomization ratio, i.e., for every one subject assigned to the control group, there are r subjects assigned to the treatment group. Let λ_0 and λ_1 denote the incidence rate parameters of the target adverse event, and n_0 and n_1 the observed number of events from the control and treatment groups, respectively. The assumption of constant (i.e., not varying with time) incidence rate is equivalent to Poisson arrivals (or exponential inter-arrival times) of adverse events. Given the total number of observed events $n = n_0 + n_1$ from both groups, the number of events n_1 from treatment group follows a binomial distribution $Bin(n, \pi)$, where $\pi = r\lambda_1/(\lambda_0 + r\lambda_1)$ is the probability of a reported event from treatment group. Then the relationship between the relative risk $R = \lambda_1/\lambda_0$ and the binomial probability π are given by

$$R = \frac{\pi}{r(1 - \pi)} \text{ and } \pi = \frac{rR}{1 + rR}. \tag{4.17}$$

Using this framework, Heyse et al. (2008) designed REST with $r = 1$ and calculated the upper boundary point for an unsafe vaccine product with respect to vaccine intussusception cases as the smallest integer ν_1 such as $\sum_{x=\nu_1}^{n} b(x; n, \pi_0) \leq 0.025$, where $b(x; n, \pi) = \binom{n}{x}\pi^x(1 - \pi)^{n-x}$ denotes the probability of observing x vaccine intussusception cases among a total of n reported cases assuming a binomial proportion $\pi_0 = 1/2 = 0.5$. On the other hand, the vaccine is considered to have an acceptable safety profile if the relative risk $R \leq 10$, a threshold that is chosen due to relatively lower background incidence rate of intussusception cases. The acceptable safety profile for stopping enrollment in accordance with the group sequential design was based on satisfying the upper bound of the 95% confidence interval on the relative risk R being ≤ 10. Under this assumption, Heyse et al. (2008) calculated the lower boundary point for a safe vaccine product with respect to the vaccine intussusception cases as the largest integer ν_2 such that $\sum_{x=0}^{\nu_2} b(x; n, \pi_1) \leq 0.025$, where $\pi_1 = 10/(1 + 10) = 0.9091$ corresponding to a relative risk of 10. Simulations showed that such a design could ensure a much lower probability (0.06) of stopping the trial early and a high probability (0.94) of successfully reaching the end of the trial if there is no increase in the risk of intussusception associated with the vaccine. On the other hand, the probability of stopping the trial early due to safety concerns increases substantially for relative risks in the range of $2.5 - 6$ (Heyse et al., 2008).

4.2.2 Sequential conditioning and an efficient sequential GLR test

The REST design basically uses a repeated significance test that terminates the study after n intussusception cases are observed and declares the vaccine to be unsafe if

$$P\left\{\text{Binomial}(n, p_0) \geq \#_n(V)\right\} \leq 0.025, \tag{4.18}$$

where $\#_n(V)$ denotes the number of vaccine cases among the n cases. The study is also terminated and declares the vaccine to be safe if

$$P\left\{\text{Binomial}(n, p_1) \leq \#_n(V)\right\} \leq 0.025, \tag{4.19}$$

where $p_1 = 10/11$, corresponding to a 10-fold increase in risk for the vaccine group. Although the nominal significance level of 0.025 in (4.18) or (4.19) does not adjust for repeated analysis of the accumulated data, Monte Carlo simulations (involving 10,000 random sequences) showed that the probability for the study to stop with a positive conclusion regarding vaccine safety is 0.94 for a vaccine with no increased risk of intussusception, and the probability for the study to declare the vaccine to be unsafe is almost 1 for relative risks of 6 or greater. This conservative approach is appropriate given the nature of the safety evaluation. Shih et al. (2010) have introduced a methodological innovation described below, for which conventional sequential tests are directly applicable to the inter-arrival observation of the adverse events; see Bartroff et al. (2013, pp. 43, 78-83) for the background of repeated significance and group sequential tests.

Consider a clinical trial in which subjects are randomized to receiving vaccine or placebo. Assume that the arrivals of adverse events follow a Poisson process, with rate λ_V for vaccine (V) and λ_C for placebo (C) recipients. This assumption will be relaxed later by allowing the rates to vary with time. When an event occurs, it is associated with either V or C and

$P(\text{V} \mid \text{event occurs at time } t \text{ after previous one})$

$$= \frac{\lambda_V e^{-\lambda_V t} \cdot e^{-\lambda_C t}}{(\lambda_V + \lambda_C)e^{-(\lambda_V + \lambda_C)t}} = \frac{\lambda_V}{\lambda_V + \lambda_C}. \quad (4.20)$$

Suppose adverse events occur at times $T_1 < T_2 < \ldots$, and the event indicator at T_i is $\delta_i = 1$ for V, or 0 for C. Let $\tau_i = T_i - T_{i-1}$. Since the Poisson interarrival times are i.i.d. exponential, it follows from (4.20) that the likelihood function of (λ_V, λ_C) based on the observations (T_i, δ_i), $1 \leq i \leq n$, is

$$\prod_{i=1}^{n} \left[\left(\frac{\lambda_V}{\lambda_V + \lambda_C} \right)^{\delta_i} \left(\frac{\lambda_C}{\lambda_V + \lambda_C} \right)^{1-\delta_i} (\lambda_V + \lambda_C) e^{-(\lambda_V + \lambda_C)\tau_i} \right]. \quad (4.21)$$

The goal of a pre-licensure randomized clinical trial is to show that the vaccine product is safe. This can be formulated as testing $H_0 : \lambda_V/\lambda_C \leq 1$ versus $H_1 : \lambda_V/\lambda_C \geq \gamma$, where $\gamma > 1$. Let $p = \frac{\lambda_V}{\lambda_V + \lambda_C}$. Then $\lambda_V/\lambda_C \geq \gamma$ if and only if $p \geq \frac{\gamma}{1+\gamma}$. Let $\pi_0 = 1/2$, $\pi_1 = \gamma/(1+\gamma)$. In view of (4.21), the likelihood ratio statistic for testing H_0 versus H_1 is $\prod_{i=1}^{n} (\frac{\pi_1}{\pi_0})^{\delta_i} (\frac{1-\pi_1}{1-\pi_0})^{1-\delta_i}$. Hence the actual event times contain no additional information about λ_V/λ_C beyond that provided by the type (V or C) of the events. This argument also applies to $\lambda_{V,i}$ and $\lambda_{C,i}$ that vary with i, since $\prod_{i=1}^{n}(\lambda_{V,i} + \lambda_{C,i})e^{-(\lambda_{V,i}+\lambda_{C,i})\tau_i}$ is cancelled out in the likelihood ratio statistic, as the δ_i are still independent Bernoulli random variables with means $\pi_i = \lambda_{V,i}/(\lambda_{V,i}+\lambda_{C,i})$. Shih et al. (2010) propose to use a sequential generalized likelihood ratio (GLR) test

$$\tau = \inf\{n \geq 1 : l_{n,0} \geq b \text{ or } l_{n,1} \leq a\}, \quad (4.22)$$

which is asymptotically efficient for testing $H_0 : p \leq p_0$ versus $H_1 : p \geq p_1$. The stopping rule (4.22) is bounded above by n^*, where n^* is the smallest integer n such that $nI(\pi^*) \geq \max(a,b)$ and $\pi^* \in (\pi_0, \pi_1)$ is the solution of the equation

$$\pi^* \log\left(\frac{\pi^*}{\pi_0}\right) + (1-\pi^*) \log\left(\frac{1-\pi^*}{1-\pi_0}\right) = \pi^* \log\left(\frac{\pi^*}{\pi_1}\right) + (1-\pi^*) \log\left(\frac{1-\pi^*}{1-\pi_1}\right).$$

4.3 Phase I–II designs for both efficacy and safety endpoints in cytotoxic cancer treatments

Gooley et al. (1994) propose to use efficacy and toxicity data and study three ad hoc designs. Thall and Russell (1998) propose a design combining binary toxicity data and trinomial (no, moderate, severe) response data into a single variable that can be modeled by proportional odds regression with a prior distribution on its parameters. Subsequent proposals to combine efficacy and toxicity outcomes include Ivanova (2003), Braun (2002), Thall and Cook (2006) and Thall et al. (2008). These designs are basically of the phase I dose-finding type but also include efficacy considerations to determine the dose for phase II efficacy testing. While the traditional phase I and phase II designs aim at finding an estimate $\widehat{\gamma}$ of the MTD γ in phase I and then testing the null hypothesis $K_0 : p(\widehat{\gamma}) \leq p_0$ in phase II, in which $p(d)$ denotes the probability of an efficacious response at dose d, Bartroff et al. (2014) propose an integrated approach in designing early-phase dose-finding trials. In their design, a joint efficacy-toxicity model is chosen to model toxicity y_i and efficacy z_i, which can be dependent, and a phase I design is chosen to estimate MTD. In phase II, a group-sequential GLR test of $H_0 : P(z = 1|x = \gamma) \leq p_0$, rather than $K_0 : p(\widehat{\gamma}) \leq p_0$ is used. The MTD estimate $\widehat{\gamma}$ is updated at each stage and always dose patients at the current estimate. If H_0 is rejected, $\widehat{\gamma}$ is updated with all phase I-II data as the recommended dose.

Section 4.1.4 has discussed adaptive designs for phase I trials to determine the doses of combination therapies for use in phase II trials. Harrington et al. (2013) point out that the need to design "smarter, faster clinical trials, appropriate for the era of molecularly targeted therapies" is particularly pressing for early phase trials of combination therapies, especially those involving targeted therapies, and advocate the development and use of adaptive designs to meet this need. Standard rule-based dose-finding designs such as up-and-down rules that only consider the last cohort to guide escalation or de-escalation to the nearest neighbor typically lead to highly sub-therapeutic doses for combination therapies that are considerably more complex than single agents. They argue that a promising future lies in model-based designs that can combine trial data (which include measurements of toxicity, efficacy, pharmacokinetics, and pharmacodynamics) with prior knowledge from the literature and previous related studies, and in particular adaptive model-based designs that allow investigators to use accumulated information during the course of the trial to learn the toxicity contour (formed by dose combinations that all have a prescribed target probability of DLT) and choose the most efficacious dose on the contour. They review some adaptive designs in this direction already developed and used, including Houede et al. (2010) and Whitehead et al. (2010), and the adaptive phase I designs of Dragalin et al. (2008) for selecting drug combinations based on efficacy-toxicity response. Moreover, the approach of Bartroff et al. (2014) can be extended to modify this kind of adaptive phase I design for combination therapies to develop seamless phase I-II designs to test for efficacy in phase II.

4.4 Summary of clinical trial safety data

Clinical trial safety data usually comprise the following categories: (a) any unwanted clinical manifestations (clinical terminal endpoints of safety), (b) laboratory test results (hematology, biochemistry, urology), (c) vital signs (e.g., blood pressure, body temperature, respiratory rate, pulse rate), and (d) others, e.g., electrocardiogram (ECG) and clinical imaging data. The following safety-related information is also collected during clinical trials: (i) patient exposure (e.g., dosage and duration), (ii) severity or grade of adverse events, outcome of adverse events (e.g., hospitalization, death), (iii) use of concomitant medications. From medical perspectives, the following information is primarily of interest to investigators and regulators: treatment-emergent AE (TEAE), drug-related AE, serious AE, higher-intensity AE, and death. In addition to reporting safety results from individual trials, regulatory agencies also require that safety and tolerability data be summarized across trials in an aggregate manner during the development activities of a compound, especially before its marketing authorization, the so-called integrated summary of safety (FDA, 1988; Temple, 1991; ICH, 1998). While safety evaluation in early phases (phases I and IIa) of clinical studies is most likely to be exploratory in nature, establishment of safety and tolerability profiles of a compound is an important objective of late-phase (phase IIb, III, and IV) clinical trials that have large sample sizes, relatively long study duration and randomized controls, although late-phase trials are usually not designed to confirm the presence or absence of major safety events. Hence, for the analysis of safety data from these trials, the ICH E9 guideline (ICH, 1998) states: "In most trials the safety and tolerability implications are best addressed by applying descriptive statistical methods to the data, supplemented by calculation of confidence intervals wherever this aids interpretation...The calculation of p-values is sometimes useful either as an aid to evaluating a specific difference of interest, or as a 'flagging' device applied to a large number of safety and tolerability variables to highlight differences worth further attention." It further notes that "if hypothesis tests are used, statistical adjustments for multiplicity to quantify the type I error are appropriate, but the type II error is usually of more concern." This is discussed further in Chapter 5.

4.4.1 Clinical adverse events

One of common reported AE categories is treatment emergent AEs (TEAEs), defined as any AEs that occur during the time period from a subject's randomization or treatment initiation to the end of treatment, or 30 (or 60) days after treatment termination; the choice of duration may differ from protocol to protocol. To illustrate, Table 4.1 shows the number N of subjects in each treatment group and the number n of those who experienced at least one AE reported as a preferred term in a primary system organ class (SOC). Such a summary table provides easy-to-grasp information on the comparison of percentages of subjects who experience the specified AEs among treatment groups. Table 4.1 shows that the percentage of subjects who experience any AE in the "Nervous system disorder" SOC for the new treatment at high dose is twice that in the low-dose or placebo group (15.4% for high dose versus 7.5% for low dose versus 7.8% for placebo). Note that a patient may be counted more than once if he or she has multiple adverse events in more than one SOC. For example, if a subject has an AE in "Gastrointestinal disorder" SOC and another AE in "Hepatobiliary disorder," then the subject is counted twice in this table. On the other hand, if a subject experiences two AEs that belong to the same SOC, he or she is only counted once. Moreover, TEAEs are often tabulated by preferred terms according to the level of incidence, e.g., only the most frequently reported adverse events with $\geq 2\%$ incidence rate in at least one group are presented in Table 4.2, in which a subject may be counted more than once if he or she has more than one AE. The crude incidence rate (in %) in Table 4.2 is defined as the number of subjects with a particular preferred term divided by the total number of subjects in each treatment group, regardless of the duration of follow-up time for each individual patient (including dropouts for any reason).

It should be pointed out that all reported AEs usually go through a Safety Endpoint Adjudication Committee who adjudicates, in a blinded manner, whether each reported AE is a true AE, and if yes, whether it is caused by or related to the study treatment. Moreover, AEs that are classified as treatment-related are also summarized in tables similar to Table 4.2. In addition to treatment-related AEs, deaths and serious TEAEs that may or may not lead to a subject's discontinuation are tabulated as in Table 4.3. The SAEs can further be presented by SOC and preferred terms for each of the study treatment, and can also be divided into groups according to gender, treatment cycle, and severity level of the AEs as in Table 4.4. Depending on the nature of the study compound, a set of adverse events of special interest that are of "scientific and medical concern specific to the sponsor's product or program, for which ongoing monitoring and rapid communication by the investigator to the sponsor can be appropriate" (FDA, 2011b), should also be presented.

4.4.2 Laboratory test results

Laboratory tests are routinely performed in clinical trials for the purpose of patient screening before trial initiation, monitoring the patient's pathophysiological conditions that may be associated with the study agent or due to disease progression, and/or diagnosis of the patient's suspected

TABLE 4.1 Treatment emergent adverse events for SOCs under high (H) and low (L) doses.

Primary system organ class	Treatment (H) N = 234		Treatment (L) N = 227		Placebo N = 230	
	n	%	n	%	n	%
Any primary system organ class	193	82.5	197	86.8	184	80.0
Infections and infestations	48	20.5	48	21.1	63	27.4
Skin and subcutaneous tissue disorder	47	20.1	33	14.5	48	20.9
Nervous system disorder	36	15.4	17	7.5	18	7.8
Gastrointestinal disorder	33	14.1	22	9.7	19	8.3
Musculoskeletal and connective tissue disorder	22	9.4	11	4.8	17	7.4
Respiratory, thoracic, and mediastinal disorder	14	6.0	12	5.3	16	7.0
Blood and lymphatic system disorder	12	5.1	5	2.2	10	4.3
Eye disorder	11	4.7	6	2.6	8	3.5
Metabolism and nutrition disorder	8	3.4	4	1.8	5	2.2
Vascular disorder	8	3.4	3	1.3	0	
Cardiac disorder	5	2.1	0		2	0.9
Hepatobiliary disorder	4	1.7	1	0.4	1	0.4
Investigations	3	1.3	3	1.3	0	
Renal and urinary disorder	3	1.3	0		2	0.9
Ear and labyrinth disorder	1	0.4	3	1.3	1	0.4
Endocrine disorder	1	0.4	3	1.3	0	
General disorders and administration site conditions	1	0.4	2	0.9	0	
Injury, poisoning, and procedural complications	0		2	0.9	1	0.4
Psychiatric disorder	0		2	0.9	0	
Reproductive system and breast disorders	0		1	0.4	1	0.4
Surgical and medical procedures	0		0		1	0.4
Neoplasms benign, malignant, and unspecified	0		1	0.4	0	

health conditions. A laboratory test refers to a clinical testing procedure in which a sample of blood, urine, other body fluid, tissue, or substance taken from a subject is examined with respect to the constitution of biochemical, cytological, microbiological, and proteomic substances in a sample, to help gather information about a person's health condition. Labo-

TABLE 4.2 Most frequent (at least 2% incidence rate in any treatment group) treatment emergent adverse events.

Preferred team	Treatment (H) N = 234		Treatment (L) N = 227		Placebo N = 230	
	n	%	n	%	n	%
Any preferred team	193	82.5	197	86.8	184	80.0
Nasopharyngitis	27	11.5	21	9.3	36	15.7
Eczema	15	6.4	10	4.4	7	3.0
Headache	15	6.4	9	4.0	9	3.9
Pharyngitis	9	3.8	12	5.3	7	3.0
Acne	6	2.6	3	1.3	8	3.5
Bronchitis	6	2.6	0		0	
Cystitis	0		3	1.3	6	2.6
Insomnia	0		6	2.6	3	1.3
Upper respiratory tract infection	0		6	2.6	0	

TABLE 4.3 Treatment emergent serious adverse events.

SAE	Treatment (H) N = 234		Treatment (L) N = 227		Placebo N = 230	
	n	%	n	%	n	%
Death	1	0.4	0		0	
TESAEs	9	3.8	9	4.0	2	0.9
TESAEs leading to discontinuation	1	0.4	3	1.3	0	

ratory tests may also be conducted for research purposes to understand the pathophysiology of a particular disease process (Wians, 2009). It is believed that changes in certain laboratory test results (or parameters) may serve as precursors of some critical organ dysfunctions or important clinical adverse manifestations. Laboratory data are usually multidimensional and involve multiple parameters, comprising test results in hematology, clinical biochemistry, urinalysis, and other study-specific categories. For example, hematology parameters may include red and white blood cell counts, hemoglobin, lymphocytes, and monocytes.; biochemistry parameters may consist of alanine transaminase (ALT), aspartate transaminase (AST), bilirubin, and creatine; urinalysis may include sugar, protein, red and white blood cells. Many of these laboratory test data are collected each time when patients visit trial sites and are presented in the form of summary statistics (such as mean, standard deviation SD, minimum, and maximum) and changes from baseline (Table 4.5). Patients with abnormal test results for key laboratory parameters, such

TABLE 4.4 Number of patients (n) with treatment emergent adverse events among totals being treated (N) by treatment group, gender, treatment cycle (cycles 1–4), and severity (grades 1–4).

Seve-rity	Treatment				Control			
	Male		Female		Male		Female	
	n/N	%	n/N	%	n/N	%	n/N	%
				Cycle 1				
1	46/140	32.9	51/135	37.8	32/137	23.4	30/126	23.8
2	31/140	22.1	26/135	19.3	22/137	16.1	9/126	7.1
3	13/140	9.3	18/135	13.3	3/137	2.2	8/126	6.3
4	4/140	2.9	5/135	3.7	3/137	2.2	2/126	1.6
				Cycle 2				
1	25/129	19.4	46/127	36.2	40/123	32.5	44/118	37.3
2	28/129	21.7	27/127	21.3	20/123	16.3	47/118	39.8
3	19/129	14.7	11/127	8.7	14/123	11.4	11/118	9.3
4	12/129	9.3	3/127	2.4	4/123	3.3	8/118	6.8
				Cycle 3				
1	15/114	13.2	37/108	34.3	33/97	34.0	38/95	40.0
2	22/114	19.3	19/108	17.6	13/97	13.4	13/95	13.7
3	32/114	28.1	23/108	21.3	11/97	11.3	10/95	10.5
4	21/114	18.4	10/108	9.3	3/97	3.1	7/95	7.4
				Cycle 4				
1	48/85	56.5	38/93	40.9	34/86	39.5	25/80	31.3
2	11/85	12.9	22/93	23.7	17/86	19.8	13/80	16.3
3	16/85	18.8	14/93	15.1	6/86	7.0	22/80	27.5
4	3/85	3.5	6/93	6.5	3/86	3.5	3/80	3.8

as ALT and AST for liver function, and serum creatine and blood urea nitrogen (BUN) for renal function, are also singled out for monitoring and listed in the final clinical trial reports.

Alternatively, patients can be grouped into different categories according to their laboratory test results falling within pre-defined ranges (e.g., "below," "within," or "above" the normal range) of critical laboratory parameters. The proportions of patients in individual categories are calculated for each group at each visit; see Table 4.6. Such summaries, often called "shift" tables, can be used to explore changes in proportions of patients in each category over time. Logistic regression models can also be used to estimate an increasing or decreasing trend of the proportions over time.

TABLE 4.5 Summary statistics (at baseline, week 12) and change magnitude of selected laboratory test results for liver function.

Parameter	Treatment			Control		
	Baseline	Wk12	Change	Baseline	Wk12	Change
ALT (U/L)						
N	234	232	-2	228	225	-3
Mean	22.3	28.9	5.6	23.4	25.6	2.3
SD*	8.7	10.9	2.2	9.0	10.3	1.9
AST (U/L)						
N	234	233	-1	228	224	-4
Mean	23.1	33.6	10.5	25.8	26.6	0.8
SD	9.3	11.7	3.9	10.0	13.3	1.4
Total bilirubin (mg/dL)						
N	234	232	-2	228	224	-4
Mean	0.67	0.80	0.13	0.73	0.83	0.10
SD	0.24	0.29	0.06	0.26	0.34	0.06

TABLE 4.6 Shift table of percentages of subjects in specific categories of laboratory test results for liver function over time.

Laboratory parameter	Treatment (N)			Placebo (N)		
	Baseline (234)	Visit 1 (232)	Visit 2 (226)	Baseline (228)	Visit 1 (225)	Visit 2 (220)
ALT (U/L)						
< 7	8.1	4.3	6.7	4.6	6.5	7.4
7 − 55	86.9	80.2	75.2	88.0	86.6	82.8
> 55	5.0	15.5	18.1	7.4	6.9	9.8
AST (U/L)						
< 8	5.3	4.8	4.0	5.9	5.7	4.3
8 − 48	90.6	82.0	78.4	88.7	82.1	86.3
> 48	4.1	13.2	17.6	5.4	12.2	9.4
Total bilirubin (mg/dL)						
< 0.1	3.3	4.5	2.1	6.7	4.8	5.6
0.1 − 1.9	90.9	83.1	76.5	86.5	82.4	88.9
> 1.9	5.8	11.4	21.4	6.8	13.8	5.5

4.4.3 Vital signs

Vital signs are measures of the human body's basic functions. There are four major types of vital signs, namely, body temperature, pulse rate, respiration rate (rate of breathing), and blood pressure (blood pressure sometimes is not considered a vital sign, but is often measured along with the vital signs). Vital signs are useful for detecting and monitoring critical health conditions, and therefore data on these vital signs are routinely collected during clinical trials. Similar to laboratory safety data as presented in Tables 4.5 and 4.6, vital sign measurements are commonly displayed using summary statistics for the change from baseline for each post-baseline visit by treatment group. Patients with newly occurring notable vital sign changes from baseline or immediate previous measurements are usually summarized by using some pre-defined criteria (Table 4.7) and shift tables (Table 4.8) are usually created to examine changes of proportions of patients (especially in the "abnormal" category) over time between treatment groups.

TABLE 4.7 Some commonly used criteria for classification of resting adults based on vital signs.

Vital sign	Categories		
Body temperature	Hypothermia	Normal	Fever
Centigrade (°C)	< 35	36–37	≥ 38
Fahrenheit (°F)	< 95	98.6	≥ 100.4
Heart rate	Bradycardia	Normal	Tachycardia
(beats per minutes)	< 60	60–100	≥ 100
Respiratory rate	Bradypnea	Normal	Tachypnea
(breaths per minutes)	< 12	12–20	≥ 20
Blood pressure (BP) (mmHg)	Hypotension	Normal	Hypertension
Systolic BP	< 90	90–140	≥ 140
Diastolic BP	< 60	60–90	≥ 90

4.4.4 Integrated summary of safety (ISS)

A compound may have more than one disease indication for which multiple clinical studies may be conducted in multiple regions or countries involving patient populations with diverse background and diseases. Combining data from individual studies into a large database allows for not only study-by-study comparisons of more common adverse events, but also pooled estimates of the incidence rates of common and rare events and adverse effects in subgroup populations. As pointed out by Temple (1991), integrated summaries of safety are not merely summaries of multiple trials, but also provide new analyses of safety information from all sources (animal models, clinical pharmacology, controlled and uncontrolled studies, epidemiologic data). The ISS consists of the following three critical components (Temple, 1991):

(a) *Extent of exposure*: Detailed descriptions of patient populations who were exposed to the drug (diagnosis, severity of illness, concomitant

TABLE 4.8 Shift table of subjects with newly notable vital sign changes from baseline.

Vital sign	Treatment (N)			Placebo (N)		
	Baseline (175)	Visit 1 (173)	Visit 2 (171)	Baseline (169)	Visit 1 (161)	Visit 2 (147)
Body temperature (°C)						
< 35	9	7	4	4	3	3
$35 - 38$	161	159	150	156	151	139
≥ 38	5	7	17	9	7	5
$\vdots$	$\vdots$	$\vdots$	$\vdots$	$\vdots$	$\vdots$	$\vdots$
Systolic blood pressure (mmHg)						
< 90	0	1	0	0	0	0
$90 - 140$	166	159	152	162	157	142
≥ 140	9	13	19	7	4	5

illness, concomitant drugs, etc.), the doses and durations of exposure, and the analyses conducted.

(b) *Common adverse events*: Comparison of the incidence rates between treatment and control, incidences of adverse effects (possibly common events with pre-defined threshold on incidence rates) in various subgroups (e.g., gender, ethnicity, young versus older adults), with the data from pediatric trials among children aged less than 17 years to be analyzed separately.

(c) *Serious adverse events*: Details on deaths and dropouts due to adverse experiences, where unexpected important adverse effects might be found in the search for "needles in the haystack."

4.4.5 Development Safety Update Report (DSUR)

The objective of a DSUR is to present a comprehensive annual review and evaluation of safety data collected from all clinical trials (completed and ongoing) conducted with the investigational product for all indications, at all dosage levels, and/or among all intended populations. In addition to safety data from clinical trials, DSUR should also include the following findings that may impact the safety and well-being of clinical trial subjects:

(a) results of preclinical studies,

(b) results of observational or epidemiological studies,

(c) manufacturing or microbiological changes,

(d) results of published studies and of clinical trials conducted by co-developers or partners.

These topics will be considered in Chapters 7 and 8, in particular (a) in Section 7.1.1, (d) in Section 7.8, (c) in Sections 8.3.4 and 8.3.5, and (b) in Sections 7.6, 7.7 and 7.8. While focusing on the investigational product, DSUR should also provide information relevant to the safety of trial participants from comparator products. DSUR should also contain information on deaths and dropouts, graphical displays of which can "provide an opportunity to convey insight about patterns, trends, or anomalies that may signal potential safety issues in ways that would be difficult to comprehend from tabular to textual presentations" (Gould, 2015b). These graphical displays are described in Section 4.6. Moreover, closely related to methodologies for graphical displays and for the analysis of laboratory data in Section 4.4.2, Chuang-Stein (1998) has advocated more statistical research in multivariate visualization, mixture of responders, and correlated test results pertaining to the analysis and presentation of laboratory safety data. She notes that in contrast to the analysis of clinical efficacy and safety endpoints, there has not been much development in safety signal detection from clinical laboratory data that are conventionally used to examine individual patients' pathophysiological conditions according to pre-defined "normal" ranges by physicians who are mostly interested in a relatively small set of patients whose laboratory test results show "abnormality" in some key parameters; the majority of patients whose laboratory data are in the "normal" ranges do not cause concern. In addition, laboratory values typically fluctuate about a stable state in the absence of toxic effects, and the regulating mechanisms of the human body act as controls to preserve the stable state in the presence of external stimuli on the corresponding organ system. If the stimulus is too strong or too large, these controls would cause some laboratory values to increase or decrease beyond what is considered to be a normal range. To incorporate these system control considerations, Rosenkranz (2009) uses stochastic processes to model potential systematic effects in the laboratory measurements in a group of subjects, using the estimated parameters of these processes to quantify the effects of drugs or other medical treatments. Southworth and Heffernan (2012a) propose to apply extreme value theory to laboratory safety data for prediction of incidence of severe adverse drug reactions by fitting the generalized Pareto distribution, with shape parameter ξ and scale parameter σ, to the data points that exceed of a suitably chosen threshold μ:

$$f(x; \xi, \mu, \sigma) = \frac{1}{\sigma} \left[1 + \frac{\xi(x - \mu)}{\sigma} \right]^{\frac{1}{\xi} - 1}, \quad x > \mu,$$

which is the conditional density of an observation given that it exceeds

μ and approximates well the distribution of laboratory test values x exceeding μ if μ is sufficiently large. Southworth and Heffernan (2012a,b) discuss applications of the generalized Pareto distribution to monitor potential safety concerns and also provide a multivariate extension to model multiple laboratory indices simultaneously for detecting unexpected extremal multivariate relationships.

4.5 Exposure-adjusted incidence rates (EAIR) and regression models

4.5.1 EAIR and confidence intervals for hazard rates

Although the crude incidence rate in Table 4.2 provides essential information on the rate of occurrence of adverse events, its validity requires the strong assumption of randomness of patient discontinuation for reasons other than AEs across groups. If this assumption is violated, as in the case of uneven patient dropout rates (due to withdrawal of consent, lack of efficacy, loss to follow up, etc.), then the number of patients being exposed at risk for any given time period after randomization may change dynamically and result in imbalanced exposure time between the control and treatment groups. A remedy for this deficiency is to calculate the exposure time of each patient and then divide the number of subjects with AEs by the total exposure time for all patients to obtain the *exposure-adjusted incidence rate* (EAIR). Specifically, let n_i and T_i denote, respectively, the total observed number of subjects experiencing a target AE and the total exposure time (in months or years) among N_i subjects in the ith group ($i = 1$ for treatment, and $i = 0$ for control) in a two-armed randomed trial. Then $\hat{\lambda}_i = n_i/T_i$ is the estimate of EAIR for the ith group. We next describe commonly used methods to construct confidence intervals for the difference $\theta = \lambda_1 - \lambda_2$ in EAIR between the two groups, assuming that conditional on T_i,

$$n_i \sim \text{Poisson}(\lambda_i T_i), \quad i = 1, 2. \tag{4.23}$$

   (a) *Confidence intervals using Wald's approximation.* Since the conditional variance of $\hat{\lambda}_i$ given T_i is λ_i/T_i and λ_i can be consistently estimated by $\hat{\lambda}_i$, Wald's approximate $(1 - \alpha)$-level confidence interval for θ is

$$\hat{\lambda}_1 - \hat{\lambda}_2 \pm \hat{\sigma} z_{1-\alpha/2}, \tag{4.24}$$

where $\hat{\sigma}^2 = \hat{\lambda}_1/T_1 + \hat{\lambda}_1/T_2$ and z_q denotes the qth quantile of the standard normal distribution.

(b) *Confidence intervals using the Miettinen–Nurminen method.* For (crude) rates of occurrence as in Table 4.2, Miettinen and Nurminen (1985, abbreviated by MN in the sequel) point out that Wald's approximation might under-estimate the standard error, resulting in poor coverage for the confidence interval when the observed number of occurrence (or non-occurrence) of events is small or moderate. Noting that better standard error estimates are used in testing the null hypothesis for which the rate difference between treatment and control is specified by the hypothesis and does not need to be estimated, they propose to construct confidence intervals by inverting likelihood ratio tests. Liu et al. (2006) have extended this method, which they call the "MN method," to construct confidence intervals for $\theta = \lambda_1 - \lambda_2$, the difference in EAIR between the treatment and control groups. Under the Poisson model (4.23), the MLE $(\tilde{\lambda}_{1,\theta}, \tilde{\lambda}_{2,\theta})$ of (λ_1, λ_2) subject the constraint $\lambda_1 - \lambda_2 = \theta$ has the form

$$\begin{cases} \tilde{\lambda}_{1,\theta} = \tilde{\lambda}_{2,\theta} + \theta \\ \tilde{\lambda}_{2,\theta} = \frac{1}{2}\left\{(\tilde{\lambda} - \theta) + \left[(\tilde{\lambda} - \theta)^2 + \frac{4n_2\theta}{T_1+T_2}\right]^{\frac{1}{2}}\right\}, \end{cases} \quad (4.25)$$

where $\tilde{\lambda} = (n_1 + n_2)/(T_1 + T_2)$ is the MLE of the overall EAIR for the combined population. On the other hand, the test statistic χ^2-test of the null hypothesis $\lambda_1 - \lambda_2 = \theta$ has the form $(\hat{\lambda}_1 - \hat{\lambda}_2 - \theta)^2/\tilde{v}_\theta$, where $\tilde{v}_\theta = \tilde{\lambda}_{1,\theta}/T_1 + \tilde{\lambda}_{2,\theta}/T_2$, which depends on θ, and the test rejects the null hypothesis at level α if the test statistic exceeds the $(1 - \alpha)$-quantile χ^2_α of the χ^2-distribution with 1 degree of freedom. Inverting this test yields the $(1 - \alpha)$-level confidence interval

$$\chi^2_\alpha = (\hat{\lambda}_1 - \hat{\lambda}_2 - \theta)^2/(\tilde{\lambda}_{1,\theta}/T_1 + \tilde{\lambda}_{2,\theta}/T_2). \quad (4.26)$$

Combining (4.25) with (4.26) yields a fourth-order polynomial equation in θ, and Liu et al. (2006) use a numerical algorithm given by Miettinen and Nurminen (1985) to solve this polynomial equation. They also introduce a conditional MN method and show that it performs better than Wald's approximate confidence intervals but worse than the MN method. Moreover, they argue that $\lambda_1 - \lambda_2$ is preferred to the risk ratio λ_1/λ_2 since it is still well defined for rare events with zero count in group 2 and is more easily computed.

(c) *Extension to stratified incidence rates.* Let $\theta = \lambda_1 - \lambda_2$ be the difference in incidence rates between treatment and control groups. Suppose that there is a stratum variable (e.g., age) with K levels across which the incidence rate changes from stratum to stratum, and that one is interested in testing $H_0 : \theta \leq \theta_0$ against $H_1 : \theta > \theta_0$. Let n_{ik} be the observed number of events given the exposure time T_{ik} for the ith group in the kth stratum. Let $n_k = n_{1k} + n_{2k}$ and $T_k = T_{1k} + T_{2k}$ be the stratum-specific total of observed event cases and of exposure time, respectively, for the kth stratum across treatment groups, and $n_i = \sum_{k=1}^{K} n_{ik}$ and $T_i = \sum_{k=1}^{K} T_{ik}$ be the group-specific total of the observed event cases and exposure time, respectively, for the ith treatment group across the K strata ($i = 1, 2$). Let λ_{ik} be the intensity rate for the ith group at the kth stratum and $\hat{\lambda}_{ik} = n_{ik}/T_{ik}$ be the maximum likelihood estimate of λ_{ik} under the Poisson model. Then the group-specific estimate of λ_i across the K strata can be estimated by the weighted average

$$\hat{\lambda}_i = \sum_{k=1}^{K} \omega_k \hat{\lambda}_{ik} \qquad (4.27)$$

of the stratum-specific intensity rates, where the weight ω_k is commonly chosen to be proportional to the exposure time T_k relative to the total exposure time, i.e., $\omega_k = T_k/\sum_{h=1}^{K} T_h$, or the Mantel-Haenszel-type weights

$$\omega_k = \frac{T_{1k}T_{2k}/(T_{1k} + T_{2k})}{\sum_{h=1}^{K} T_{1h}T_{2h}/(T_{1h} + T_{2h})}. \qquad (4.28)$$

Using (4.27) to estimate θ by $\hat{\lambda}_1 - \hat{\lambda}_2$, one can apply the Wald's approximation to obtain an approximate $100(1 - \alpha)\%$ confidence intervals $\hat{\theta} \pm \hat{\sigma}_\theta z_{1-\alpha/2}$, where $\hat{\sigma}_\theta^2 = \sum_{k=1}^{K} \omega_k^2 \left(\hat{\lambda}_{1k}/T_{1k} + \hat{\lambda}_{2k}/T_{2k} \right)$. Alternatively, the MN method can also be extended to give confidence intervals for θ; see Supplement 1 of Section 4.7.

4.5.2   Poisson regression and negative binomial models

As in the preceding section, suppose that conditional on the exposure time T_i, the observed number n_i of event cases for the ith group follows a Poisson distribution $n_i \sim \text{Poisson}(\lambda_i T_i)$, and that the intensity rate λ_i is estimated by $\hat{\lambda}_i = n_i/T_i$. Therefore, $E(n_i) = \mu_i = \lambda_i T_i$. In the presence of explanatory variables $\mathbf{x}_i = (x_{i1}, \ldots, x_{iJ})$, the Poisson regression model for the expected incidence rate is given by

$$\log(\mu_i/T_i) = \log(\mu_i) - \log(T_i) = \alpha + \sum_{j=1}^{J} \beta_j x_{ij}. \qquad (4.29)$$

The term $-\log(T_i)$ is called an offset to the log link of the mean

$$\mu_i = T_i \exp \left(\alpha + \sum_{j=1}^{J} \beta_j x_{ij} \right), \qquad (4.30)$$

which is equivalent to (4.29); see Agresti (2013). More generally, suppose that there are J strata across I treatment groups and the observed number of events is n_{ij} with exposure time T_{ij}, for the ith treatment group in the jth stratum. Then the expected mean of n_{ij} is given by $\mu_{ij} = \lambda_{ij}T_{ij}$ which can be expressed in a Poisson regression model as

$$\log(\mu_{ij}/T_{ij}) = \alpha + \beta_1 x_i + \beta_2 x_j, \tag{4.31}$$

where x_i and x_j can be chosen as indicator variables representing the ith treatment group and jth stratum, respectively, assuming no interaction between treatment group and stratum (Frome, 1983; Frome and Checkoway, 1985).

A well-known issue in fitting Poisson regression models is overdispersion, which occurs when the estimated variance $\sigma^2 = \text{Var}(n)$ exceeds its expected mean μ. For example, suppose there are $n = \sum_{i=1}^{N} y_i$ observed events among a total of N subjects who have the same exposure time, where $y_i = 1$ if an event occurs and $y_i = 0$ otherwise. Suppose $P(y_i = 1) = \pi$ and $\text{Cov}(y_i, y_j) = \rho$. Then the mean of n is equal to $N\pi$ and its variance σ^2 is given by

$$\text{Var}(n) = \text{Var}\left(\sum_{i=1}^{N} y_i\right) = N\pi(1-\pi)\left[1 + \rho(N-1)\right], \tag{4.32}$$

which is larger than the expected value $N\pi(1-\pi)$ if $\rho > 0$ (overdispersion) or smaller than the expected value $N\pi(1-\pi)$ if $\rho < 0$ (underdispersion). Overdispersion usually results from non-independence of the events due to clustering effects. A method to address overdispersion in Poisson regression is to regard λ as a random variable having a gamma distribution with density function

$$f(\lambda; \alpha, \mu) = \frac{(\alpha/\mu)^\alpha \lambda^{\alpha-1}}{\Gamma(\alpha)} \exp\left(-\alpha\lambda/\mu\right), \tag{4.33}$$

where μ is the mean and α is the shape parameter. Then y_i has the negative binomial distribution

$$p(y; \alpha, \mu) = \frac{\Gamma(\alpha+y)}{\Gamma(\alpha)\Gamma(y+1)}\left(\frac{\alpha}{\alpha+\mu}\right)^\alpha\left(\frac{\mu}{\alpha+\mu}\right)^y, \quad y = 0, 1, \ldots, \tag{4.34}$$

with mean μ and variance $\mu(1+\mu/\alpha)$. The dispersion parameter is defined as $\phi = 1/\alpha$. In the presence of explanatory variables $\mathbf{x} = (x_{i1}, \ldots, x_{iJ})$, the analog of (4.31) has the form

$$\log(\mu_i) = \beta_0 + \sum_{j=1}^{J} \beta_j x_{ij} \tag{4.35}$$

and maximum likelihood can be used to estimate $\beta_0, \beta_1, \ldots, \beta_J$; see Hilbe (2011) and Cameron and Trivedi (2013) for details.

4.5.3   Rare events data analysis and statistical models for recurrent events

Many adverse events, especially serious adverse events with low incidence rates, are not commonly observed or observed with small number of events during clinical trials and post-marketing observational studies. According to the Council for International Organizations of Medical Sciences (CIOMS, 1999), an adverse drug reaction may be considered rare if its incidence rate is less than 1 per 1000 person-years. Some examples of rare events are anaphylaxis, hemolytic anemia, liver necrosis, and sudden death in general population. Statistical issues in dealing with rare events include lack of statistical power for early detection of signals and for testing the difference in incidence rates between groups, overdispersion when fitting Poisson or negative binomial regression models caused by excessive zeros, and biased estimates of regression coefficients in fitting generalized linear models which include logistic and Poisson regression models and which are widely used in the analysis of adverse event data.

Exact or bias-corrected logistic regression. To address the bias of the MLE due to low counts of the rare events, Mehta and Patel (1995) use the following exact logistic regression method to obtain parameter estimates of β in the model $\text{logit}(\pi_i) = \beta_0 + \sum_{j=1}^{p} \beta_j x_{ij}$, in which $\pi_i = P(y_i = 1)$. Let $\mathbf{t} = \sum_{i=1}^{n} y_i \mathbf{x}_i$ be the sufficient statistic with density function

$$f(t_0, t_1, \ldots, t_J) = \frac{c(\mathbf{t}) \exp(\mathbf{t}^T \boldsymbol{\beta})}{\sum_{\mathbf{u}:c(\mathbf{u}) \geq 1} c(\mathbf{u}) \exp(\mathbf{u}^T \boldsymbol{\beta})}, \qquad (4.36)$$

where $c(\mathbf{t}) = |S(\mathbf{t})|$, the cardinality of the set

$$S(\mathbf{t}) = \left\{ (y_1, \ldots, y_n) : \sum_{i=1}^{n} y_i = m, \sum_{i=1}^{n} y_i x_{ij} = t_j, j = 1, \ldots, p \right\}.$$

The conditional density of t_p given $t_1, \ldots, t_{p-1}$ depends only on β_p and is given by

$$f(t_p | \beta_p) = \frac{c(t_0, t_1, \ldots, t_p) \exp(\beta_p t_p)}{\sum_u c(t_0, t_1, \ldots, t_{p-1}, u) \exp(\beta_p u)}, \qquad (4.37)$$

with the summation in the denominator taken over all u for which $c(t_1, \ldots, t_{p-1}, u) \geq 1$. The exact logistic regression estimate of β_p is the value that maximizes this conditional likelihood. Leitgöb (2013) has reported that the exact logistic regression works well for $n < 200$ and a small number of (discrete) covariates (preferably dichotomous).

As an alternative, King and Ryan (2002) propose a bias-corrected logistic regression method that is based on McCullagh's approximation of the bias of the MLE when the sample size or the total Fisher information is small; see McCullagh (1987, p. 210) and Cordeiro and McCullagh (1991). King and Zeng (2001) note that for rare events data, the probability $P\{Y_i = 1\}$ tends to be underestimated and hence propose a method to correct the estimated probabilities by $P\{Y_i = 1\} \approx \tilde{\pi}_i + C_i$, where $\tilde{\pi}_i = 1/\left[1 + \exp\left(\mathbf{X}\widehat{\boldsymbol{\beta}}\right)\right]$, $C_i = (0.5 - \tilde{\pi}_i)\tilde{\pi}_i(1 - \tilde{\pi}_i)\mathbf{X}V(\widehat{\boldsymbol{\beta}})\mathbf{X}^T$, and $V(\widehat{\boldsymbol{\beta}})$ denotes the covariance matrix of β.

Zero-inflated Poisson or negative binomial regression. The zero-inflated Poisson (ZIP) regression model takes the form

$$f(y_i; \mathbf{x}_i, \mathbf{z}_i) = \begin{cases} \omega(\mathbf{z}_i) + [1 - \omega(\mathbf{z}_i)]g(y_i = j), & \text{if } j = 0 \\ [1 - \omega(\mathbf{z}_i)]g(y_i), & \text{if } j > 0 \end{cases} \qquad (4.38)$$

where $0 < \omega < 1$ is a zero-inflation parameter,

$$g(y_i) = \frac{[\lambda(\mathbf{x}_i)]^{y_i}}{y_i!} \exp\left[-\lambda(\mathbf{x}_i)\right] \qquad (4.39)$$

is the standard Poisson distribution, $\mathbf{x}_i$ and $\mathbf{z}_i$ are two sets of covariates that can be disjoint, overlapping, or identical (Baetschmann and Winkelmann, 2013). As in the Poisson regression model, the canonical link function for $\lambda(\mathbf{x}_i)$ is given by $\lambda(\mathbf{x}_i) = \exp\left(\alpha + \beta\mathbf{x}_i\right)$, or by

$$\lambda(\mathbf{x}_i) = \exp\left[\alpha + \beta\mathbf{x}_i + \eta\log(T_i)\right] \qquad (4.40)$$

when the exposure time T_i is also involved. The zero-inflation parameter is modeled through its logit link function $\text{logit}\left[\omega(z_i)\right] = \exp\left(\alpha' + \beta'\mathbf{z}_i\right)$. Baetschmann and Winkelmann (2013) also add log exposure time as an explanatory variable to the logistic regression model

$$\omega(\mathbf{z}_i, T_i) = \frac{\exp\left[\alpha' + \beta'\mathbf{z}_i + \eta'\log(T_i)\right]}{1 + \exp\left[\alpha' + \beta'\mathbf{z}_i + \eta'\log(T_i)\right]}. \qquad (4.41)$$

The zero-inflated negative binomial (ZINB) regression model has the same form as in (4.38) but with $g(y_i)$ replaced by the negative binomial model in (4.34); see also Rose et al. (2006) and Liu (2013) for details and examples.

Statistical models for recurrent events. During the time course of a clinical trial, some adverse events may occur multiple times on the same patient. One may be interested in the cumulative number of events over time, event rate per unit time, time to successive events, time elapse between successive events, or a combination of these. We first define the *mean cumulative function* $M(t)$ of a recurrent event process in the time interval $[0, t]$ and the estimator $\hat{M}(t)$, following the counting process approach of Ghosh and Lin (2000) and using their notation. Let D denote the survival time and $N^*(t)$ denote the number of recurrent events that occur in $[0, t]$. Naturally, subjects who die cannot experience any further recurrent events so that the counting process $N^*(\cdot)$ does not jump after D. Let C denote the follow-up or censoring time, which is assumed to be independent of both D and $N^*(\cdot)$. However, Ghosh and Lin (2000) make no assumptions regarding the dependence among the recurrent events or the dependence between D and $N^*(\cdot)$. Because of censoring, D and $N^*(\cdot)$ may not be fully observed. Instead, one observes $\{N(\cdot), X, \delta\}$, where $N(t) = N^*(t \wedge C)$, $X = D \wedge C$, and $\delta = I(D \leq C)$. The observations $\{N_i(\cdot), X_i, \delta_i\}$, $i = 1, \ldots, n$, for the n subjects are assumed to be independent replicates of $\{N(\cdot), X, \delta\}$. It is also assumed for technical reasons that there exists a constant τ such that $P(X \leq \tau) > 0$. The mean cumulative function is defined as $M(t) = E(N^*(t))$. This is the marginal expected number of recurrent events up to t per subject, acknowledging the fact that *no subject can experience any further recurrent event after death*. "This quantity has a clear clinical meaning and is interpretable regardless of what the distributions of D and $N^*(\cdot)$ are," and the italicized fact is what distinguishes the Ghosh-Lin approach from previous works which assume that "recurrent events are not terminated by death during the study". Hence $M(t) = \int_0^t S(u) dR(u)$, where $S(t) = P(D \geq t)$ and $dR(t) = E(dN^*(t)|D \geq t)$. Let $0 < t_1 < \ldots < t_K$ be the times of occurrence of the event in the sample, and let d_j be the number of events occurring at t_j and n_j be the number of subjects at risk just prior to t_j. Then, $R(t)$ can be estimated by the Nelson-Aalen estimator

$$\hat{R}(t) = \sum_{t_j \leq t} \frac{d_j}{n_j}, \qquad (4.42)$$

and $S(t)$ can be estimated by the Kaplan-Meier estimator

$$\prod_{t_j \leq t} \left(1 - \frac{D_j}{n_j}\right), \qquad (4.43)$$

where D_j is the number of deaths occurring at t_j. Hence $M(t)$ can be estimated by $\hat{M}(t) = \int_0^t \hat{S}(u) d\hat{R}(u)$. Ghosh and Lin (2000) show that $\left\{\sqrt{n}\left[\hat{M}(t) - M(t)\right], 0 \leq t \leq \tau\right\}$ converges weakly to a zero-mean Gaussian process and also derive a consistent estimate of its covariance function. An approximate $100(1 - \alpha)\%$ confidence interval for $M(t)$ is $\hat{M}(t) \pm z_{1-\alpha/2}\hat{\sigma}(t)$, which can be improved for moderate sample sizes through the log transformation

$$\hat{M}(t) \exp\left[\pm z_{1-\alpha/2}\hat{\sigma}(t)/\hat{M}(t)\right]; \qquad (4.44)$$

see also Pena et al. (2001), Nelson (2003), Cook and Lawless (2007), Kuramoto et al. (2008), Rondeau (2010), Amorim and Cai (2015), and Hengelbrock et al. (2016). Supplement 2 in Section 4.7 describes regression models for recurrent events.

4.6 Graphical displays of safety data

To communicate safety data and relevant information to clinical investigators, "a picture is worth a thousand tables" (Krause and O'Connell, 2012). Depending on the product and the nature of safety data, which may be proportions (adverse event rate), or counts over time (number of patients with an event of interest over time), or continuous variables such as laboratory data (e.g., liver function test results), different graphical approaches may be adopted to provide insights into patterns, associations, magnitude, time to event, or any other features of adverse event occurrence. Friendly (2000), Chen et al. (2007), and Krause and O'Connell (2012) have provided comprehensive discussions on data visualization and some commonly used graphics for visual summarization of safety data and communication of their analysis to clinical investigators.

4.6.1 Graphical displays of proportions and counts

Perhaps the most frequently encountered safety data are incidence rates of treatment groups for pre-defined adverse events, e.g., TEAEs with at least 3 reported cases or a crude incidence rate of at least 5% for each event term in each treatment group. Such data can be easily displayed in a *forest plot* in which the common TEAEs are plotted in some pre-defined order, as in Figure 4.1 that plots the crude incidence rates for treatment and control (left panel), rate differences (middle panel) and relative risks of treatment over control (right panel), for common TEAEs with at least 3 reported cases for each AE term in either group. The TEAE terms are plotted in decreasing order of the rate differences between groups, thereby showing clearly the magnitude of treatment effect on selected terms. Plotting the differences and relative risks in incidence rates in a same graphical display enables the forest plot to reveal the consistency of using these measures to quantify the treatment effects of the TEAEs.

The crude incidence rate does not take into consideration the information of time to event and patient dropouts, which may lead to imbalanced exposure of patients, especially when dropout rates differ between groups. To address this issue, one can use instead piecewise constant incidence rates that take into account the number of patients being exposed at each short time interval, as in Figure 4.2 showing for some non-recurrent adverse event of interest the number of patients at risk at the beginning of every 3-month time interval (top panel), the incidence rates of the treat-

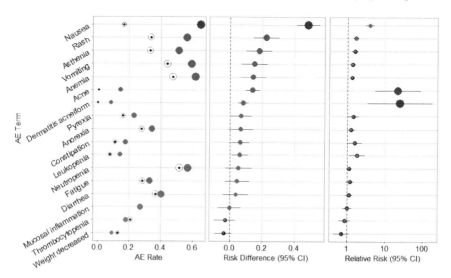

FIGURE 4.1 Crude incidence rates (left panel with • denoting treatment group and ⊙ control group, and the size of symbols representing the magnitude of incidence rate), rate differences with 95% confidence intervals (middle panel), and relative risks with 95% confidence intervals (right panel) for common treatment-emerging adverse events with crude incidence rate at least 5% in either group.

ment and control groups and their differences (middle panel), and the cumulative incidence rates (bottom panel). Note that every decline in the plot of the top panel represents patients who experience the event already in previous time interval and patients who drop out of the study for whatever reasons (e.g., intolerability to adverse event, loss to follow up, lack of efficacy), and that the incidence rate for treatment increases faster than that of control over time. The middle panel shows that the confidence interval for the rate difference (estimated using normal approximation) becomes wider at the time close to the end of the trial because of fewer number of patients . The cumulative incidence C_i at the ith time interval is estimated by

$$C_i = 1 - \prod_{j=1}^{i} \left(\frac{n_j - d_j}{n_j} \right),$$

where n_j (respectively, d_j) denotes the number of patients at risk at the beginning of (respectively, having the event in) the jth interval (Hansen et al., 2017), which is basically 1 minus the Kaplan-Meier estimate (4.43) of the survival function except that D_j is replaced by d_j and the incidence rates are assumed to be constant over the prespecified time intervals.

The bottom panel shows that the cumulative incidence rate for treatment increases faster than that for control which also increases over time.

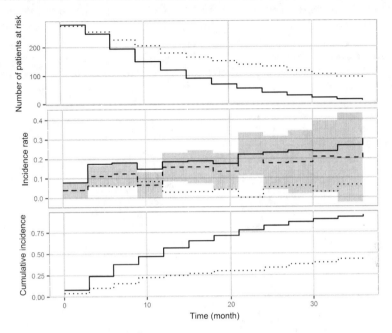

FIGURE 4.2 Numbers of patients at risk, incidence rates and rate difference between groups over time and cumulative incidence rate. Solid lines denote the treatment group and dotted lines the control group. The dashed line and the shaded area in the middle panel represent the rate difference and its 95% confidence interval, respectively.

For patients treated with multiple treatment cycles, TEAEs are recorded and categorized according to event severity in each treatment cycle as in Table 4.4, for which the TEAEs include all recurrent events. Using the data in Table 4.4, one can evaluate whether the treatment causes excessive TEAEs as compared with the control across treatment cycles by collapsing the data to generate a *four-fold plot* in Figure 4.3 for adverse event indicator (yes or no for AE) versus group (treatment "trt" or control "cntl") for each cycle. In this display for a given cycle, the frequency n_{ij} in each cell is shown by a quarter circle whose radius is proportional to $\sqrt{n_{ij}}$ so that the shaded area is proportional to the cell count, using the sample odds ratio $\hat{\phi} = n_{11}n_{22}/(n_{12}n_{21})$ for scaling the four shaded areas. An association between the two dichotomous variables, represented by group (treatment or control) and adverse event (yes or no, irrespective of the level of severity of an AE), is shown by the tendency of diagonally opposite cells in one direction to differ in size from those in the other direction.

Confidence rings are provided for the observed odds ratios to visualize the results of testing the null hypothesis that the odds ratios are equal to 1; the rings for adjacent quadrants overlap if the observed counts are consistent with the null hypothesis (Friendly, 1994a). The joint 95% confidence rings in Figure 4.3 do not overlap, indicating that the observed odds ratios differ from 1, for cycles 1, 3, and 4. The odds ratios are estimated to be $\hat{\phi}_1 = 3.32$, $\hat{\phi}_2 = 1.09$, $\hat{\phi}_3 = 2.10$, and $\hat{\phi}_4 = 2.75$ for cycles 1, 2, 3, and 4, respectively.

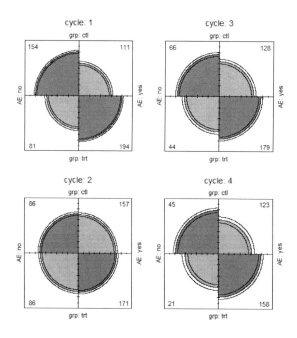

FIGURE 4.3 Four-fold plots for group ("trt" or "ctl") and adverse event ("AE:yes" versus "AE:no") by treatment cycle.

4.6.2 Mosaic plots comparing AE severity of treatments

We begin by considering an $I \times J$ table with cell counts n_{ij} and probabilities $p_{ij} = n_{ij}/n_{..}$ for the ith row (representing the treatment group) and jth column (representing the severity level of AEs), $i = 1, \ldots, I$ and $j = 0, \ldots, J - 1$, in which level 0 is tantamount to non-occurrence of AE. Denote by $n_{i.} = \sum_{j=0}^{J-1} n_{ij}$ the total frequency for the ith row, $n_{.j} = \sum_{i=1}^{I} n_{ij}$ the total frequency of the jth column and $n = \sum_{i=1}^{I} n_{i.} = \sum_{j=0}^{J-1} n_{.j}$ the grand total. Then under the null hypothesis of independence, the expected frequencies of n_{ij} can be estimated by $\hat{m}_{ij} = n_{i.}n_{.j}/n$, which leads to the Pearson residual $d_{ij} = (n_{ij} - \hat{m}_{ij})/\sqrt{\hat{m}_{ij}}$. The d_{ij} are asymptotically normal with mean 0, but their asymptotic variances are less than 1, with an average variance equal to $(I-1)(J-1)/(IJ)$. Therefore, the use of conventional standard normal quantiles may be too conservative for rejecting actual departure from the null hypothesis. One solution is to standardize the Pearson residual by

$$r_{ij} = \frac{n_{ij} - \widehat{m}_{ij}}{\sqrt{\widehat{m}_{ij}(1 - p_{i\cdot})(1 - p_{\cdot j})}},$$

where $p_{i\cdot} = n_{i\cdot}/n$ and $p_{\cdot j} = n_{\cdot j}/n$, so that r_{ij} is asymptotically standard normal under the null hypothesis of independence; see Agresti (2013, pp.80–81). The expected frequencies in the $I \times J$ table under the independence assumption can be represented graphically using a *mosaic plot* that consists of rectangles with widths proportional to the marginal row frequencies $n_{i\cdot}$ and heights proportional to the marginal column frequencies $n_{\cdot j}$; hence the area of each rectangle is proportional to the expected frequency $\widehat{m}_{ij}$; see Friendly (1994b).

For the data in Table 4.4, one can fit a logistic regression model using treatment group and treatment cycle as explanatory variables and the number of patients experiencing AE of level j as the outcome variable. A mosaic plot of the standardized Pearson residuals is given in Figure 4.4 which uses the intensity of grey color (e.g., a large absolute value is in dark color) and the line type on the edges (with solid lines indicating positive values and dashed lines indicating negative values of the tiles) for visualization of departure from the independence model. Figure 4.4 shows that a positive standardized Pearson residual (between 4 and 4.5) for severity level 4 in the treatment group at treatment cycle 3, whereas a negative standardized Pearson residual of considerably large magnitude is observed for the control group in the same treatment cycle. We can also include gender as an additional explanatory variable in the logistic regression model. A mosaic plot of the standardized Pearson residuals is given in Figure 4.5, which clearly indicates that for treatment cycle 3, male patients experience more grade 4 TEAEs in the treatment group than in the control group.

4.6.3   Graphical displays for continuous data

Figures 4.6 and 4.7 provide typical examples of graphical displays of continuous safety data for visualization of time trends and distributional differences of measurements, or changes in measurements from baseline, between treatment and control. The data used in the figures are laboratory test results of blood samples taken from patients at baseline and every post-baseline visit during a clinical trial of an investigational drug, for which the safety issue is whether there are pathophysiological adverse effects on key organs such as liver and kidney. Blood concentrations of alanine transaminase (ALT), aspartate transaminase (AST), and total

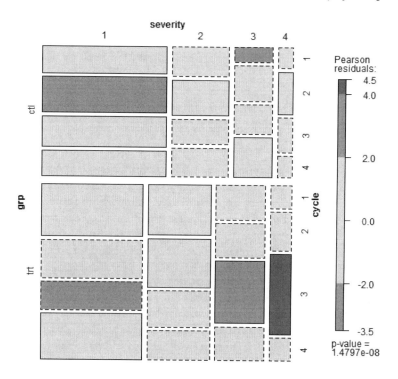

FIGURE 4.4 Mosaic plot of standardized Pearson residuals in the logistic regression model with treatment group, AE severity, and treatment cycle as explanatory variables.

bilirubin (TBL) are commonly used indicators for liver function. A higher-than-normal blood concentration for any one of the three may indicate some degree of liver damage. The top panel of Figure 4.6 gives boxplots for ALT at baseline, visit 1 and visit 2, denoted by ALT0, ALT1 and ALT2, respectively, and AST0, AST1, AST2, TBL0, TBL1, TBL2, for the control and treatment groups. Patients in the treatment group show increasing trends over time for all three laboratory parameters, but patients in the control group exhibit an increasing trend in ALT and relatively flat AST and TBL from baseline to visits 1 and 2. The bottom panel of Figure 4.6 plots the histograms and cumulative distribution functions of the ALT for the control and treatment groups at both baseline and visit 2, using reverse histograms for the control group. It shows that the ALT levels at baseline are comparable for the two groups and that the cumulative density curves are very close to each other at baseline. However, the ALT

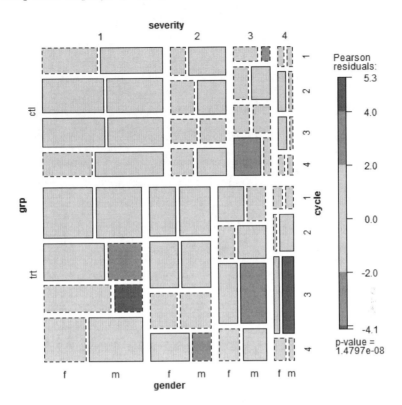

FIGURE 4.5 Mosaic plot of standardized Pearson residuals in the logistic regression model with treatment group, AE severity, treatment cycle, and gender as explanatory variables.

measurements shift to the right in both groups at visit 2, and the shift is larger in the treatment group. The top panel of Figure 4.7 plots the histograms, for the treatment and control groups, of the differences in ALT measurements between visit 2 and baseline from the same patient. A scatterplot in the bottom panel provides another way to visualize an increasing or decreasing trend of laboratory measurements between baseline and any post-treatment visit. It shows the relationship between ALT measurements at baseline and visit 2; data points above the 45 degree line indicate that ALT increases from baseline to visit 2. The plot also includes patient ID numbers at the upper right corner to indicate the ALT values above the normal range.

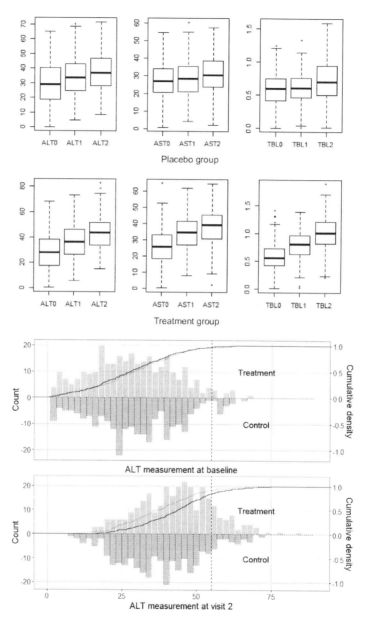

FIGURE 4.6 Top panel: Boxplots of ALT, AST and TBL at baseline and visits 1 and 2. Bottom panel: Histogram and cumulative density of ALT measurements at baseline and visit 2 for treatment (solid curve) and control (dotted curve).

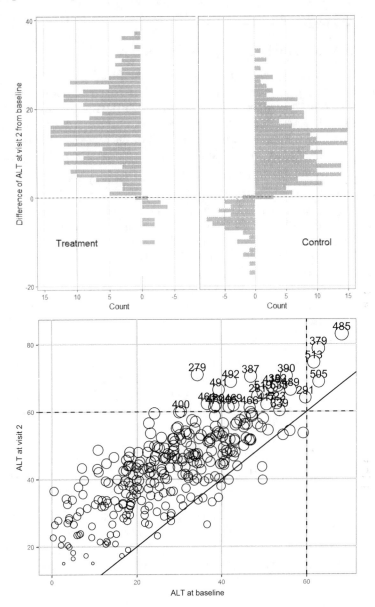

FIGURE 4.7 Top panel: Histograms of differences of ALT measurements at visit 2 from baseline for treatment group and corresponding reverse histogram for control group. Bottom panel: Scatterplot of ALT measurements at baseline and visit 2 for treatment group.

4.7   Supplements and problems

1. *The Miettinen-Nurminen method.* The seminal paper by Miettinen and Nurminen (1985) introduces a method to construct confidence intervals in the "comparative analysis" of two Bernoulli populations. Let p_1 and p_2 denote the respective success probabilities of the two populations, and n_1 and n_2 be the respective sample sizes. The paper considers three comparative metrics: rate difference RD $= p_1 - p_2$, rate ratio RR $= p_1/p_2$, and odds ratio OR $= \left(\frac{p_1}{1-p_1}\right) / \left(\frac{p_2}{1-p_2}\right)$, and points out that typical comparative analyses take the form of testing the null hypothesis of no treatment difference in some chosen comparative metric, or point and confidence interval estimation of the metric, leading to the MN method for constructing confidence intervals by inverting likelihood ratio tests. It then extends the method to "stratified pairs of proportions", assuming K strata so that the RD metric now has the form $\sum_{k=1}^{K} w_k(\hat{p}_{1k} - \hat{p}_{2k})$, with weights w_k that sum to 1. Appendix I of their paper gives closed-form expressions for the constrained MLE of p_{1k} and p_{2k} under the constraint $\sum_{k=1}^{K} w_k(p_{1k} - p_{2k}) = 0$. Corresponding results for the RR and OR metrics are also given.

2. *Regression models for recurrent events.* Kuramoto et al. (2008) describe several regression models which focus on different aspects of safety concerns with recurrent events. Let $x_i = 1$ or 0 be the indicator function representing treatment or control group, and λ_0 be the baseline hazard rate. The Poisson regression model $\lambda_i = \lambda_0 \exp(\beta x_i)$ assumes that λ_i is a constant over time and does not depend on either event history or time t. Let $Y_i(t) = 1$ if subject i is at risk over the interval $[t, t + \Delta]$ and 0 otherwise (e.g., censored). Allowing time-varying hazard rates, the basic Poisson model can be generalized to

$$\lambda_i(t) = Y_i(t)\lambda_0(t) \exp(\beta x_i) \tag{4.45}$$

for subject i, where $\lambda_0(t)$ is the baseline hazard rate (e.g., the hazard rate for control group). Another generalization is the gamma-frailty model

$$\lambda_i(t) = Y_i(t)\mu_i \exp(\beta_0 + \beta_1 x_i) \tag{4.46}$$

for subject i, in which μ_i has a gamma distribution that is used to model unobserved frailties of the patients. Details can be found in the references cited after (4.44).

Generalized extreme value regression models. Wang and Dey (2010) propose to use the generalized extreme value (GEV) distribution with cumulative distribution function of the form

$$G(x) = \exp\left\{-\left[1 + \tau\frac{(x-\mu)}{\sigma}\right]_+^{-1/\tau}\right\} \tag{4.47}$$

where $y_+ = \max(y,0)$, μ is the location parameter, $\sigma > 0$ is the scale parameter, and τ is the shape parameter that controls the tail behavior of the distribution. The GEV distribution (4.47) becomes the Gumbel distribution with $G(x) = \exp\{-\exp[(x-\mu)/\sigma]\}$ when $\tau \to 0$, and corresponds to the Weibull distribution when $\tau < 0$ and to the Frechet distribution when $\tau > 0$ (Kotz and Nadarajah, 2000). For a binary response variable Y and a set of explanatory variables x, let $\pi(\mathbf{x}) = P\{Y = 1|\mathbf{X} = \mathbf{x}\}$. Wang and Dey (2010) propose to use (4.47) as a functional form for $\pi(\mathbf{x})$, i.e., $\pi(\mathbf{x}) = G\left(\boldsymbol{\beta}^T\mathbf{x}\right)$. In particular, choosing G to be the Gumbel distribution with $\sigma = 1$ and $\mu = -\alpha$ yields

$$\log[-\log(\pi(\mathbf{x}))] = \alpha + \boldsymbol{\beta}^T\mathbf{x}_i, \tag{4.48}$$

which is the log-log link proposed by Agresti (2013, pp. 255-257) who notes that logistic or probit regression uses a link function that is symmetric about $\pi(\mathbf{x}) = 1/2$ and is inappropriate for considering the right tail of Y whose mean is near 0. Since the response variable belongs to the exponential family, maximum likelihood can be used to estimate the regression and GEV parameters; see Kotz and Nadarajah (2000), Wang and Dey (2010), and Calabrese et al. (2011). Embrechts et al. (1997) have shown the close connection between the GEV and generalized Pareto distributions in the last paragraph of Section 4.4.5.

3. *Exercise.* Consider a clinical trial with a high dose (H), a low dose (L), and one control group. The data on the number of AEs of special interest (cardiac disorders) and the patient exposure time are summarized by age groups in Table 4.9.

   (a) Fit a Poisson regression model.
   (b) Estimate the expected event incidence rate for each cell.
   (c) Estimate the relative risks of the two treatment groups (H and L) over the control group after accounting for age.
   (d) Draw conclusions on treatment effect and age effect on the incidence of cardiac disorders.

4. *Exercise.* Fit the zero-inflated Poisson regression model (4.38) and the generalized extreme value regression model (4.47) to the data in Table 4.9. Interpret the results from both models and explain their differences from those obtained in Problem 3.

TABLE 4.9 The number of reported cases of cardiac disorders and exposure time (person-month) by treatment group and age stratum.

age	Treatment (H)			Treatment (L)			Control		
	no. cases (n_{ij})	exp. time (T_{ij})	crude rate $(\lambda_{ij}, \%)$	no. cases (n_{ij})	exp. time (T_{ij})	crude rate $(\lambda_{ij}, \%)$	no. cases (n_{ij})	exp. time (T_{ij})	crude rate $(\lambda_{ij}, \%)$
20–29	1	1568	0.06	0	1940	0	1	2306	0.04
30–39	2	943	0.21	1	1377	0.07	0	1788	0
40–49	8	742	1.08	2	963	0.21	1	1556	0.06
50–59	5	332	1.51	9	462	1.95	2	970	0.21

TABLE 4.10 Angioedema cases and exposure time by duration after new prescription among patients initiating ACE or other antihypertensive (OAH) medications for US veterans between April 1999 and December 2000.

Time duration	ACE ($N = 195,192$)			OAH ($N = 399,889$)		
	Person-years	Cases	Incidence (per 1000)	Person-years	Cases	Incidence (per 1000)
Before use	89,547	42	0.47	297,194	180	0.61
< 31 days	16,266	120	7.38	33,324	33	0.99
$31 - 60$ days	15,367	43	2.80	30,162	16	0.53
$61 - 90$ days	14,877	29	1.95	28,913	12	0.42
$90 - 180$ days	37,955	60	1.58	73,920	27	0.37
$181 - 270$ days	32,398	40	1.23	63,084	24	0.38
$271 - 360$ days	26,760	27	1.01	52,588	22	0.42
≥ 361 days	35,465	33	0.93	67,901	45	0.66
After discont.	46,892	40	0.85	91,164	51	0.56

5. *Exercise.* Miller et al. (2008) studied the incidence of angioedema among US veterans who initiated antihypertensive medications including angiotensin-converting enzyme (ACE) inhibitors that were known to be potentially associated with angioedema, a subcutaneous non-spitting edema typically of sudden onset and short duration. The reported angioedema cases and exposure time in person-years for ACE and OAH (other antihypertensive medications) groups by treatment duration are given in Table 4.10, which shows a decreasing trend in exposure-adjusted incidence rates of angioedema over treatment duration for ACE patients. In addition to crude and exposure-adjusted incidence rates, the authors also used multiple Poisson regression models to estimate the adjusted relative risk of angioedema for ACE use, relative to the use of OAH. After adjusting for calendar year, age, sex, race, and diagnoses of congestive heart failure, coronary artery disease, and diabetes in the Poisson regression model, Miller et al.

(2008) concluded that the relative risk for new ACE patients to new OAH users was 3.56 (95% confidence interval 2.82 - 4.44). Fit a negative binomial regression model, and draw a conclusion on whether ACE is associated with excessive cases of angioedema relative to OAH, after adjusting for treatment duration.

5

Multiplicity in the Evaluation of Clinical Safety Data

The collection of safety and tolerability data in all clinical trials goes well beyond the data collected to address specific safety hypotheses, which may be developed from the chemical or biological properties of the product, or possibly from observations from early-phase nonclinical and clinical trials. Adding to the complexity, the set of possible adverse effects is very large and new unanticipated effects are always possible. Moreover, confirmatory clinical trials to test the efficacy hypotheses usually have large sample sizes, and this may result in many more adverse event types, most of which were not expected based on the pharmacological profile of the product, preclinical experiments in animals, or in vitro studies. Hence there is potential for drawing false positive conclusions and the need for understanding the multiplicity aspects in safety signal detection. Safety assessment continues into the post-marketing phase initially with clinical trials designed specifically to address possible safety issues, and later with pharmacovigilance based on large databases of patient electronic health records and systems that collect spontaneous reports of adverse events. While the multiplicity considerations differ during different phases of drug development, they are always an important component in the analysis and interpretation of clinical safety data. In their discussion of safety analysis in the pre-marketing phases, Chuang-Stein and Xia (2013) identify multiplicity as a key issue that needs to be included in the planning. In this chapter we consider multiplicity in the planning and interpretation of safety assessment throughout the drug and vaccine development process. We describe both frequentist error-controlling methods and Bayes (in particular, empirical Bayes) methods that have been developed to address multiplicity in the evaluation of clinical safety data. In Chapter 7 we continue the discussion of multiplicity in the data mining post-marketing environment for safety signal detection and pharmacovigilance, which have been noted by Gould (2007) and others.

5.1   An illustrative example

This example considers adverse event data from a safety and immuno-genicity trial of a measles, mumps, rubella, varicella (MMRV) combination vaccine trial; see Mehrotra and Heyse (2004a). The study population includes healthy toddlers, $12 - 18$ months of age. The comparison of interest is between Group 1: MMRV + PedvaxHIB® on Day 0 and Group 2: MMR + PedvaxHIB® on Day 0, followed by an optional varicella vaccination on Day 42. The safety follow-up includes local and systemic reactions over Days 0-42 for N = 148 subjects in Group 1, and N = 132 subjects in Group 2 over Days 42-84. The follow-up duration of 42 days is standard for live virus vaccines such as varicella. The question of interest, which involves the varicella component of MMRV, is whether the safety profile differs between its administration in a combination and giving it 6 weeks later as a monovalent vaccine. Section 5.1.1 gives some general background about these data and Section 5.1.2 describes the multiplicity issues that arise in the analysis of the data to address this question.

5.1.1   A three-tier adverse event categorization system

The Safety Planning, Evaluation, and Reporting Team (SPERT) (Crowe et al., 2009) describes a 3-tier system for the analysis of adverse events. Originally proposed by Gould (2002), the 3-tier safety reporting system was implemented in two large biopharmaceutical companies that instituted a standard formal process for evaluating clinical safety data; see Chuang-Stein and Xia (2013). Dealing with multiplicity when evaluating adverse event associations starts with the planning of the clinical trials program through the use of a program safety analysis plan (PSAP), applying a system for categorizing adverse events according to three tiers. Such categorization allows the statistical analysis to potentially use different approaches as deemed appropriate for each tier or set of adverse events to reduce false positive safety findings.

- *Tier 1* is associated with specific hypotheses that are defined by the clinical team as an adverse event of special interest.

- *Tier 2* is the large set of adverse events encountered as part of the systematic collection and reporting of safety data. The MMRV data summarized above is an example of Tier 2 adverse events.

- *Tier 3* includes the rare spontaneous reports of serious events that require further clinical and epidemiological evaluation.

An adverse event can belong to both Tier 1 and Tier 3, as illustrated below. In 1998, a tetravalent rhesus-human reassortant rotavirus vaccine (RRV-TV; RotaShield®, Wyeth Laboratories) was licensed and recommended by the Advisory Committee for Immunization Practices (ACIP) for routine immunization of infants in the United States. A slight increase in intussusception, the telescoping or prolapse of one portion of the bowel into an immediately adjacent segment, was observed in the prelicensure studies, but did not raise the safety concern. However, post-marketing surveillance studies (Murphy et al., 2001) showed a temporal association between RRV-TV and intestinal intussusception. Intussusception is an uncommon illness with a background incidence of 18 to 56 cases per 100,000 infant years during the first year of life in the US. No definitive association between RRV-TV and intussusception was observed in clinical studies conducted prelicensure. As a result of this finding in post-marketing surveillance studies, the RRV-TV vaccine was voluntarily withdrawn from the market in October, 1999, and two weeks later the ACIP rescinded its recommendation for universal vaccination. At the time the intussusception issues arose around the RRV-TV, clinical development of RotaTeq®, a pentavalent human-bovine reassortant rotavirus vaccine (PRV) developed by Merck & Co., Inc., Kenilworth, NJ, USA, was in Phase II trials. The PRV clinical development program was immediately expanded to include the Rotavirus Efficacy and Safety Trial (REST), which was undertaken to specifically address the safety question on the association between vaccination with the candidate PRV and intussusception. REST was a placebo-controlled study including approximately 70,000 subjects, making it one of the largest clinical trials ever conducted prelicensure. The details of the study are given by Vesikari et al. (2006), and the statistical methods and results have been described in Section 4.2.1 and 4.2.2. The clinical importance of REST is discussed in a recent paper by Rosenblatt (2017) that highlights the importance and complexity of safety evaluation in clinical development programs for novel drugs and vaccines. Intussusception, therefore, is an example of an adverse event that was considered Tier 3 because it is serious but uncommon in its natural history. Too few cases of intussusception were observed in the original prelicensure trials of the RRV-TV vaccine to reach a conclusion that could alter the benefit-risk trade-off of an important new vaccine. The association with rotavirus vaccines was established subsequently in post-marketing studies that led to the treatment of intussusception as a Tier 1 adverse event for the subsequent vaccine PRV, for which studies were designed specifically to address the issue prospectively in hypothesis-driven clinical trials.

The focus of research on multiplicity issues in the analysis of clinical safety data is related to Tier 2 adverse events, for which the clinical trial data for these are typically summarized by using risk differences, risk ratios or odds ratios, and the statistical analysis includes confidence intervals and/or p-values. The methods used for the analysis need to be specified in advance in the statistical analysis plan. To achieve a good balance between false positive and false negative findings, SPERT (Crowe et al., 2009) recommends using the Double False Discovery Rate procedure and a Bayesian hierarchical mixture model that will be described in Sections 5.3 and 5.4. To illustrate the complexities in evaluating Tier 2 adverse events, we consider safety and immunogenicity trial by Kaplan et al. (2002) to compare a combination vaccine, labeled A, to one of its individual component vaccines, labeled B, in an infant population. The analysis of the adverse event data identifies UHPC (Unusual High Pitched Crying) as the single event with an individual P-value < 0.05; the incidence of UHPC for group A was 6.7% compared to 2.3% for group B, yielding a two-sided P-value of 0.016 unadjusted for multiplicity. However, UHPC was just one of 92 adverse experience types in the study, and there was no medical rationale for this finding, nor were there additional data suggesting such a relationship from the already approved and marketed components of the combination vaccine. To address the multiplicity issue, the study team undertook a confirmatory study requested by regulators. The large follow-up trial concluded that the original result was a false positive signal, hence a significant amount of time and money was expended on chasing down what easily could have been identified as a false positive signal by using appropriate multiplicity adjustments for Tier 2 adverse events in the original analysis.

5.1.2   The MMRV combination vaccine trial

We now return to adverse event data from the safety and immunogenicity trial of the MMRV combination vaccine. There are 40 Tier 2 adverse event types that were categorized by using a standard dictionary into 8 body systems; see Mehrotra and Heyse (2004a) whose data summary consists of counts of infants with the specific adverse event type, the between-group difference in percent, and a 2-sided P-value computed using Fisher's exact test. Two graphical representations have been used to visualize the data. Figure 5.1 is a "volcano plot" (Supplement 1 in Section 5.5) that plots -log(P) versus the difference (in %) of infants who experienced the adverse event. The plot shows that 4 adverse event types gave unadjusted P-values less than 0.05. A Q-Q (Quantile-Quantile) plot of the 40 ordered P-values versus the quantiles of the Uniform$(0, 1)$ distribution is given in Figure 5.2 that shows that generally the unadjusted P-values track along the diagonal line, indicative of P-values generated under the null hypothesis. There are 4 adverse event types with unadjusted P-values ≤ 0.05, and 7 event types with common P-value of 1. This is indicative of P-values computed from discrete binary data with low incidence rate. The 4 adverse event types with 2-sided p-values ≤ 0.025 are flagged in 3 different body systems and are listed in Table 5.1. These data will be used in the subsequent sections to describe and illustrate the

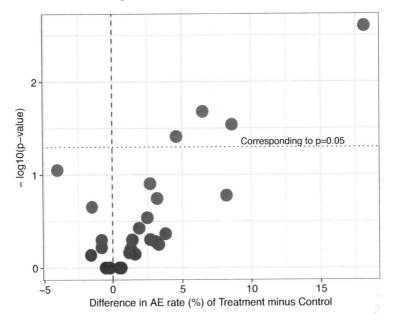

FIGURE 5.1 Volcano plot of $-\log(p)$ versus difference (%) in incidence rates between treatment and control for MMRV adverse event data.

multiplicity issues encountered in evaluating adverse event data that are routinely collected in randomized controlled trials.

TABLE 5.1 Adverse event types and counts with unadjusted two-sided p-value ≤ 0.05.

Body System	Adverse Event	Group 1 $N_1 = 148$	Group 2 $N_2 = 132$	Difference Group	2-sided p-value
08	Irritability	75	43	18.1%	0.0025
10	Rash	13	3	6.5%	0.0209
03	Diarrhea	24	10	8.6%	0.0289
10	Rash, Measles/ Rubella-Like	8	1	4.6%	0.0388

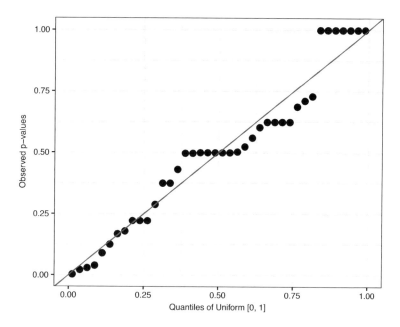

FIGURE 5.2 Q-Q plot of ordered p-values (vertical axis) against uniform quantiles (horizontal axis).

5.2   Multiplicity issues in efficacy and safety evaluations

Almost all clinical trials are designed with the objective of evaluating the efficacy of a pharmaceutical, biological, or vaccine product. Evaluating safety is also recognized as a primary objective but the study design, endpoint selection, and sample size determination are usually based on the primary efficacy hypothesis. For safety, unless at least one Tier 1 adverse event has been identified before the trial, there is no specific safety hypothesis to test for the clinical trial design. The study plan still collects, and analyzes adverse experiences reported by the study participants, and data should be carefully catalogued and summarized using standard coding dictionaries such as MedDRA. Crowe et al. (2009) have pointed out the potential for too many false positive safety signals if the multiplicity problem is ignored, and Kaplan et al. (2002) has given an example of how false positive signals can impact the interpretation of the safety profile of the drug or vaccine.

The ICH E-9 Guideline (ICH, 1998) discusses this issue and recommends descriptive statistical methods supplemented by individual confidence intervals. It points out that if hypothesis tests are used, statistical adjustments of the type I error for multiplicity may not be appropriate because the type II error is usually of greater concern, and individual P-values may be useful as a flagging device applied to a large number of safety variables to highlight differences worthy of further attention. Hence, the challenge lies in a proper balance between no adjustment and too much adjustment for multiplicity. This balance has led to a preference for methods that control the *false discovery rate* (FDR) over those that control the familywise error rate (FWER) which is important for efficacy claims. Since Mehrotra and Heyse (2004a) who were among the first to propose the use of FDR control for clinical adverse event data, application of multiplicity adjustment procedures has grown steadily in the evaluation of clinical safety data. The next paragraph gives the definitions and background of FWER and FDR.

Let $\{H_i, i = 1, \cdots, m\}$ denote a family of null hypotheses. In the current setting of adverse event types in a clinical trial, true null hypotheses are those associated with adverse event types for which the incidence is the same between the treatment and control groups. The familywise error rate (FWER) is defined as the probability that some true null hypothesis is rejected. Noting that FWER control may be too conservative for many applications, Benjamini and Hochberg (1995) propose to control instead the false discovery rate FDR $= E(V/R)$, which is the expected proportion of rejected hypotheses that are incorrectly rejected and in which R is the number of rejected null hypotheses and V is the number of incorrectly rejected H_i. When no hypothesis is rejected (i.e., $R = 0$), the FDR is defined to be 0. Soric (1989) has called rejected hypotheses "statistical discoveries." The random variable V/R is called "false discovery proportion" by Genovese and Wasserman (2004, 2006). Since V is the number of false positives, FWER control provides assurance that $P(V \geq 1)$ does not exceed a prescribed rate α. FDR controls the expected proportion of discoveries that are actually false. Note that FWER $= P(V \geq 1) \leq E(V/R) =$ FDR. A modification of FDR is the *positive false discovery rate* pFDR $= E(V/R|R > 0)$ proposed by Storey (2002, 2003) who shows that pFDR can be written as a Bayesian posterior probability when the test statistics come from a random mixture of the null and alternative distributions. The application of FDR control procedures has increased dramatically in recent years due to the prevalence of large-scale inference problems in genomics research.

5.3   P-values, FDR, and some variants

Associated with the m hypotheses in $H_1, H_2, \cdots, H_m$ are corresponding unadjusted P-values $P_1, P_2, \cdots, P_m$; the P-value (or attained signif-

icance level) of a test is the smallest significance level at which the
test rejects the null hypothesis. If the test of the null hypothesis H
is based on a test statistic $T = T(\mathbf{X}_1, \ldots, \mathbf{X}_n)$, then the P-value is
$P_H\{T(\mathbf{X}_1^*, \ldots, \mathbf{X}_n^*) \geq T \mid T\}$, in which $(\mathbf{X}_1^*, \ldots, \mathbf{X}_n^*)$ is a sample generated
under H independently of the sample $(\mathbf{X}_1, \ldots, \mathbf{X}_n)$. Let $P_{(1)} \leq P_{(2)} \leq \cdots \leq P_{(m)}$ be the ordered P-values with $H_{(i)}$ corresponding to the hypothesis aligned with $P_{(i)}$. Benjamini and Hochberg (1995) control the
FDR at a prespecified rate α by the step-down procedure that rejects
$H_{(1)}, H_{(2)}, \cdots, H_{(J)}$, where $J = \max\{i : P_{(i)} \leq \alpha i/m\}$, assuming the P_i to
be independent. When the above set is empty, no hypotheses are rejected;
on the other hand, all hypotheses are rejected if $J = m$. Supplement 2 of
Section 5.5 shows that a similar step-down procedure with $\alpha i/m$ replaced
by $\alpha/(m + i - 1)$ can control FWER. For $i = 1$ and $i = m$, i/m is equal to
$1/(m + i - 1)$, otherwise i/m is larger and therefore the FDR control procedure has greater power than the FWER control procedure in detecting
the true positives. It is convenient to implement the procedure using the
adjusted P-values

$$P_{[m]} = P_{(m)}, P_{[j]} = \min\{P_{[j+1]}, (\frac{m}{j})P_{(j)}\} \text{ for } j \leq m - 1, \qquad (5.1)$$

rejecting $H_{[j]}$ if $P_{[j]} \leq \alpha$. Table 5.2 lists these adjusted P-values next to
the unadjusted ones for the adverse events associated with body system
10 (skin) in Table 5.1.

5.3.1 Double false discovery rate and its control

Mehrotra and Heyse (2004a) propose a two-step procedure labeled DFDR
(double false discovery rate) by Tukey, for "flagging Tier 2 adverse ex-
perience" that are grouped by body systems. The first stage uses $P_b^* = \min(P_{b,1}, \ldots, P_{b,m_b})$ as the "flagging" P-values of the bth body system, with
m_b adverse event types, for $b = 1, \ldots, B$. These P-values are used to test
the intersection null hypothesis $H^{(b)}$ that treatment and control have no
differences in the m_b adverse event types. They are adjusted for multiplicity (for $1 \leq b \leq B$) using the Benjamini-Hochberg procedure leading
to the adjusted P-values $\tilde{P}_b^*$ and the group-level rejection criterion for the
first step:
    Step 1. Reject $H^{(b)}$ if $\tilde{P}_b^* \leq \alpha_1$, for $b = 1, \ldots, M$.
The second step of DFDR applies the Benjamini-Hochberg procedure to
the reduced set of null hypothesis $\mathcal{H} = \{H_i^{(b)} : H^{(b)} \text{ is rejected and } 1 < i \leq m_b\}$, leading to adjusted P-value $\tilde{P}_i^{(b)}$ and the final rejection criterion for
individual adverse events within the body systems whose hypotheses are
rejected in the first step:
    Step 2. Reject $H_i^{(b)} \in \mathcal{H}$ if $\tilde{P}_i^{(b)} \leq \alpha_2$.
Mehrotra and Heyse (2004a) propose to choose α_1 and α_2 by bootstrap
resampling so that $E_{H_0}(V/R) \leq \alpha$, where H_0 denotes the intersection

null hypothesis $\cap_{b=1}^{B} H^{(b)}$. Instead of a two-dimensional search, they fix $\alpha_1 = \alpha_2$ or $\alpha_1 = \alpha_2/2$ and carry out a grid search over $\alpha_2 \leq \alpha$.

TABLE 5.2 Unadjusted 2-sided P-values and adjusted P-values for the skin-related AEs.

Adverse Event	Group 1 N_1 = 148	Group 2 N_2 = 132	2-sided P-value	Adjusted P-value
Rash	13	3	0.0209	0.1745
Rash, Measles/ Rubella-Like	8	1	0.0388	0.1745
Bite/Sting	4	0	0.1248	0.3743
Urticarial	0	2	0.2214	0.4980
Rash, Diaper	6	2	0.2885	0.5193
Eczema	2	0	0.4998	0.7498
Viral, Exanthema	1	2	0.6033	0.7731
Rash, Varicella	4	2	0.6872	0.7731
Pruritus	2	1	1.0000	1.0000

TABLE 5.3 Smallest B&H adjusted p-values from each of the 8 body systems.

BS	# AEs	Representative AE Description	Group 1 N_1 = 148	Group 2 N_2=132	Unadjusted p-value	Adjusted p-value
01	5	Asthenia/Fatigue	57	40	0.1673	0.6248
03	7	Diarrhea	24	10	0.0289	0.2026
05	1	Lymphadenopathy	3	2	1.0000	1.0000
06	1	Dehydration	0	2	0.2214	0.2214
08	3	Irritability	75	43	0.0025	0.0075*
09	11	Bronchitis	4	1	0.3746	0.9447
10	9	Rash	13	3	0.0209	0.1745
11	3	Conjunctivitis	0	2	0.2214	0.6641

Noting that including the bootstrap in each candidate α_2 in the search layer of the procedure may seem too cumbersome to some users, Mehrotra and Heyse (2004a) consider setting $\alpha_2 = \alpha$ without resampling, which amounts to the modified second step:

Step 2'. Reject $H_i^{(b)} \in \mathcal{H}$ if $\tilde{P}_i^{(b)} \leq \alpha$.

Mehrotra and Adewale (2012) report two simulation studies on this modified DFDR procedure (defined by Step 2'), one of which shows the FDR of this procedure (with $\alpha_1 = \alpha/2$) has FDR values exceeding the nominal value α. They consider another choice $\alpha_1 = \alpha$ that shows all FDR values below α, and point out "potential theoretical issues" with the bootstrap resampling procedure in Mehrotra and Heyse (2004a). Table 5.3 and 5.4 illustrate how this two-step procedure works for the Tier 2 adverse event types in the MMRV combination safety vaccine trial of Section 5.1.2, using $\alpha_1 = \alpha_2 = \alpha = 0.1$. Note that body system 08 has only three adverse event types, and Step 2 of this procedure identifies Irritability as the only significant adverse event. Supplement 2 in Section 5.5 provides further discussion of these results and their theoretical issues, together with recent work by Lai et al. (2018a) on an alternative new approach to the "divide-and-conquer" idea underlying DFDR for multiple testing.

TABLE 5.4 Final flagging - clinical adverse event counts for body system 08.

Adverse Event	Group 1 N1 = 148	Group 2 N2 = 132	Percent Difference	Unadjusted p-value	Adjusted p-value
Irritability	75	43	18.1	0.0025	0.0075*
Crying	2	0	1.4	0.4998	0.7497
Insomnia	2	2	-0.2	1.0000	1.0000

5.3.2   FDR control for discrete data

The Q-Q plot of the MMRV data in Figure 5.2 shows a distinctive pattern of a discrete distribution for the reported P-values. Heyse (2011) proposes a modification of the Benjamini-Hochberg (B&H hereafter) procedure to enhance its power for discrete data. Suppose m_0 of the m null hypotheses $H_1, ..., H_m$ are true. He notes that for continuous P-values, which are uniformly distributed under the null hypotheses, $P\{P_{(j)} \leq \alpha j/m\} = \alpha j/m$ for $j = 1, ..., m_0$. For discrete P-values, the probability $P\{P_{(j)} \leq \alpha j/m\}$ becomes $P\{P_{(j)} < \alpha j/m\}$ when $\alpha j/m$ is not one of the values achievable by $P_{(j)}$. Accordingly, Heyse (2011) defines $Q_i(p)$ to be the largest achievable P-value $\leq p$ for hypothesis $i = 1, \ldots, m$, setting $Q_i(p) = 0$ if no such P-value exists. The adjusted P-values for the discrete case replace (5.1) by

$$P_{<m>} = P_{(m)}, P_{<j>} = \min\left\{P_{[j+1]}, \sum_{i=1}^{m} Q_{(i)}(P_{(j)})/j\right\}, \text{ for } j \leq m-1. \quad (5.2)$$

In particular, the last column of Table 5.3, with (5.2) in place of (5.1), becomes

$$0.5865, 0.0801^*, 1.0000, 0.2214, 0.0025^*, 0.8485, 0.0534^*, 0.5122,$$

giving smaller (or equal) adjusted P-values than the corresponding last column of Table 5.2. Note that two more body systems become significant (with adjusted P-value < 0.10) when adjustments for discrete P-values are made. There are 19 (instead of 3 in Table 5.4) adverse event types resulting from this increase in significant body systems. As a consequence, for body system 08, the discrete adjusted P-value for the averse event "Irritability" rises from 0.0075 to 0.0119 despite $Q_i(P_{(j)}) \leq P_{(j)}$ in (5.2). Heyse (2011) attributes the discrete adjustment idea to Tarone (1990) and Gilbert (2005).

5.4 Bayesian methods for safety evaluation

5.4.1 Berry and Berry's hierarchical mixture model

Berry and Berry (2004) (abbreviated by B&B hereafter) propose a Bayesian approach to the analysis of Tier 2 adverse event data in Mehrotra and Heyse (2004a). They discuss the underlying motivation:

> The question is which if any AEs should be flagged as probably due to the drug. The multiplicity of AEs makes this problem difficult, and this is so regardless of one's statistical philosophy (frequentists and Bayesians alike). Random variability means that the rates of some AEs will be markedly higher in the drug group than in the placebo group, even if the drug is harmless... ignoring multiplicity gives a much higher than planned overall size of type I error. On the other hand, adjusting for multiplicities using a standard technique such as Bonferroni may fail to flag important differences... In assessing safety, type II errors are at least as important as type I errors... There are at least four considerations in deciding which types of AEs that are significantly higher on drug than on control, with $p < 0.05$, should be flagged. The first two (i.e., the actual significance level and the total number of types of AEs being considered) are standard considerations in the frequentist approach to multiple comparisons. The second two (i.e., the rates for those AEs not considered for flagging and the biological relationships among the various AEs) are not, but they are relevant in the Bayesian approach... We take a Bayesian approach and so we consider all four of the above considerations.

For the biological relationship consideration, B&B assign AEs "based on biological or regulatory grounds and not on empirical observation," which is similar to Mehrotra and Heyse (2004a) in their double FDR approach to adjust the frequentist P-values. They model AEs in the same body system as exchangeable random variables in the Bayesian approach that uses the posterior probabilities to determine which AEs should be flagged. The model incorporates information from all observed adverse event types within and across body systems in a way that is consistent with the biological rationale of adverse event generation. It handles multiplicity by borrowing information across adverse event types, which reduces the influence of extreme observations. The probability of no treatment effect is derived by using a mixture component of the model on log odds ratio

$$\theta_{bi} = \log\left(\frac{p_{bi}}{1 - p_{bi}} \cdot \frac{1 - p'_{bi}}{p'_{bi}}\right) = \text{logit}(p_{bi}) - \text{logit}(p'_{bi}), b = 1, ..., B, i = 1, ..., m_b,$$

(5.3)

where p_{bi} (respectively, p'_{bi}) is the probability of AE of type i in body system b for the treatment (respectively, control) and $\text{logit}(p) = \log(p/(1-p))$. The Bayesian model assumes independent prior distributions

$$\theta_{bi} \sim \pi_b I_{\{0\}} + (1 - \pi_b) N(\mu_b, \sigma_b^2).$$

(5.4)

Thus, θ_{bi} is degenerate at 0 with probability π_b and is normally distributed with probability $1 - \pi_b$. The use of this mixture model, with an atom at 0 representing no difference between treatment and control that corresponds to the null hypothesis $H_i^{(b)}$ in the Mehrotra and Heyse (2004a) (MH) double FDR approach, is the basis specification in B&B's Bayesian counterpart of the MH frequentist testing model. For prespecified values of the hyperparameters π_b, μ_b, and σ_b^2, the posterior distribution of θ_{bi} can be computed by Markov chain Monte Carlo (MCMC). B&B call this procedure "Solo Bayesian", which considers the individual type of AEs "in isolation" and can vary markedly with different choices of the hyperparameters. They propose to specify the hyperparameters as random variables that have their own prior distributions, culminating in a 3-level hierarchical Bayesian model.

The first level is the mixture model (5.4) for the log odds ratio θ_{bi}, but with independent prior distributions for the hyperparameters given by

$$\pi_b \sim \text{Beta}(\alpha, \beta), \mu_b \sim N(\mu, \nu), \sigma_b^2 \sim \text{IG}(\gamma_0, \lambda_0),$$

(5.5)

which constitute the second level of the hierarchical model. The hyperparameters α, β, μ, and ν are random variables that have prior distributions, but the shape parameter γ_0 and scale parameter λ_0 of the inverse gamma (IG) distribution are assumed to be prespecified hyperparameters. The third level of hierarchical model specifies the prior distribution of α, β, μ, ν:

$$\mu \sim N(\mu_0, \nu_0), \nu \sim \text{IG}(\gamma_0', \lambda_0'), \alpha \sim \text{TrunExp}(\lambda_1), \beta \sim \text{TrunExp}(\lambda_1'),$$

(5.6)

in which $\mu_0, \nu_0, \gamma_0', \lambda_0', \lambda_1$, and λ_1' are prespecified hyperparameters, and TrunExp denotes the truncated exponential distribution with density function $f_\lambda(t) = \lambda e^{-\lambda t} I_{\{t \geq 1\}} / e^{-\lambda}$. B&B explain why they choose 1 as the truncation threshold for α and β, noting that the Beta(α, β) density function (5.5) is infinite at 0 if $\alpha < 1$, and at 1 if $\beta < 1$. They also point out that choosing $\lambda_1 = \lambda'_1$ implies that θ_{bi} has prior probability 1/2 of being equal to 0. Supplement 4 in Section 5.5 gives further details and background about MCMC computations of posterior quantities that are reported by B&B. In particular, they contrast the unadjusted 2-sided P-values in Table 5.1 with the corresponding posterior probability $P(\theta_{bi} > 0|\text{Data})$:

$$0.780, 0.190, 0.231, 0.126$$

for Irritability, Rash, Diarrhea and Rash (Measles/Rubella-Like), respectively, using the 3-level hierarchical mixture model. Table 5.5 gives a complete comparison over all observed adverse events and the associated body systems.

Xia et al. (2011) have provided a comparison of the operating characteristics of the unadjusted Benjamini and Hochberg FDR (B&H FDR), the Double FDR (DFDR), and the three-stage hierarchical model (B&B). Additionally, they have also provided an extension of the B&B hierarchical model of the evaluating adverse event rates using a Poisson distribution. Their results show that the B&H FDR has the lowest false discovery rate but also lowest power. The DFDR procedure has satisfactory power except for uncommon event rates, for which it has lower power compared to the hierarchical model. They recommend the DFDR procedure from a practical perspective because it is relatively easy to implement and addresses the multiplicity well.

5.4.2 Gould's Bayesian screening model

Gould (2008) emphasizes that the problem of clinical safety analysis is not one of testing hypotheses and introduces a Bayesian screening model for (a) identifying the drug-adverse event associations that should be evaluated further; and (b) quantifying the strength of the evidence for an association. The first goal is addressed by using a Bayesian screening technique, and the second by using a posterior distribution of the some measure of association (e.g., odds ratio) given the available data. The question of interest is not whether the incidence of an adverse event for the treatment is increased relative to the control, but rather whether there is evidence of a sufficiently large increase to justify more definitive evaluations, based on observed clinical safety data from different adverse event types. Gould (2018) introduces a unified Bayesian screening approach to evaluating potential elevated adverse event risk in clinical trials and large observational databases, which provides "a direct assessment of the likelihood of no material drug-event association" and quantifies "the strength of the observed association" with self-adjustment for multiplicity. For the ith adverse event type ($i = 1, \ldots, m$), counts x_i (respectively, y_i) are observed among n_C control (respectively, n_T treatment) patients. The model assumes that $x_i \sim \text{Bin}(n_c, p'_i)$ and $y_i \sim \text{Bin}(n_T, p_i)$

TABLE 5.5 Fisher's 2-sided P-values (with asterisks if $p < 0.1$) and posterior probabilities (boldfaced next to P-value with asterisks) under the 3-level hierarchical Bayesian model.

b	i	Type of AE	2-sided P-value	Posterior probability $\theta_{bi} > 0$	$\theta_{bi} = 0$
1	1	Astenia/fatigue	0.167	0.211	0.762
1	2	Fever	0.561	0.122	0.827
1	3	Infection, fungal	0.500	0.101	0.796
1	4	Infection, viral	0.625	0.100	0.813
1	5	Malaise	0.525	0.116	0.826
3	1	Anorexia	0.179	0.117	0.821
3	2	Cendisiasis, oral	0.500	0.083	0.835
3	3	Constipation	0.500	0.101	0.812
3	4	**Diarrhea**	0.029*	**0.231**	0.743
3	5	Gastroenteritis	0.625	0.093	0.823
3	6	**Nausea**	0.089*	**0.050**	0.805
3	7	Vomiting	0.730	0.076	0.849
5	1	Lymphadenopathy	1.000	0.136	0.717
6	1	Dehydration	0.221	0.087	0.666
8	1	Crying	0.500	0.185	0.655
8	2	Insomnia	1.000	0.153	0.661
8	3	**Irritability**	0.003*	**0.780**	0.214
9	1	Bronchitis	0.375	0.059	0.900
9	2	Congestion, nasal	0.375	0.058	0.901
9	3	Congestion, respiratory	0.603	0.040	0.896
9	4	Cough	0.497	0.062	0.906
9	5	Infection, upper respiratory	0.431	0.083	0.897
9	6	Laryngotracheobronchitis	1.000	0.047	0.898
9	7	Pharyngitis	0.497	0.061	0.906
9	8	Rhinorrhea	1.000	0.051	0.904
9	9	Sinusitis	0.625	0.051	0.903
9	10	Tonsillitis	1.000	0.042	0.905
9	11	Wheezing	0.625	0.050	0.907
10	1	Bite/sting	0.125	0.087	0.859
10	2	Eczenma	0.500	0.070	0.860
10	3	Pruritis	1.000	0.062	0.868
10	4	**Rash**	0.021*	**0.190**	0.784
10	5	Rash, diaper	0.288	0.099	0.852
10	6	**Rash, measles/rubella-like**	0.039*	**0.126**	0.836
10	7	Rash, varicella-like	0.687	0.076	0.862
10	8	Urticaria	0.221	0.048	0.852
10	9	Viral exanthema	0.603	0.055	0.855
11	1	Conjunctivitis	0.221	0.079	0.721
11	2	Otitis media	0.711	0.102	0.757
11	3	Otorrhea	1.000	0.121	0.749

are independent, $p_i' \sim \text{Beta}(\alpha, \beta)$ and

$$p_i \sim (1 - \gamma_i)\text{Beta}(\alpha + x_i, \beta + n_c - x_i) + \gamma_i\text{Beta}(\alpha_1, \beta_1), \qquad (5.7)$$

in which $\gamma_i \sim \text{Bernoulli}(\pi)$ is a Bernoulli random variable that is independent of the two independent Beta random variables indicated, where $\pi \sim \text{Beta}(1+\zeta, 1)$. The use of Beta priors gives a conjugate family for which posterior analysis can be carried out by updating the parameters of the Beta distribution. Details are given in Supplement 3 of Section 5.5, where Gould's choice of the hyperparameters $\alpha, \beta, \alpha_1, \beta_1$ and ζ is also described. The use of the Beta conjugate family results in simpler Bayesian analysis than B&B and does not require MCMC for its implementation. Gould (2013) proposes a further simplification that uses the Poisson approximation to the binomial distributions $\text{Bin}(n_c, p_i')$ and $\text{Bin}(n_T, p_i)$, leading to

$$x_i \sim \text{Poi}(\lambda_i'), \ y_i \sim \text{Poi}(\rho\lambda_i), \qquad (5.8)$$

where ρ is the allocation ratio for the test group relative to the control. The conjugate family for λ_i' is Gamma (a, b) with scale parameter b, for which the posterior distribution of λ_i' is Gamma $(a + x_i, b + 1)$.

For the Poisson family, Gould (2013) uses the risk ratios $R_i = \lambda_i/\lambda_i'$ as the metric to compare the AE rate of the treatment group to that of the control group. The analog of the mixture model (5.7) for the Poisson family is

$$\lambda_i \sim (1 - \gamma_i) \, \text{Gamma} \, (a + x_i, b + 1) + \gamma_i \, \text{Gamma} \, (c_i, d_i). \qquad (5.9)$$

Let $d_i = b + 1$, and $b_\rho = (b + 1)/(b + 1 + \rho)$. Assuming this distribution for the Poisson rates λ_i and λ_i', the conditional distribution of $R_i/(R_i + b_\rho)$ given (γ_i, x_i, y_i) is

$$(1-\gamma_i)f(y_i; a+x_i, \rho)\text{Beta}(a+x_i+y_i, a+x_i)+\gamma_i f(y_i; c_i, b_\rho) \, \text{Beta}(c_i+y_i, a+x_i),$$
$$(5.10)$$

where $f(\cdot; n, p)$ is the density function of the negative binomial distribution for the number of Bernoulli trials until n successes when the probability of success in a single trial is p; see Supplement 3 in Section 5.5. Gould (2013) uses these posterior calculations to evaluate the sensitivity and specificity (under the Bayesian mixture model) of a screening rule that flags the ith adverse event type if $R_i > R^*$. The parameters a, b and c_i are chosen on the basis of these sensitivity and specificity evaluations; see Supplement 3 of Section 5.5.

For the original binomial model $x_i \sim \text{Bin} \, (n_c, p_i')$ and $y_i \sim \text{Bin}(n_T, p_i)$, with the priors $p_i' \sim \text{Beta} \, (\alpha, \beta)$ and (5.7) for p_i, Gould (2008) uses the odds ratio $\psi_i = \left(\frac{p_i}{1-p_i}\right) / \left(\frac{p_i'}{1-p_i'}\right)$ as the metric to compare the treatment and control AE rates. He derives a formula similar to, but more complicated than, (5.10) for the posterior distribution of ψ_i. This formula is used to determine α, β, and then α_1, β_1 that satisfy certain properties of the screening rule $\psi_i > \psi^*$; details are given in Supplement 3 of Section 5.5.

5.4.3   Compound statistical decisions and an empirical Bayes approach

To elucidate how the hierarchical Bayes models of Berry and Berry (2004) and Gould (2008, 2013, 2018) work and their connection to the frequentist approach to multiple testing via FDR control, Lai and Miao (2017) have recently built upon the works of Efron (2003, 2004, 2007) on local false discovery rate (lfdr). They note the similarity of Efron's model to these hierarchical mixture models, and also trace back to Robbins (1951, 1964) seminal works on compound decision theory and empirical Bayes approach to compound decision problem. Although the posterior probabilities in the results of Berry and Berry (2004) appear to be very different from the FDR values of Mehrotra and Heyse (2004a), it turns out that this can be mostly explained by the weight that the 3-level mixture model assigns to π_b. If one knows *a priori* that there are relatively few AE types associated with the drug (i.e. $1 - \pi_b$ close to 0) and incorporates this prior information in the model, then the posterior probability of $\theta_b > 0$ would not be so dissimilar to the adjusted P-values, as shown by Lai and Miao (2017).

Robbins' seminal paper on the empirical Bayes methodology (Robbins, 1964) and his earlier paper on the related subject of compound decision theory (Robbins, 1951) were acclaimed by Neyman (1962) as "two breakthroughs in the theory of statistical decision making." Consider the simple problem of estimating a parameter θ based on the observed datum X, whose probability density function $p(x|\theta)$ depends on θ. The Bayesian approach assumes the existence of a prior distribution G for θ; and the Bayes estimate minimizing squared error loss, $E[t(X) - \theta]^2 = \int E_\theta[t(X) - \theta]^2 \, dG(\theta)$, is given by the posterior mean $t(X) = E[\theta|X]$. The difficulty with implementing the Bayesian approach is specification of the prior distribution, which may be impossible in practice. In many applications, however, one is faced with n structurally similar problems of estimating θ_i from X_i $(i = 1, 2, ..., n)$, where X_i has probability density function $p(x; \theta_i)$ and the θ_i can be assumed to have the same distribution as G. As a concrete example, Robbins (1964) describes the case in which the ith automobile driver in a certain sample is observed to have X_i accidents in a given year, $i = 1, ..., n$. Assuming that X_i is a Poisson with density $p(x; \theta_i) = e^{-\theta_i}\theta_i^x/x!, (x = 0, 1, ...)$, he first shows that if we want to estimate the "accident-proneness" parameter θ_i for each of the n drivers. If the distribution G of accident proneness in the population of drivers were known, then the Bayes estimate of the accident process parameter θ_i of the ith driver is the posterior mean $t(X_i)$, which can be expressed as

$$t(x) = (x + 1)f(x + 1)/f(x). \tag{5.11}$$

Since G is essentially never known, he notes that f can be consistently estimated by the empirical density of the n observations $X_1, ..., X_n$, and then uses this estimate as a substitute for the unknown f in (5.11), leading to an empirical Bayes estimate of the form $t(x; X_1, ..., X_n)$. This kind of idea plays an important role in the development of empirical Bayes methods for the analysis of Spontaneous Reporting Systems in Chapter 7. The same ideas are applicable to the "compound statistical decision problems," in which the θ_i are regarded as unknown constants rather than an unobservable random sample from a distribution G, and the overall loss function is the sum of the loss functions of the individual problems. This was introduced by Robbins (1951) who derived "asymptotically subminimax" solutions to these compound decision problems in the case of testing n simple hypotheses $H_{0i} : \theta_i = 0$ versus $H_{1i} : \theta_i = 1$ based on statistics X_i from independent $N(\theta_i, 1)$ populations $(i = 1, .., n)$. Hannan and Robbins (1955) subsequently showed that the optimal test of H_{0i} based on X_i that minimizes the compound loss would depend on the proportion $\bar{\theta}_n = n^{-1} \sum_{i=1}^{n} \theta_i$ of 1's among the θ_i and that one could use all the data $X_1, \ldots, X_n$ to obtain an estimate that is $\bar{\theta}_n + o_p(1)$, similar to the empirical Bayes decision rule in the preceding paragraph. Lai and Miao (2017) and Lai et al. (2018b) have recently developed this idea much further for the complicated multiple testing problems.

5.5 Supplements and Problems

1. *Volcano and Q-Q plot.* A volcano plot is a scatter-plot of the significance level (expressed as the negative log of the P-value) on the vertical axis versus the difference (in % or in the log scale) between the treatment and control outcomes (which are the incidence rates of adverse events in Figure 5.1 or microarray gene expression levels in DNA microarray experiments) on the x-axis. In genetics, such a plot relates the measure of statistical significance from a statistical test to the magnitude of the change from the control to treatment gene expression levels, over thousands of genes in DNA microarray experiments. Data points with low P-values (hence high $- \log$ P-values) appear at the top of the plot and far to the left- or right-hand sides (corresponding to large-magnitude changes from control to treatment expression levels), enabling visual identification of the genes with large-magnitude changes that are also statistically significant. To handle a large number of genes for which many data points overlap in the plot, the R package ggplot2 can be used to control the transparency and size of the point by using the "alpha" and "size" options.

   The Q-Q plot of a distribution G versus another distribution F plots the pth quantile y_p of G against the pth quantile x_p of F for $0 < p < 1$. The R function qqplot(x, y) plots the quantiles of two samples x

and y against each other. The function `qqnorm(x)` replaces the quantiles of one of the samples by those of a standard normal distribution. Under the normality assumption, the Q-Q plots should lie approximately on a straight line. Instead of the standard normal distribution, Figure 5.2 considers the uniform distribution because the P-values are uniformly distributed under the null hypothesis.

2. *FWER, FDR, double FDR and post-selection multiple testing.* In the context of testing m null hypotheses $H_1, \ldots, H_m$, the *familywise error rate* (FWER) is defined as the probability of rejecting H_i for some $i \in I$, in which $I \subset \{1, \ldots, m\}$ is the index set of true null hypotheses. To control FWER, the simplest way is to use Bonferroni correction, testing each H_i at significance level α/m. This is very conservative for large m, and Holm (1979) has developed the step-down procedure that rejects $H_{(i)}$ if $P_{(i)} \leq \alpha/(m+1-i)$, otherwise accepts $H_{(i)}$ and all other hypotheses that have not been rejected already. This step-down method has FWER $\leq \alpha$. Subsequent extensions by Shaffer (1986) and Holland and Copenhaver (1987) choose other thresholds than $\alpha/(m+1-i)$, and Lehmann and Romano (2006, pp. 352–353) give a generic form of these step-down methods to control FWER. Note that the Benjamini-Hochberg step-down procedure in the first paragraph of Section 5.3 uses the threshold $\alpha i/m$ for $P_{(i)}$ to control FDR. Simes conjectures that this step-down procedure also controls FWER "for a large family of multivariate distributions" as suggested by his simulations. Sarkar and Chang (1997) and Sarkar (1998) prove that the conjecture is true for multivariate totally positive distributions of order 2 (MTP$_2$). The MTP$_2$ class, which includes equicorrelated multivariate normal with positive correlations, absolute-valued equicorrelated multivariate normal, multivariate gamma, and multivariate t, is characterized by

$$f(\mathbf{x})f(\mathbf{y}) \leq f(\min\{\mathbf{x}, \mathbf{y}\}) f(\max\{\mathbf{x}, \mathbf{y}\}) \text{ for all } \mathbf{x} \text{ and } \mathbf{y}, \qquad (5.12)$$

where f is a joint density function belonging to this class and the minimum and maximum are evaluated componentwise. A large class of joint distributions (containing MTP$_2$ as a subset) is PRDS (positive regression dependency on each one from a subset I), which is characterized by the following property for increasing set D: $P(\mathbf{X} \in D | X_i = x)$ is *nondecreasing in x for every $i \in I$. D is called increasing if

$$\mathbf{x} \in D \text{ and } \mathbf{y} \geq \mathbf{x} \text{ (componentwise inequality)} \Rightarrow \mathbf{y} \in D.$$

Benjamini and Yekutieli (2001) have proved the following results:

(a) *If the joint distribution of the test statistics is PRDS on the index set of the true null hypotheses, then the Benjamini-Hochberg step-down procedure controls the FDR at level less than or equal to $\alpha m_0/m$, where m_0 is the number of true null hypotheses.*

(b) *The modified Benjamini-Hochberg step-down procedure that re-*
places α by $\tilde{\alpha} = \alpha/\left(\sum_{i=1}^{m} i^{-1}\right)$ always controls FDR at level less
than or equal to $\alpha m_0/m$, without any dependency assumption on
the test statistics.

Mehrotra and Heyse (2004b) find that FDR is as high as 51.2% for
no multiplicity adjustment, 4.8% for full FDR adjustment, and satisfactory FDR control for DFDR with various choices of α_1 and α_2.
They investigate the impact of various choices of α_1 and α_2 on the
FDR and note that the value $\alpha_1 = \alpha_2/2$ is a reasonable choice for
controlling the FDR at a level α for the dataset in their illustration.
Lai et al. (2018a) have recently developed a novel approach to (a) the
long-standing problem of the actual P-values after test-based variable
selection and (b) the closely related problem of post-selection multiple
testing.

3. *Bayesian inference and Gould's Bayesian screening of AEs.* The model
   proposed by Gould (2008) is associated with m adverse event types
   and binomial random variables $y_i \sim \text{Bin}(n_T, p_i)$ and $x_i \sim \text{Bin}(n_c, p_i')$
   for the ith adverse event type, as explained in Section 5.4.2. The Beta
   prior distribution Beta (α, β) for p_i' yields a conjugate family, for which
   the posterior distribution is Beta $(\alpha + x_i, \beta + n_c - x_i)$. The prior distribution of p_i is specified via a Bernoulli random variable γ_i so that it can
   be written as the form (5.7). We first consider the use of the Poisson
   approximation (5.8) to simplify the posterior analysis and make the
   argument easier to understand, returning to the original Bernoulli
   case at the end of this supplement.

   The essential Bayesian framework for the Poisson counts (5.8) has
   been described in the second paragraph of Section 5.4.2. Here we focus on Gould's (2013) approach to the choice of a, b, and c_i. Since a, b
   are the shape and scale parameters of the gamma prior distribution
   for λ_i', it is natural to choose them based on x_i alone. With the even-
   tual goal of the screen rule $R_i > R^*$ in mind, Gould (2013) suggests
   to choose a and b so that the specificity of the rule (evaluated under
   the Bayesian null model $\gamma_i = 0$) is maintained at some level x, e.g.,
   $x = 0.95$ or 0.99, prior to observing y_i so that (5.10) reduces to Beta
   $(a + x_i, a + x_i)$, whose distribution function is the incomplete beta
   function $B(t; \tilde{a}, \tilde{b}) = \int_0^t u^{\tilde{a}-1}(1-u)^{\tilde{b}-1}\,du$, with $\tilde{a} = \tilde{b} = a + x_i$. This
   corresponds to the conditional distribution of $R_i/(R_i + 1)$ given x_i and
   $\gamma_i = 0$ (corresponding to $\rho = 0$ as the treatment group has not yet been
   observed). Since $R_i \leq R^*$ is equivalent to $R_i/R_i + 1 \leq R^*/R^* + 1$),
   Gould (2013) defines a by $B(R^*/(R^* + 1), a, a) = \tilde{\kappa}$ and b via a and $\hat{\lambda}$ by

   $$G(\hat{\lambda}; a, b) = \kappa, \text{ with } G(\hat{\lambda}; \hat{a}, \hat{b}) = \kappa, \qquad (5.13)$$

   where $\tilde{\kappa}$ is closer to 1 than κ, $G(\cdot; a, b)$ is the distribution function of

Gamma (a, b), and $(\hat{a}, \hat{b})$ is the maximum likelihood estimate of the negative binomial distribution NB $(a, b/(1 + b))$ for x_i in the Bayesian model with specified hyperparameters a and b. Making use of (5.10) for the case $\gamma_i = 1$ (still before y_i is observed), he defines c_i by

$$B(R^*/(R^* + 1); c_i, a + x_i) = \kappa', \qquad (5.14)$$

with the goal of maintaining the sensitivity (evaluated under the Bayesian non-null case $\gamma_i \neq 0$) of the screening rule at level x'. Thus, Gould (2013) actually begins with a screening rule with a "presumably clinically meaningful value" R^* for risk ratios and analyzes the diagnostic properties (including the false discovery rate and missed discovery rate) in an analytically tractable Bayesian mixture model; see Section 2.3 of Gould (2013).

For the original binomial model, $x_i \sim \text{Bin}(n_c, p_i')$ and $y_i \sim \text{Bin}(n_T, p_i)$, Gould (2008) considers the odds ratio ψ_i; see the last paragraph of Section 5.4.2. In the Bayesian mixture model $p_i' \sim \text{Beta}(\alpha, \beta)$ and (5.7) for p_i, Supplement 3 shows how a formula similar to (5.10) can be derived for the conditional distribution of ψ_i given (γ_i, x_i, y_i). With this formula, the arguments used by Gould (2008, Section2.4) to determine the hyperparameters α, β and then α_i, β_i, allowing (α_1, β_1) to determine on i via x_i, are similar to those above for the Poisson case.

4. *Markov chain Monte Carlo (MCMC) computations.* The ultimate objective of Bayesian data analysis is to calculate the posterior distributions of parameters of interest. Given the hierarchical structure of priors and hyper priors, e.g., the three-level hierarchical priors in Berry and Berry (2004), there is generally no closed form of posterior distributions whose determination usually relies on special computational techniques, such as numerical integration and Monte Carlo methods, of which the most important is Markov chain Monte Carlo (MCMC); see Carlin and Louis (2000, Chapter 5) for details. There are several MCMC approaches including Metropolis-Hastings sampling, Gibbs sampling and slice sampling, each of which employs different algorithms to approximate the posterior distributions. For instance, suppose that the joint posterior distribution of $\theta = (\theta_1, \ldots, \theta_K)$ given the data $\mathbf{X}$, denoted by $p(\theta|\mathbf{X})$, is available (e.g., Berry and Berry (2004, page 425)) and one can use Gibbs sampling method to estimate the marginal posterior distribution $p(\theta_k|\mathbf{X})$ through iteratively sampling θ_k from the conditional distribution $p(\theta_k|\theta^{(-k)}, \mathbf{X})$ where $\theta^{(-k)} = \theta\backslash\theta_k$. Specifically, let $\theta_k^{(i)}$ be the ith draw (sample) of θ_k from the conditional distribution, $i = 1, \ldots, I$. The Gibbs sampling algorithm proceeds as

follows

$$\text{Draw } \theta_1^{(i)} \sim p(\theta_1|\theta_2^{(i-1)}, \ldots, \theta_K^{(i-1)}, \mathbf{X}),$$
$$\text{Draw } \theta_2^{(i)} \sim p(\theta_2|\theta_1^{(i)}, \theta_3^{(i-1)}, \ldots, \theta_K^{(i-1)}, \mathbf{X}),$$
$$\vdots$$
$$\text{Draw } \theta_K^{(i)} \sim p(\theta_K|\theta_1^{(i)}, \ldots, \theta_{K-1}^{(i)}, \mathbf{X}),$$

where $\theta_k^{(0)}$ is an initial value assigned to θ_k. After I iterations with I_0 ($< I$) "burning-in" runs (during which the samples may not be representative of the posterior distribution and hence are discarded), one approximates the marginal distribution of θ_k as

$$\hat{p}(\theta_k|\mathbf{X}) = \frac{1}{I - I_0} \sum_{i=I_0+1}^{I} p(\theta_k|\theta_1^{(i)}, \ldots, \theta_{k-1}^{(i)}, \theta_{k+1}^{(i)}, \ldots, \theta_K^{(i)}). \qquad (5.15)$$

The theory of MCMC guarantees that the stationary distribution generated from Gibbs sampling algorithm after "burning-in" runs converges to the target posterior distribution of interest (Gilks et al., 1995) and for this reason an MCMC algorithm usually requires a large number of iterations to ensure convergence.

Exercise. Consider a Bayesian hierarchical model that results in a bivariate normal distribution of parameters θ_1 and θ_2

$$\begin{pmatrix} \theta_1 \\ \theta_2 \end{pmatrix} \sim N \left(\begin{pmatrix} \mu_1 \\ \mu_2 \end{pmatrix}, \begin{pmatrix} \sigma_1^2 & \rho\sigma_1\sigma_2 \\ \rho\sigma_1\sigma_2 & \sigma_2^2 \end{pmatrix} \right) \qquad (5.16)$$

where $\mu_1, \mu_2, \sigma_1^2, \sigma_2^2$ and ρ are known. Write a program that uses the Gibbs sampling algorithm described above with $I = 500$ and $10,000$ to calculate the posterior means and variances of θ_1 and θ_2 for the following sets of values of $\mu_1, \mu_2, \sigma_1^2, \sigma_2^2, \rho$:

(a) $\mu_1 = \mu_2 = 0$, $\sigma_1^2 = \sigma_2^2 = 1$ and $\rho = 0$,

(b) $\mu_1 = \mu_2 = 0$, $\sigma_1^2 = 1$, $\sigma_2^2 = 5$ and $\rho = 0$,

(c) $\mu_1 = 0$, $\mu_2 = 1$, $\sigma_1^2 = 1$, $\sigma_2^2 = 5$ and $\rho = 0$,

(d) repeat steps (a) - (c) but with $\rho = 0.25, 0.5, 0.75, 0.99$

(e) discuss the impact of different values of $\mu_1, \mu_2, \sigma_1^2, \sigma_2^2, \rho$ on the performance of Gibbs sampling.

6

Causal Inference from Post-Marketing Data

Post-marketing data from clinical trials and observational studies are important for regulatory agencies "to monitor the safety of drugs after they reach the marketplace and to take corrective action if drugs risks are judged unacceptable in light of their benefits" (Institute of Medicine, 2012). Section 6.1 describes data from phase IV clinical trials and observational data from spontaneous reporting of adverse events by users of approved drugs. There are many challenges, which have in turn spurred the development of new methodologies, to analyze and infer from post-marketing data. The preceding chapter has considered challenges due to multiplicity and methods to address them for Tier 2 clinical data. In this chapter we consider challenges in, and approaches to, causal inference from post-marketing data. Section 6.2 begins with an introduction to causal inference from experimental studies and associated statistical models and methods. Section 6.3 focuses on non-experimental (observational) studies and causal inference methods in these studies. Section 6.4 addresses unmeasured confounding in observational studies by using instrumental variables (IVs) and study designs that provide natural substitutes for instruments. Section 6.5 introduces recent developments in structural causal models and symbolic causal calculus. The supplements and problems in Section 6.6 provide additional background for causal inference from experimental and non-experimental studies.

6.1 Post-marketing data collection

Upon regulatory approval, a medical product is continuously investigated and/or monitored through post-marketing studies and surveillance. Depending on the type and amount of evidence used for regulatory approval and specific therapeutic areas for which the product is approved, the objective and design considerations of post-marketing studies could differ substantially. For example, if a product targeting a rare disease for which no efficacious therapies are available is approved based on a limited amount of evidence on clinical efficacy and safety, then the regulatory agency may require the manufacturer to conduct a randomized controlled trial as a post-marketing commitment study to further confirm the product's benefit and risk. "Post-marketing commitments" (PMCs) are studies that the manufacturer of an approved medical product has agreed to conduct but may not be required by the regulatory agency to do so. On the other hand, if a product with a well-established safety profile in clinical trials is approved based on fairly convincing evidence of efficacy or benefit-risk ratio, then a post-marketing surveillance program consisting of non-interventional epidemiological observational studies may be required to demonstrate long-term safety. In general, post-marketing studies can be categorized as prospective and retrospective, based on the nature of data collection, on whether intervention is applied, and on whether randomization is employed. The US Food and Drug Administration Amendments Act (FDAAA, 2007) makes a distinction between "study" and "clinical trial," by defining *clinical trials* as "any prospective investigations in which the applicant or investigator determines the method of assigning the drug product(s) or other interventions to one or more human subjects" and *studies* as "all other investigations, such as investigations with humans that are not clinical trials as defined above (e.g., observational epidemiologic studies), animal studies, and laboratory experiments." In addition, Section 901 of the FDAAA (2007) authorizes the FDA to require post-marketing studies and/or clinical trials for assessing a known serious risk and/or signals of the serious risk related to the use of the product, or for identifying an unexpected serious risk when available data indicate the potential of such risk.

6.1.1 Clinical trials with safety endpoints

After marketing authorization, the FDA may require an adequately powered-randomized controlled clinical trial (RCT) with pre-specified safety endpoints, depending on the adequacy of pre-marketing evidence on efficacy and safety of a drug to support benefit-risk claim, potential drug-drug interactions, and drug effect on specific sub-populations (e.g., children, pregnant women, specific ethnic groups), and specific safety concerns (e.g., long-term safety, safety on specific organs, safety among specific sub-populations such as children, pregnant women, particular ethnic groups, and immuno-compromised patients); see FDA (2012) and FDA (2013a)for such examples and Chapter 4 for the design and analysis of clinical trials with safety endpoints.

6.1.2 Observational pharmacoepidemiologic studies using registries

Under the FDAAA, PMR (post-marketing requirement) observational studies are designed to "assess a serious risk associated with a drug exposure or to quantify risk or evaluate factors that affect the risk of serious toxicity, such as drug dose, timing of exposure, or patient characteristics," while PMC studies are those designed to "examine the natural history of a disease or to estimate background rates for adverse events in a population not treated with the drug that is subject to the marketing application" (FDA, 2012). Pharmacoepidemiologic studies in the PMR category either test pre-defined hypotheses, with or without a control group, or describe safety analyses such as providing upper bounds of detectable risks. The designs for the PMR and PMC studies should be tailored to their primary objectives. Among prospective observational studies, registry studies deserve special attention because of their unique features in study design and study population. A registry for product safety registers patients whose demographic variables, medical conditions, treatment received, and outcomes experienced are recorded in designated clinical settings for the purpose of safety monitoring, risk adjustment, and/or continual benefit-risk assessment of a medical product. Registries have become increasingly appealing in post-marketing studies and safety surveillance of medical products (Willis et al., 2012). In some cases, registry studies are the only source to provide relatively comprehensive safety information for approved products in special subsets of population. For example, because pregnant women are routinely excluded from pre-marketing clinical trials due to the fear of unwanted adverse effects on the mother and/or the fetus, most products are marketed with limited information on safety during pregnancy and hence are not recommended for use by pregnant women. However, health conditions are commonly encountered in pregnant women, who often require medications. Hence, it becomes essential to evaluate adverse effects of medical products among pregnant women using pregnancy registries (Dellicour et al., 2008). Registries can give a representative picture of a target population with certain conditions who receive the medical product of interest as well a range of concurrent medications. They are useful for providing reliable information for estimation of the incidence rates of adverse events and possibly drug-drug interactions because of their large sample sizes. However, caution should be exercised when using registry data for causal inference in drug-related safety investigation as registries often do not include sound control groups of patients who are in similar conditions but do not receive the medication under investigation. Registries are most often employed for surveillance of specialized medications (Willis et al., 2012).

6.1.3   Prospective cohort observational studies

Prospective (cohort) observational studies start with a cohort of subjects
from a pre-identified population and follow them over a time period for
inference on the incidence rates of outcomes of interest. They typically
pre-identify a subset of the population with exposure (i.e., use of the approved product) and another subset of the population without exposure
(i.e., no use of the approved product), and make comparisons between the
two sets of the population with respect to the incidence of serious adverse
events, after adjusting for confounding factors, if any, upon completion of
the follow-up period. If there is an ethical issue to have a concurrent control group or if the study population is relatively stable in the incidence
rate of adverse events of interest, then the historical data from the study
population can be used as a control. Since the information of exposure duration for each individual and the number of reported adverse events are
available, the exposure-adjusted incidence rate (EAIR) can be calculated
from the collected data. In addition, attributable risk based on the absolute difference (or relative risk) in the EAIRs of particular adverse events
can also be calculated to indicate how much excessive risk is associated
with the product under investigation. In case of imbalanced risk factors
between comparative groups, a risk-adjusted regression approach can be
used to ensure the effect of potential risks has been adjusted out when
comparing the incidence rates between groups; see Section 4.5. Moreover,
because of its longitudinal nature, a prospective observational study allows for collection of recurrent adverse events, for which Section 4.5.3
describes related statistical methods.

6.1.4   Retrospective observational studies

Retrospective observational studies are studies in which the information
of exposure to a product by a patient, with or without an adverse event
of interest, is traced back to a certain time point to infer the association
of the product under investigation with the event. Although retrospective observational studies are not included in the FDA (2013a) guideline
for post-marketing studies and clinical trials, they are important study
designs in pharmacoepidemiology for studying possible association of a
product with an important event, e.g., the matched case-control study
to investigate the association of intussusception among infants with the
tetravalent rhesushuman reassortant rotavirus vaccine (Murphy, 2001).
Depending on how study populations are selected and the data on their
medical condition and product exposure are collected, retrospective observational studies are categorized as cohort studies, case-control studies,
and case series studies.

Retrospective cohort studies start with a subset of a population, with
or without a serious adverse event, and look backwards into the history

of exposure to some risk factor (e.g., use of a product) for each individual within the selected cohort. Examples of retrospective cohort studies are the evaluation of possible association of sitagliptin use with an increased risk of heart failure-related hospitalization among patients with type 2 diabetes who had pre-existing heart failure, using a commercially insured claims database (Weir et al., 2014), and the use of electronic medical records of a pediatric population to monitor their past drug exposure and safety outcomes (Bie et al., 2015). It should be pointed out that even though retrospective cohort studies allow the temporal sequence of risk factors and adverse outcomes to be assessed and are usually less time-consuming, they suffer from the following drawbacks. First, selection bias may occur when the selected population does not represent the target population and therefore generalization may be problematic. Second, there may be information-recording bias, because the medical records are not collected for the purpose of evaluating the association of the medical product with a set of particular events, hence the recorded history may not reflect the complete picture of the cohort's adverse experiences. Third, as in any other typical non-randomized observational studies, retrospective cohort studies can only establish an association between drug exposure and an adverse event, and no causation can be inferred because it is often impossible to measure, even through statistical modeling, the risk factors that might have affected the event outcome (Sedgwick, 2014).

6.2 Potential outcomes and counterfactuals

6.2.1 Causes of effects in attributions for serious adverse health outcomes

Dawid et al. (2016) describe an ongoing legal case concerning an anti-diabetic drug Mediator, also known as Benfluorex, which had been widely used off-label as an appetite suppressant until the French Health Agency CNAM announced its finding in 2010 that 500 deaths in France over a 30-year period could be attributed to Mediator, based on extrapolation of results in two scientific studies of the effects of the drug on valvular heart disease. As the news spread through the media, the French authorities withdrew the drug from the market and hundreds of individuals who had used Mediator jointly filed a lawsuit against the manufacturer. The trial "has been under way since May 2012" and "whether Mediator was in fact the cause of the heart disease in any of those who brought the lawsuit had yet to be addressed, and no expert scientific testimony had been presented to the court" at the time of preparation of Dawid et al. (2016) that also gives a brief summary of the aforementioned scientific studies. One study was a matched case-control study that involved 27 cases of valvular heart disease and 54 controls, and examined whether the patients had or had not used Mediator. It used logistic regression to adjust for potential confounding factors that include body mass index, diabetes, and dexfenfluramine use, and reported a significant odds ratio. The other study examined the records of over a million diabetic patients in a cohort study and reported a significantly higher hospitalization rate for valvular heart disease in Mediator users.

Dawid et al. (2016) distinguish between "causes of effects" (CoE) as in the preceding example about assigning responsibility (cause) for heart disease (undesirable effect) that "Lawyers and the Courts are more concerned with" and "effects of causes" (EoC) that studies the consequences of possible actions/causes, as exemplified by the following question: "Ann has a headache. She is wondering whether to take aspirin. Would that cause her headache to disappear (within, say, 30 minutes)?" In contrast, the corresponding CoE question would be: "Ann had a headache and took aspirin. Her headache went away after 30 minutes. Was that caused by the aspirin?" They point out that "EoC can be addressed by using experimental design and statistical analysis, but it is less clear how to incorporate statistical or epidemiological evidence into CoE reasoning."

Holland (1986) gives further examples of CoE in health outcomes, beginning with Fisher's criticism of Doll and Hill's studies of lung cancer in relation to smoking, which all appeared in the *British Medical Journal* in 1950, 1952, 1956, and 1957. The data that led to this debate are "purely associational" and "ascertained only smoking status and lung cancer status on sets of subjects," and "Fisher argued that smoking might only be indicative of certain genetic differences between smokers and nonsmokers and that these genetic differences could be related to the development or not of lung cancer." In a subsequent letter to the editor of the same journal in 1957, McCurdy pointed out, however, "that lung cancer rates increase with the amount of smoking and that subjects who stopped smoking had lower lung cancer rates than those who did not," thereby reinforcing the causal link of smoking. Holland (1986) also gives another example establishing specific bacteria as the cause of certain infectious diseases. He notes, however, that "medicine is more difficult when the biological theory is less developed," and describes suggestions by Hill (1965) for deciding whether an observed association can be interpreted as causation.

6.2.2 Counterfactuals, potential outcomes, and Rubin's causal model

Counterfactual theories of causation in philosophy are based on counterfactual conditionals of the form "If A were the case, C would be the case"; see Lewis (1973). A counterfactual conditional is a conditional whose antecedent is false and whose consequence describes how the world would have been if the antecedent had been true. Dawid et al. (2016) argue that some form of counterfactual reasoning "appears unreasonable" in CoE analysis and propose to use "probability of causation defined using counterfactual logic" for such analysis. Let E be a binary variable with $E = 1$ representing "exposure" (as in treatment with aspirin) and $E = 0$ non-exposure, and let Y represent the response variable (e.g. whether Ann's headache disappears after 30 minutes or not); see the penultimate paragraph of Section 6.2.1. The concept of "counterfactual contrast" rests on potential outcomes that split Y into two variables $Y(0)$ and $Y(1)$ associated with $\{E = 0\}$ and $\{E = 1\}$, respectively, which "are regarded as existing prior to the determination of E." Since in this example Ann had in fact taken aspirin because of her headache, $Y(0)$ is a counterfactual reponse, which would have been observed had Ann in fact not taken aspirin. If $Y(0) = 1$, then Ann's headache would also have disappeared even if she had not taken the aspirin. Hence Dawid et al. (2016) define the probability of causation as the conditional probability

$$PC = P\{Y(0) = 1 | E = 1, Y(1) = 1, X\}, \qquad (6.1)$$

in which X denotes all concomitant information (about Ann in this example). We describe in the next subsection methods to estimate (6.1).

The outcomes $Y(0)$ and $Y(1)$ are called *potential outcomes*, which play a fundamental role in Rubin's causal model and in his approach to causal inference summarized in Rubin (2005). He says that although some authors "call the potential outcomes 'counterfactuals,' borrowing the term from philosophy," he prefers not to do so because "these values are not counterfactual until after treatments are assigned, and calling all potential outcomes 'counterfactuals' certainly confuses quantities that can never be observed (e.g., your height at age 3 if you were born yesterday in the Arctic) and so are truly a priori counterfactual, with unobserved potential outcomes that are not a priori counterfactual." Since its introduction by Rubin (1974), potential outcomes and the associated causal model described in the next paragraph have undergone many developments and extensions. The version we use here is closely related to applications to adverse outcomes after drug exposure.

The potential outcomes for the ith unit (subject) of a study, $i = 1, ..., n$, are denoted by $Y_i(\tau), \tau \in \mathcal{J}$, where $\mathcal{J}$ is the set of treatments (or causes) to which the units may be exposed; the terms "cause" and "treatment" are used interchangeably in Rubin's causal model. Each unit is potentially exposable to any one of these treatments before exposure, and has received only one treatment post-exposure. Much of the literature considers the case $\mathcal{J} = \{t, c\}$ consisting of two elements t (for treatment) and c (for control). We consider here more general $\mathcal{J}$, which is a finite set allowing for different levels for the treatment t (as in dose levels of a drug or amount of smoking for cigarette smokers). The assignment variable T_i assigns to the ith unit the treatment (or cause) in $\mathcal{J}$ that acts on it. The actual observations, therefore, are $\{(Y_i(T_i), \mathbf{X}_i), i = 1, ..., n\}$, in which $\mathbf{X}_i$ is the pre-exposure covariate of the ith unit. Causal inference is about comparison of the distributions of potential outcomes $Y_i(\tau), \tau \in \mathcal{J}$, for what Rubin (2005) calls a "common set of units" (denoted by $i \in \{1, \ldots, n\}$), under the following two assumptions:

- *Stable Unit Treatment Value Assumption (SUTVA).* Given the observed covariates $\mathbf{X}_1, ..., \mathbf{X}_n$, the distribution of potential outcomes of one unit is independent of the potential treatment assignments for the other units.

- *Ignorability*: T_i has the same conditional distribution given $\{(\mathbf{X}_i, Y_i(\tau)) : \tau \in \mathcal{J}, 1 \le i \le n\}$ as that given $\mathbf{X} = (\mathbf{X}_1, ..., \mathbf{X}_n)$, and $P(T_i = \tau|\mathbf{X}) \ge \epsilon$ for some $\epsilon > 0$ and all $\tau \in \mathcal{J}$ and $1 \le i \le n$.

Regarding the common set of units as a sample (with or without replacement) from a population, causal inference on potential outcomes from the observed Y_i's can be carried out by conditioning on the covariates under the preceding assumptions, as will be explained in the next subsection. For a randomized controlled trial comparing treatment t versus control c, these assumptions are clearly satisfied, and in fact, the notion of potential outcomes $Y_i(t)$ and $Y_i(c)$ was first introduced by Neyman (1923) in conjunction with unbiased estimation of its mean difference

$$E\{Y(t) - Y(c)\} \text{ by } \overline{Y}(t) - \overline{Y}(c), \text{ where } \overline{Y}(t) = \sum_{i=1}^{n}(Y_i(t)\mathbb{1}_{\{T_i=t\}})/n_t, \overline{Y}(c) =$$

$\sum_{i=1}^{n}(Y_i(c)\mathbb{1}_{\{T_i=c\}})/n_c$, $n_t = \sum_{i=1}^{n} \mathbb{1}_{\{T_i=t\}}, n_c = n - n_t$. In this randomized experiment setting for potential outcomes, Neyman (1923) also showed that the usual variance estimates $s_t^2/n_t + s_c^2/n_c$ is a conservative (i.e., positively biased) estimate of $\mathrm{Var}(\overline{Y}(t) - \overline{Y}(c))$. Moreover, randomization removes the effects of the covariates on the observed responses. In non-randomized experiments such as observational studies, the effect of the covariates cannot be ignored. Without the SUTVA and ignorability assumptions on the treatment assignment mechanism, adjustments for possible confounding have to be made, as will be explained in Section 6.3.

6.2.3 Frequentist, Bayesian, and missing data approaches

We first extend the argument in the preceding paragraph to derive unbiased estimates of the mean potential outcomes $\mu(\tau) = \mathrm{E}(Y(\tau))$, assuming SUTVA for the treatment assignments and that all units have the same expected potential outcomes. For $\tau \in \mathcal{J}$, let $n_\tau = \sum_{i=1}^{n} \mathbb{1}_{\{T_i=\tau\}}, \overline{Y}(\tau) =$

$\sum_{i=1}^{n}(Y_i(\tau)\mathbb{1}_{\{T_i=\tau\}})/n_\tau$, and note that

$$
\begin{aligned}
\mathrm{E}(\overline{Y}(\tau)) &= \mathrm{E}\left\{\mathrm{E}\left[n_\tau^{-1}\sum_{i=1}^{n}Y_i(\tau)\mathbb{1}_{\{T_i=\tau\}}\middle|\mathbf{X}\right]\right\} \\
&= \mathrm{E}\left\{\mathrm{E}\left[n_\tau^{-1}\mathrm{E}(Y(\tau)|\mathbf{X})\sum_{i=1}^{n}\mathbb{1}_{\{T_i=\tau\}}\middle|\mathbf{X}\right]\right\} = \mathrm{E}\{\mathrm{E}(Y(\tau)|\mathbf{X})\} = \mu(\tau).
\end{aligned}
$$

$$(6.2)$$

The second equality above follows from the SUTVA. Hence $\overline{Y}(\tau)$ is an unbiased estimate of $\mu(\tau)$. Thus, the frequentist approach to causal inference uses the usual tools of consistent and asymptotically normal estimators of the means of potential outcomes, from which confidence intervals for the mean causal effects can be derived. Further details are given in Supplement 1 of Section 6.5, which also considers another direction along this line of research called *partial identification*. A parameter is partially identified if the sampling mechanism and postulated assumptions imply that the parameter lies in a set that is larger than a single point (corresponding to the identifiable case) but smaller than the entire parameter space; see Manski (2003). Dawid et al. (2016) give an example of bounding the probability of causation (6.1) by this approach, in which the bounds are functions of $\mathrm{P}(Y=1|E=1,X)$ and $\mathrm{P}(Y=1|E=0,X)$ that can be estimated from the sample of n subjects who have the same covariate value as that of the subject (unit).

Dawid et al. (2016) also introduce a Bayesian approach to inference on (6.1). In principle, this approach begins with a prior distribution of a multivariate parameter comprising the probabilities of the four configurations of $(Y(0),Y(1))$ conditioned on X (since $Y(0)$ and $Y(1)$ are binary outcomes) and then derive a fully determined posterior distribution for (6.1). However, they point out that this is problematic because $Y(0)$ and $Y(1)$ are never simultaneously observable and therefore the parameter describing the joint distribution of $(Y(0),Y(1))$ given X is not identifiable from the data, making the Bayesian inference highly sensitive to the specific prior assumptions made. They therefore assign a joint prior distribution for the estimable probabilities $\mathrm{P}(Y=1|E=1,X)$ and $\mathrm{P}(Y=1|E=0,X)$ that provide inequalities for (6.1). Hence their Bayesian inference has the form of a random interval asserted to contain (6.1). Rubin (1978, 2005) uses full prior specification in his Bayesian approach to causal inference but emphasizes the importance of ignorable treatment assignment mechanism for the causal inference to be insensitive to the prior distribution. In particular, the concept of ignorable treatment assignment is introduced in the 1978 paper in which he says:

In an experiment, one assignment of treatments is chosen and only the values under that assignment can be observed. Bayesian inference for causal effects follows from finding the predictive distribution of the values under the other assignments of treatments. This perspective makes clear the role of mechanisms that sample experimental units, assign treatments, and record data. Unless these mechanisms are ignorable (known probabilistic functions of recorded values), the Bayesian must model them in the data analysis and, consequently, confront inferences for causal effects that are sensitive to the specification of the prior distribution of the data.

Rubin (2005) also embeds Bayesian causal inference in the broader framework of Bayesian imputation methods for missing data.

We next give a brief introduction to statistical methods for missing data in the context of unobserved potential outcomes in causal inference. Supplement 2 in Section 6.5 gives a brief overview of methods for missing data. In the context of potential outcomes $Y(t)$ and $Y(c)$ corresponding to $\mathcal{J} = \{t, c\}$, Rubin (2005) says that the Bayesian missing data approach "directly confronts the fact that at least half of the potential outcomes are missing by creating a posterior predictive distribution" for the vector $\mathbf{Y}_{mis}$ of missing potential outcomes of the n units with $\mathbf{Y}_{obs}$ as the vector of observed outcomes. Let $\mathbf{T} = (T_1, ..., T_n)$ be the vector of treatment assignments. Assuming $\mathbf{X}_i, Y_i(t)$, and $Y_i(c)$ to be discrete, this posterior predictive distribution is given by

$$\mathrm{P}(\mathbf{Y}_{mis}|\mathbf{X}, \mathbf{Y}_{obs}, \mathbf{T}) \propto \mathrm{P}(\mathbf{Y}_{mis}|\mathbf{X}, \mathbf{Y}_{obs}) \qquad (6.3)$$

under ignorable assignment mechanisms, for which $\mathrm{P}(\mathbf{T}|\mathbf{X}, \mathbf{Y}_{obs}, \mathbf{Y}_{mis}) = \mathrm{P}(\mathbf{T}|\mathbf{X})$. In particular, for model-based inference that assumes a parametric model for $\mathrm{P}(Y_i(t), Y_i(c)|\mathbf{X}_i)$ with parameter θ, the likelihood function is

$$L(\theta|\mathbf{X}, \mathbf{Y}_{obs}) \propto \prod_i f_\theta(Y_{i,obs}, \mathbf{X}_i) = \prod_{T_i=t} f_\theta(Y_i(t), \mathbf{X}_i) \prod_{T_i=c} f_\theta(Y_i(c), \mathbf{X}_i). \quad (6.4)$$

Therefore the posterior distribution of θ given $(\mathbf{X}, \mathbf{Y}_{obs})$ is the above likelihood function multiplied by $d\pi(\theta)$, where π is the prior distribution of θ. Rubin (1978) uses exchangeability and deFinetti's theorem to argue why it is natural to assume $(Y_{i,obs}, \mathbf{X}_i)$ to be conditionally i.i.d. given θ in (6.4). The posterior distribution of θ and the model for the assignment mechanism can then be used to compute the posterior predictive distribution (6.3). Little and Rubin (2000) say that this Bayesian missing data approach to model-based inference is "the most general and conceptually satisfying," and Rubin (2005) points out the "central role" of (6.3) and (6.4) in Bayesian inference for causal effects and important role of deFinetti's theorem underlying (6.4): Exchangeability of $(\mathbf{X}_i, Y_i(t), Y_i(c))$ in the Bayesian model implies that they are conditionally i.i.d., hence parametric models for Bayesian causal inference should have likelihood functions satisfying (6.4).

6.3 Causal inference from observational studies

Freedman (2005) says: "When using observational (non-experimental) data to make causal inferences, the key problem is confounding. Sometimes this problem is handled by subdividing the study population...and sometimes by modeling. These strategies have various strengths and weaknesses." He goes on to point out:

> In an observational study, it is the subjects who assign themselves to the different groups. The investigators just watch what happens.... Heart attacks, lung cancer, and many other diseases are more common among smokers. There is strong *association* between smoking and disease.... Generally, association is circumstantial evidence for causation. However, the proof is incomplete. There may be some hidden confounding factor that makes people smoke and also makes them sick.... Confounding means a difference between the treatment and control groups — other than the treatment — which affects the response being studied. Typically, a confounder is a third variable, which is associated with exposure and influences the risk of disease.

6.3.1 Matching, subclassification, and standardization

Matching, or more precisely *matched sampling*, refers to forming a sample of size n from the set of observed $(X_i, Y_i(c)), i = 1, ..., rn$, from the control group (with $r \geq 1$) so that the covariate values X_i's match (in some way) the $\tilde{X}_j$'s in the observations $(\tilde{X}_j, Y_j(t)), j = 1, ..., n$, from the treatment group. Rothman (1986, p.237) points out difficulties in carrying out matching for some complex observational studies:

> The topic of matching in epidemiology is beguiling: What at first seems clear is seductively deceptive. Whereas the clarity of an analysis in which confounding has been securely prevented by perfect matching of the compared series seems indubitable and impossible to misinterpret, the intuitive foundation for this cogency attained by matching is a surprisingly shaky structure that does not always support the conclusions that are apt to be drawn. The difficulty is that our intuition about matching springs from knowledge of experiments or follow-up studies, whereas matching is most often applied in case-control studies, which differ enough from follow-up studies to make the implications of matching different and counterintuitive... In case-control studies the effectiveness of matching as a methodological tool derives from its effect on study efficiency, not on validity.

Case-control studies identify subjects by outcome status in the study design. Suppose the outcome is whether the subject is diagnosed with a disease during the course of the study. The cases are those who have the disease during the period, and the inclusion and exclusion criteria for their selection should be specific about the stage of disease and other covariates to ensure homogeneity among cases. The control group should come from the same source of population that is at risk for the disease. Matching attempts to ensure comparability between cases and control and thereby to reduce variability and systematic differences due to background variables. In contrast, follow-up or cohort studies are longitudinal studies in which two or more groups of subjects that are free of the disease at the outset and that differ according to the extent of exposure to a potential cause of the disease are compared with respect to incidence of the disease in each of the groups.

Subclassification is another method of adjustment for confounding. The treatment and control groups are divided into subclasses or strata on the basis of the covariate X, so that each subclass can be regarded as having approximately the same values of X. Although the method is natural for discrete X that takes on a relatively small number of values, it encounters major difficulties when the covariate vector X is continuous and has a large number of components. In Section 6.3.3 we resolve this difficulty by using the potential score $e(\mathbf{X})$ instead of X to carry out subclassification.

Standardization refers to reweighting the observations for confounder control. Chapter 5 at Rothman (1986) describes this basic concept in the context of comparing rates among different populations. Although the problem appears to be straightforward, it is subject to distortions in practice, as illustrated in his example, which compares the 1962 mortality in Sweden with that in Panama, Sweden, with a population of 7,496,000, had 73,555 deaths for an annual mortality rate of 0.0098, whereas Panama, with a population of 1,075,000, had 7,781 deaths[1] for an annual mortality rate of 0.0072. Although this seems to suggest that Panamanians live longer than Swedes, Rothman (1986) says:

> Apparently the mortality rate in Sweden was a third greater than that in Panama. Before concluding that life in Sweden in 1962 was considerably more risky than life in Panama, we should examine the mortality rates according to age.... For people under age 60, the mortality rate was greater in Panama; for people age 60 or older, it was 10 percent greater in Sweden than in Panama. The age-specific comparisons, showing less mortality in Sweden until age 60, after which mortality in the two countries is similar, presents an extremely different impression than the comparison of the over-

---

[1]There is a typo that showed 7,871 on Rothman (1986, p.41), which should be 7,781 according to his Table 5.1.

all mortality without regard to age.... The mortality experience of Panamanians in 1962 was dominated by the 69 percent of them who were under age 30, whereas in Sweden only 42 percent of the population was under 30. The lower mortality rate for Panama can be accounted for by the fact that Panamanians were younger than Swedes, and younger people tend to have a lower mortality rate the older people.

Standardization provides a way to address the distortion introduced by the different age distributions, and there are "direct" and "indirect" standardization methods in biostatistics and epidemiology.

For mortality rates, suppose there are k age groups, with death rates $\alpha_1, ..., \alpha_k$ in the study population and $\beta_1, ..., \beta_k$ in the standard population. Let $A_1, ..., A_k$ be the sample sizes in the study populations and $B_1, ..., B_k$ be those in the standard population. Hence $\sum_{i=1}^{k} A_i \alpha_i$ is the total number of deaths in the study population, unadjusted for the age distribution. Indirect standardization applies the age-specific death rates for the standard (unexposed) population to the age distribution of the study (exposed) population, yielding the counterfactual number of deaths in the study population if the rates were the same as those in the standard population. It yields the *standardized mortality ratio*

$$\text{SMR} = \frac{\sum_{i=1}^{k} A_i \alpha_i}{\sum_{i=1}^{k} A_i \beta_i}, \tag{6.5}$$

which basically applies *indirect standardization* to the denominator. In contrast, direct standardization takes a weighted average of the age-specific rates of the exposed population, with the weights given by the unexposed distribution. It yields the *direct standardized rate*

$$\text{SR} = \sum_{i=1}^{k} \left(\frac{B_i}{\sum_{j=1}^{k} B_j} \right) \alpha_i = \frac{\sum_{i=1}^{k} B_i \alpha_i}{\sum_{i=1}^{k} B_i}. \tag{6.6}$$

Keiding and Clayton (2014) point out that for binary outcomes and exposures, "each individual may be thought of as having a different risk for each exposure state, even though only one state can be observed in practice" (as in potential outcomes). They point out that if risks depend on a discrete confounder (e.g., age group) besides exposure, then the *causal risk ratio* for the exposed population can be estimated by the SMR, and the death rate in the unexposed population of subjects had they been exposed can be estimated by SR.

6.3.2 Propensity score: Theory and implementation

Rosenbaum and Rubin (1983) introduce the concept of balancing scores and the propensity score (PS) in particular. A *balancing score* b($\mathbf{X}$) is a function of the observed covariate vector $\mathbf{X}_i$ such that the conditional distribution of $\mathbf{X}_i$ given $\mathbf{b}(\mathbf{X}_i)$ is conditionally independent of the treatment assignment variable T_i, written $\mathbf{X}_i \perp\!\!\!\perp T_i | \mathbf{b}(\mathbf{X}_i)$. Rosenbaum and Rubin (1983) consider the case of binary T, taking the values 0 and 1, and define the *propensity score* by

$$e(\mathbf{X}_i) = \mathrm{P}(T_i = 1 | \mathbf{X}_i), \tag{6.7}$$

hence $\mathrm{P}(T_1, ..., T_n | \mathbf{X}_1, ..., \mathbf{X}_n) = \prod_{i=1}^{n} \{e(\mathbf{X}_i)\}^{T_i} \{1 - e(\mathbf{X}_i)\}^{1-T_i}$. They call a treatment assignment mechanism *strongly ignorable* if $(Y_i(0), Y_i(1)) \perp\!\!\!\perp T_i | \mathbf{b}(\mathbf{X}_i)$, noting that in this case of binary T_i, there are two potential outcomes $Y_i(0)$ and $Y_i(1)$. More generally, the treatment assignment is strongly ignorable given $\mathbf{b}(\mathbf{X}_i)$ if $(Y_i(0), Y_i(1)) \perp\!\!\!\perp T | \mathbf{X}_i$. They derive the following properties of balancing scores and the propensity score:

(a) The propensity score is a balancing score; moreover, $\mathbf{b}(\mathbf{x}) = \mathbf{x}$ is the finest balancing score and the propensity score is the coarsest.

(b) If a treatment assignment is strongly ignorable given $\mathbf{X}_i$, then it is strongly ignorable given any balancing score $\mathbf{b}(\mathbf{X}_i)$.

(c) For any strongly ignorable assignment, pair-matching or subclassification using a balancing score b gives an unbiased estimate of the treatment effect $\mathrm{E}\{Y(t) - Y(c)\}$.

Since the propensity score (6.7) is a probability given the covariate vector, it can be estimated from the observed data $(T_i, \mathbf{X}_i), i = 1, ..., n$, by fitting the logistic regression model

$$\mathrm{P}(T_i = 1 | \mathbf{X}_i) = \frac{1}{1 + e^{-(\alpha + \boldsymbol{\beta}^T \mathbf{X}_i)}} = 1 - \mathrm{P}(T_i = 0 | \mathbf{X}_i), \tag{6.8}$$

which is most commonly used because of the wide availability of statistical software to implement logistic regression.

6.3.3 Control for confounding via estimated PS

This section describes how the estimated propensity score can be used in each of the three approaches to control for confounding in Section 6.3.1.

Matching. As noted in Section 6.3.1, although matching is a popular method to select control subjects to match the treated subjects on potentially confounding covariates, it encounters difficulties when there are many covariates. For multivariate covariates, Mahalanobis metric matching uses the Mahalanobis distance $d(i, j) = (\mathbf{X}_i - \mathbf{X}_j)^T \mathbf{C}^{-1}(\mathbf{X}_i - \mathbf{X}_j)$ to match a treated subject i and control subject j, where $\mathbf{C}$ is the sample covariance matrix of the covariates from the control subjects, and the matching scheme chooses subject j with minimum distance $d(i, j)$ from the existing pool of control subjects and then removes the subject from the pool after matching with treated subject i, repeating the procedure until matches are found for all treated subjects. After introducing the propensity score to address issues of matching using the Mahalanobis metric when there are many covariates, Rosenbaum and Rubin (1985) describe the following methods that use the estimated propensity score to construct a matched sample:

(i) Nearest available matching on the estimated propensity score: First randomly order the treated and control subjects. Then select the first treated subject and find the control subject j with the smallest $\hat{q}(\mathbf{X}_j) := \log[(1 - \hat{e}(\mathbf{X}_j))/\hat{e}(\mathbf{X}_j)] = -\text{logit}(\hat{e}(\mathbf{X}_j))$.

(ii) Nearest available Mahalanobis metric matching within calipers defined by the propensity score: After randomly ordering the treated subjects, the first treated subject is selected and labeled i. All control subjects within a preset amount (or *caliper*) of the treated subject's $\hat{e}(\mathbf{X}_i)$ are then selected for computing the Mahalanobis distances from the treated subject's $\mathbf{X}_i$. The closest control subject and the treated subject are removed from the pool, and matching is then repeated for the remaining subjects. By defining calipers based on the propensity score, this method resembles blocking in experimental designs.

Stuart (2010) summarizes further developments of matching methods using propensity scores. She points out that previous methods can basically be characterized by the "distance measure" between treated subject i and control subject j. Besides the Mahalanobis distance $d(i,j)$ above, she also mentions $d_1(i,j) = |\hat{e}(\mathbf{X}_i) - \hat{e}(\mathbf{X}_j)|$ or $d_2(i,j) = |\text{logit}(\hat{e}(\mathbf{X}_i)) - \text{logit}(\hat{e}(\mathbf{X}_j))|$. Moreover, Mahalanobis matching within propensity score calipers in method (ii) above corresponds to the distance measure

$$d_3(i,j) = \begin{cases} d(i,j) & \text{if } d_2(i,j) \le c \\ \infty & \text{if } d_2(i,j) > c, \end{cases}$$

in which c is the caliper. Concerning the choice of c, she says:

When the variance of the linear propensity score in the treatment groups is twice as large as that in the control group, a caliper of 0.2 standard deviation removes 98% of the bias in a normally distributed covariate. If the variance in the treatment group is much larger than that in the control group, smaller calipers are necessary.

By linear propensity score, she means that given by the generalized linear model, as in $\alpha + \beta^T \mathbf{X}$ in (6.8). With the distance measure specified, matching methods like those in (i) and (ii) above are basically greedy nearest neighbor matching. She also points out variants of these methods, such as $k : 1$ nearest neighbor matching, ratio matching, and matching with replacement.

Stuart (2010, Section 4) emphasizes the importance of diagnosing the quality of the resulting matched samples in using matching methods, saying that "all matching should be followed by an assessment of covariate balance in the matched groups, where balance is defined as the similarity of the empirical distributions of the full set of covariates in the matched treated and control groups." Although comparing the multidimensional histograms of the covariates in the matched treated (t) and control (c) groups is an obvious diagnostic, she notices that "multidimensional histograms are very coarse and/or will have many zero cells", hence "balance metrics" based on lower-dimensional summaries of the multivariate joint distributions. One set of metrics is the standardized difference $\left(\bar{X}_{t_i} - \bar{X}_{c_i}\right)/s_t$ in means of each covariate (labeled by i), where s_t is the "standard deviation in the full treated group". She also describes another set of balance metrics, proposed by Rubin (2001) using propensity scores: (a) standardized difference of means of the propensity score in the treated and control groups, (b) ratio of variances of the propensity score, and (c) ratio of the variance of residuals orthogonal to the propensity score in the treated and control groups, for each covariate. She argues that commonly used hypothesis tests and p-values "should not be used as measures of balance" because "they often conflate changes in balance with changes in statistical power" and because "balance is inherently an in-sample property, without reference to any broader population or super-population." She also discusses the usefulness of graphical diagnostics for getting a visual assessment of covariate balance, saying:

> With many covariates it can be difficult to carefully examine numeric diagnostics for each...A first step is to examine the distribution of the propensity scores in the original and matched groups; this is also useful for assessing common support... For continuous covariates, we can also examine quantilequantile (QQ) plots, which compare the empirical distributions of each variable in the treated and control groups, ... (checking whether the plotted quartiles are close) to the 45 degree line... Finally, a plot of the standardized differences of means (of individual covariates, in the same figure) gives us a quick overview of whether balance has improved (after matching) for individual covariates

Stuart et al. (2013, Figure 1) introduce a new way, different from Figure 2 of Stuart (2010), of plotting and labeling the individual standardized differences of means before matching (using the hollow circles) and after matching (using solid red circles). They also recommended carrying out sensitivity analysis to unobserved confounding: "To assess how sensitive results are to an unobserved confounder, ... ask questions such as: How strongly related to treatment and to outcome would some unobserved have to be to change my results" or "posit an unobserved confounder and obtain adjusted impact estimates if that confounder existed, given its assumed characteristics (e.g., its prevalence, its associations with treatment, etc.)."

Stratification. Section 6.3.1 has pointed out difficulties with subclassification (or stratification) when the number of continuous covariates increases, resulting in an exponential growth of the corresponding number subclasses. The propensity score $e(\mathbf{X}_i)$, which is a scalar summary of the covariates, can be used in lieu of $\mathbf{X}_i$ for stratification. Rosenbaum and Rubin (1983, Theorem 1) have shown that treatment assignment and the observed covariates are conditionally independent given the propensity score. Hence subclassification on the population propensity score $e(\mathbf{X})$ balances $\mathbf{X}$ in the sense that within subclasses that are homogeneous in $e(\mathbf{X})$, the distribution of $\mathbf{X}$ is the same for the treated and control units. In practice, $e(\mathbf{X})$ is not known and one has to stratify based on the estimated propensity score $\hat{e}(\mathbf{X})$. Rosenbaum and Rubin (1984) illustrate that replacing $e(\mathbf{X})$ by $\hat{e}(\mathbf{X})$ can remove over 90% of the bias with 5 strata. One can use quantiles of the estimated propensity score $e(\mathbf{X}_i)$, $1 \le i \le n$, to be the subclass boundaries.

Weighting. Stratification (or weighting adjustments as discussed in Section 6.3.1) can also make use of propensity scores. An issue mentioned by Stuart (2010) in applying propensity scores is that of "common support". In some situations there may not be complete overlap of the propensity score distributions in the treated and control groups. Although nearest neighbor matching with calipers automatically uses subjects (units) in the area of common support, the subclassification and weighting methods typically use all units regardless of the overlap of the distributions. Dehejia and Wahba (1999) propose to restrict to units in the region of common support. We have considered so far the propensity score in the setting of binary treatment assignment mechanism, i.e., $\mathcal{J} = \{t, c\}$. Dehejia and Wahba (2004) have generalized the propensity score, which is the conditional probability density function (with respect to some measure in $\mathbb{R}$ or $\mathbb{R}^p$) of the treatment assignment mechanism, to the case where $\mathcal{J}$ is categorical, ordinal, or subintervals of $\mathbb{R}$ or $\mathbb{R}^p$. They call the generalization a *propensity function* and propose using a parametric family of density functions to specify $e(\mathbf{X}; \theta) \in \mathcal{J}$ so that estimation can be carried out via maximum likelihood.

Lee et al. (2010) argue for the use of machine learning in lieu of fitting the logistic regression model (6.8) in estimating the propensity score for PS weighting:

Propensity scores are generally estimated using logistic regression. However, parametric models require assumptions regarding variable selection, the functional form and distributions of variables, and specification of interactions. If any of these assumptions are incorrect, covariate balance may not be achieved by conditioning on the propensity score, which may result in a biased effect estimate... Machine learning is a general term for a diverse number of classification and prediction algorithms... Machine learning tries to extract the relationship between outcome and predictor through a learning algorithm without an *a priori* data model.... Because decision trees are common in medical research for diagnostic and prognostic purposes and are intuitive to visualize and understand, they are a natural starting point for a discussion of machine learning algorithms. Decision trees partition a data set into regions such that within each region, observations are as homogeneous as possible.... of the splits.

They refer to earlier simulation studies by Setoguchi et al. (2008) showing the superiority of CART and neural networks over logistic regression in using propensity scores to select matched samples and also use bagging and gradient boosting to enhance CART; see Section 2.1.3 and Supplement 2 of Section 2.7 for the background of these and other machine learning methods. Their simulation studies show that "regardless of sample size or the extent of non-additivity or non-linearity", random forest, bagged CART and boosted CART propensity score models "provided excellent performance in terms of covariate balance and (treatment) effect estimation" that is "consistently superior" over logistic regression. They also say:

> One criticism of machine learning is 'black box' nature of the algorithms obscures the relationship between predictors and outcome. However, etiologic inference is not a necessary component of propensity score estimation. Therefore, machine learning techniques may be well suited to the task of creating propensity scores from high-dimensional data, where improper parametric specification of relationships may lead to biased estimates.

6.3.4 Inverse probability weighting

Inverse probability weighting (IPW) is a standardization technique that reweights each observation in the sample by taking the reciprocal (hence inverse) of the sampling probability of the observation from a target population. A classic example is the *Horvitz-Thompson estimator* $\sum Y_i/\pi_i$ (in which $\sum$ denotes the sum over distinct values of a sample $Y_1, ..., Y_n$) of the sum $\sum_{j=1}^{J} \mu_j$ of a finite population, where π_i represents the probability that the sampling scheme selects μ_k if $Y_i = \mu_k$. Dividing Y_i by π_i yields an unbiased estimator. Another important class of IPWEs (in which E stands for "estimator") arises from comparing event rates (such as death rates) for exposed and unexposed populations in the presence of other risk factors (covariates). In the first and third paragraphs of Section 3.5.2, we have already mentioned the Robins-Rotnitzky inverse probability weighted estimator (Robins and Rotnitzky, 1992) for missing data processes.

Keiding and Clayton (2014, section 6) connect IPW for survival data to model-based analysis of the standardized mortality ratios, dating back to Kilpatrick (1962) in using the standardized mortality ratio SMR (see Section 6.3.1) to compare the mortality rates of the study treatment population to those in the study control population, adjusting for age via maximum likelihood under the assumption of a Poisson model for age-specific death rates in the standard population and a constant mortality ratio (across age groups) of treatment to control. Keiding and Clayton (2014, pp. 546, 500) say that "Kilpatrick had opened the way to a fully model-based analysis of (indirectly standardized) rates" and that two landmark papers of this approach were Mantel (1966) who regarded the comparison of survival between two groups as "analysis of a $2 \times 2 \times K$ table in which the K trials are defined by the time points at which deaths occurred in the study (other time points being uninformative)", and Cox (1972) who generalized this idea by using a log-linear regression model for the "instantaneous risk, or hazard" so that hazard ratios can incorporate the "effects of each risk factor". Keiding and Clayton (2014, p. 551) then highlight the next development to address "time-dependent confounding" in Cox's hazards regression model:

> Kalbfleisch and Prentice (1980, pp. 124–126) pointed out a serious difficulty (of Cox's regression model) in dealing with "internal" (endogenous) time-dependent covariates.... A censoring scheme that depends on the level of a time dependent $z(t)$ ... not independent if $z(t)$ is not included in the model... Put in another way, to ignore such a variable in the analysis is to disregard its confounding effect, but its inclusion in the conditional probability model could obscure some of the true causal effect of treatment. While Kalbfleisch and Prentice have identified a fundamental problem with the conditional approach to confounder adjustment, they offered no convincing remedy. This was left to Robins (1986).

Marginal structural models, g-estimation algorithm and IPWE. As pointed out by Robins et al. (2000), marginal structural models (MSMs) are "causal models for the estimation, from observational data, of the causal effect of a time-dependent exposure in the presence of time-dependent covariates that may be simultaneously confounders and intermediate variables" and the MSM parameters can be consistently estimated by IPWE. They also say that "MSMs are an alternative to improvement of structural nested models, the parameters of which are estimated through the methods of g-estimation." We first describe how Robins (1986) uses *measured causally interpreted structured tree graphs* (MCISTGs) to adjust for time-dependent confounding in survival analysis; these structured tree graphs (STGs) are the "structural nested models" in the preceding quote. The basic underlying idea is to identify an observational study with a "double-blind randomized trial with data on treatment protocol missing (but with available) data on date of death, observed exposure history and date of leaving treatment protocol." Under some mild temporal assumptions (which are not empirically testable from the available data) on each individual i in such a trial, Robins (1986, Section 2C) notes that by not conditioning on i, the population relationships in the temporal assumptions take the following identifiable (i.e., empirically verifiable) form:

(a) Treatments differ only through exposure concentrations.

(b) An individual who leaves protocol will not return.

(c) Treatment protocols do not depend on time-dependent covariates after time of randomization.

Robins (1986, Figure 3.4) illustrates how these temporal assumptions hold in a subgraph, which corresponds to high exposure concentration in a randomized trial on occupational mortality and which is an MCISTG, with time points t_1 (time of hire) $< t_2$ (observation time when some subjects have left job) $< t_3$ (another observation time before study termination):

> At t_1, the (trial) investigator gives (these) individuals high exposure. Nature determines survival and employment status through t_2. For individuals at work at t_2, the investigator again gives each high exposure; nature then determines their survival and employment status through t_3. For individuals off work at t_2, nature gives each zero exposure at t_2, and then determines their survival and employment status through t_3. For those at work at t_3, the investigator gives each high exposure.

He notes the essential difference between this sustained exposure and the "point exposure" of Rubin (1978) and Rosenbaum and Rubin (1983, 1984) is that "in a sustained exposure study, covariates measured at times after the start of follow-up may also be treatments." He defines the population g-causal parameter comparing two treatment protocols G_1 and G_2 of an MCISTG as the difference between the population survival curves for G_1 and G_2, and develops a G-computation algorithm to compute the probability of survival (to any observation time t) in a "fully randomized" MCISTG, as in the randomization performed by nature in his Figure 3.4.

Robins et al. (2000, pp. 552-554) assume that "the study subjects are a random sample from a large, possibly hypothetical, source population", from whom the causal effect of a dichotomous treatment A_0 (taking the value of 1 for new treatment and 0 for standard /control) on a binary outcome Y is measured by the mean causal risk difference $P(Y = 1|A_0 = 1) - P(Y = 1|A_0 = 0)$, or causal risk ratio $P(Y = 1|A_0 = 1)/P(Y = 1|A_0 = 0)$, or causal odds ratio

$$\frac{P(Y = 1|A_0 = 1)}{P(Y = 0|A_0 = 1)} \Big/ \frac{P(Y = 1|A_0 = 0)}{P(Y = 0|A_0 = 0)}. \tag{6.9}$$

These probabilities are counterfactual when conditional on individual subjects who can only receive either new or standard treatment, and Robins et al. (2000) use the linear model $P(Y = 1|A_0) = \psi_0 + \psi_1 A_0$, or log-linear model $\log P(Y = 1|A_0) = \theta_0 + \theta_1 A_0$, or linear logistic model

$$\text{logit} P(Y = 1|A_0) = \beta_0 + \beta_1 A_0, \tag{6.10}$$

to express the causal effects in terms of the parameters of these models, which they call *saturated MSMs*:

> They are *marginal* models, because they model marginal distribution of the counterfactual random variables $Y_{A_0=1}$ and $Y_{A_0=0}$ rather than the joint distribution ... They are *structural* models because they model the probabilities of counterfactual variables (which are often referred to as structural models in the economic and social science literature). Finally, they are *saturated* because (they are) two parameters for the two unknown probabilities $P(Y_{A_0=1} = 1)$ and $P(Y_{A_0=0} = 1)$.

They use $Y_{A_0=1}$ (respectively, $Y_{A_0=0}$) to denote the binary outcome variable of the subject who receives the new treatment (respectively, the standard treatment). They then explain how inverse probability weighting can be used to estimate the causal parameters ψ_0, ψ_1 (or $\theta_0, \theta_1; \beta_0, \beta_1$) when there are no unmeasured confounders given data on the measured covariates:

> Using the weight statement (i.e., option SCWGT) in PROC GENMOD (of SAS), each subject i is assigned a weight w_i equal to the inverse of the conditional probability of receiving his or her own treatment... Why does this approach work? The effect of weighting in PROC GENMOD is to create a pseudopopulation consisting of w_i copies of each subject i... This new pseudopopulation has the following two important properties. First, in the pseudopopulation, unlike the actual population, A_0 is unconfounded by the measured covariates. Second, $P(Y_{A_0=1} = 1)$ and $P(Y_{A_0=0} = 1)$ in the pseudopopulation are the same as in the true study population... Hence, it follows that we can unbiasedly estimate the causal effects... But this is exactly what our inverse-probability of treatment weights estimator (IPTW) does.

Robins et al. (2000, pp. 557, 560) show that IPWE is biased "and thus MSMs should not be used in studies in which at each time k there is a covariate level such that all subjects with that level of the covariate are certain to receive the identical treatment A_k." They also say that "Nevertheless, g-estimation of structural nested models can always be used to estimate exposure effects, even in studies in which MSMs cannot be used."

Doubly robust estimators of causal effects. As noted by Funk et al. (2011), doubly robust estimation "combines outcome regression (to adjust for confounding in epidemiological analysis) with weighting by propensity score" such that only one of the two approaches needs to be "consistent (and therefore asymptotically unbiased)" and therefore doubly robust as originally introduced by Robins et al. (1994, 1995). Let $X = 1$ (or 0) if exposed (or unexposed) to the treatment, and let $\mathbf{Z} = (Z_1, \ldots, Z_k)$ be the vector of covariates, measured at baseline (prior to exposure). The regression approach relates outcome Y to $(X, \mathbf{Z})$ by

$$E(Y|X, \mathbf{Z}) = \alpha + \beta_0 X + \beta_1 Z_1 + \ldots, +\beta_k Z_k, \qquad (6.11)$$

in which β_0 can be interpreted as the mean difference in Y due to exposure, adjusted for the other covariates in the model. If there are no additional unmeasured covariates and the regression model (6.11) is correctly specified, consistent estimates of β_0 address the confounding issue; see Section 6.5 for further background and details of this approach. Alternatively, one can estimate the propensity score (PS) by fitting

$$\mathrm{logit} P(X = 1|\mathbf{Z}) = \beta + b_1 Z_1 + \ldots + b_k Z_k, \qquad (6.12)$$

and weight an exposed individual by 1/PS and an exposed individual by 1/(1 - PS), as in inverse probability weighting. Robins et al. (2007) point out that the inverse probability weights can be highly variable in the sense that "a small subset of the sample will give extremely large weights relative to the remainder of the sample" if (6.12) is misspecified or if the model parameters are not well estimated. In this case IPWE performs poorly, but "augmenting" it by the regression model (6.11) can still have reasonable performance. The *augmented inverse probability weighted estimator* (AIPWE) of the causal effect $\Delta = E\left(Y_{A_0=1}\right) - E\left(Y_{A_0=0}\right)$, also called the *doubly robust* (DR) estimator for which Funk et al. (2011) have developed a SAS© macro DR, can be expressed in the form

$$\hat{\Delta}_{\mathrm{DR}} = \frac{1}{n} \sum_{i:X_i=1} \left\{ \frac{Y_i}{\hat{e}_n(\mathbf{Z}_i)} - \frac{1 - \hat{e}_n(\mathbf{Z}_i)}{\hat{e}_n(\mathbf{Z}_i)} \hat{Y}_{1,i} \right\}$$

$$- \frac{1}{n} \sum_{i:X_i=0} \left\{ \frac{Y_i}{1 - \hat{e}_n(\mathbf{Z}_i)} - \frac{\hat{e}_n(\mathbf{Z}_i)}{1 - \hat{e}_n(\mathbf{Z}_i)} \hat{Y}_{0,i} \right\},$$

in which $\hat{e}_n(\mathbf{Z_i})$ is the estimated propensity score (by fitting the logistic regression model (6.12) to $\{(X_i, \mathbf{Z}_i), 1 \leq i \leq n\}$ and $\hat{Y}_{1,i}$ (respectively, $\hat{Y}_{0,i}$) is the predicted outcome given $X_i = 1$ (respectively, $X_i = 0$) using the fitted model for $E(Y|X, \mathbf{Z})$ assuming (6.11) or more general regression models. Note that $Y_i/\hat{e}_n(\mathbf{Z}_i)$ for $X_i = 1$ (or $Y_i/\{1 - \hat{e}_n(\mathbf{Z}_i)\}$ for $X_i = 0$) corresponds to IPWE, and $-(1 - \hat{e}_n(\mathbf{Z}_i))\hat{Y}_{1,i}/\hat{e}_n(\mathbf{Z}_i)$ for $X_i = 1$ (or $-\hat{e}_n(\mathbf{Z}_i)\hat{Y}_{0,i}/\{1 - \hat{e}_n(\mathbf{Z}_i)\}$ for $X_i = 0$) corresponds to the augmentation in AIPWE, which basically uses the sample average $n^{-1}\sum_{i:X_i=1}\{\ldots\}$ to estimate $E(Y_{A_0=1})$ and $n^{-1}\sum_{i:X_i=0}\{\ldots\}$ to estimate $E(Y_{A_0=0})$.

6.3.5 Structural model for latent failure time

Robins (1992) illustrates confounding due to "treatment by indication" in survival analysis with the following example from an observational study of the effect on survival of AZT (zidovudine) for the treatment of AIDS (acquired immunodeficiency syndrome) in HIV-infected subjects, saying that AZT has toxic effects that can worsen the anemia in anemic patients who are at increased risk of death. Thus, "anemia is both a risk factor for death and a predictor of subsequent treatment with AZT" as an HIV-infected subject who is not (respectively, who is) currently treated with AZT must decide with the physician whether to initiate (respectively, to discontinue or modify the dose for) AZT treatment. Suppose measurements on the covariates are recorded at times $k = 0, 1, \ldots$. Let T_i be the survival time, $L_{0,i}$ be the vector of time-independent covariates (such as race, sex) of subject i, and $L_{k,i}$ the vector of time-dependent covariate measurements at time k. Let $A_{k-1,i}$ be the dosage rate in the time interval from time $k - 1$ to k (when the dose is reset). Let $\bar{L}_{k,i} = (L_{0,i}, \ldots, L_{k,i})$ and $\bar{A}_{k-1,i} = (A_{0,i}, \ldots, A_{k-1,i})$. Following Rubin (1978), Cox and Oakes (1984), and Robins (1987), Robins (1992) assumes that (a) there exists a latent failure time U_i for survival time of subject i if the AZT treatment had always been withheld from the subject and that

$$U_i \perp\!\!\!\perp A_{k,i} \text{ conditional on } (\bar{L}_{k,i}, \bar{A}_{k-1,i}, T_i > k), \qquad (6.13)$$

and that (b) V_i is related to $A_i(t)$, the dosage rate at time u, by

$$U_i = \int_0^{T_i} e^{\psi_0 A_i(t)} dt, \qquad (6.14)$$

where $\psi_0 \in \mathbb{R}$ is an unknown parameter, "following Cox and Oakes (1984, §5.2)". Robins and Tsiatis (1992) consider a more general vector $\mathbf{Z}_i(t) \in \mathbb{R}^p$ of time-dependent covariates than $A_i(t) \in \mathbb{R}$, and use $\bar{\mathbf{Z}}_i(t) = \{Z_i(s), 0 \leq s \leq t\}$ to denote the "history of the covariate process through time t" and a more general function $h(\mathbf{Z}_i(t), \beta)$ than $\exp\left(\beta^T \mathbf{Z}_i(t)\right)$ in defining the latent failure time. Using the transformation $u = \psi\left(\bar{\mathbf{Z}}(t), \beta\right) = \int_0^t h\left(\mathbf{Z}_i(s), \beta\right) dt$, which means that "an individual who lived T_i years with a specific history of exposure would have lived U_i years if unexposed", they note that $du/dt = h\left(\mathbf{Z}_i(t), \beta\right)$ represents the "relative rate at which baseline time is being used up compared to the actual time as a function of the history of exposure, $\bar{Z}(t)$, up to that time." To allow for right censoring, let C denote the subject's potential censoring time so that one observes $\left(\delta_i, T_i \wedge C_i, \bar{Z}(T_i \wedge C_i)\right)$, where $\delta_i = I_{(T_i \leq C_i)}$. A rank-preserving structural modeling approach that uses linear rank tests censored data has been developed by Tsiatis (1990); see also Lai and Ying (1991). Robins and Tsiatis (1992) use these methods and results for testing $\beta = \beta_0$ and constructing confidence intervals for β.

6.4 Unmeasured confounding: Instrumental variables and research designs

6.4.1 Instrumental variables

When the data do not appear to capture all inputs that predict both the treatment and the outcome, it could be due to unobserved variables that are causing outcome differences across groups. The method of instrumental variables controls confounding as it allows consistent parameter estimation in the presence of correlation between explanatory variables and residual errors. Baiocchi et al. (2014) discuss some common sources of instrumental variables for health studies. Consider the linear model $Y = \beta X + \epsilon$ where Y is the outcome variable, X the treatment variable, and ϵ the error term. X is exogenous if X and ϵ are uncorrelated. On the other hand, X is endogenous if it is correlated with the error term ϵ. Here, ϵ is affecting X and therefore indirectly affecting Y. An instrumental variable, Z, is associated with X but not with Y. It randomly induces variation in X and assumes that (a) Z is correlated with X; (b) Z is uncorrelated with ϵ, the error term (the exclusion restriction); and (c) Z is not a direct cause of Y, which can be represented graphically as in Figure 6.1. Section 6.5 gives further details and background of graphical models of causal effects, and of "conditional independence" which has already been introduced in Section 6.3.2 in the definition of strong ignorability.

An instrumental variable (IV) therefore only affects the outcome through its effect on the treatment. In practice, it is often challenging to find instruments since many of them do not satisfy the exclusion restriction (b). To estimate β in the IV-regression model $Y = \beta X + \epsilon$, a standard method is two-stage least squares (2SLS). In the first stage, the treatment variable is regressed on the instrument and a set of covariates to obtain coefficients that reflect the amount of variation in treatment attributable to the instrument. The predicted values from the first-stage regression

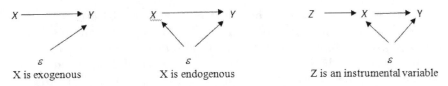

FIGURE 6.1 Illustration of an exogenous, endogenous, and instrumental variable.

are then used in the second stage to obtain an estimate of the relation of treatment to outcome. The coefficient of the second-stage model is the estimate of the causal effect of the treatment of the instrumental variable on the outcome. This two-stage estimation strategy is especially useful for more complicated versions of the model, e.g., when multiple instruments are included. The parameter estimates thus generated are consistent but can be biased. Angrist and Pischke (2014) discuss the following issues concerning standard errors and bias of the 2SLS procedure. The IV-regression model is said to be *just-identified* if there is one instrument for each endogenous variable. In this case, the estimator is unbiased. The model is *under-identified* if there are fewer instruments than endogenous variables. These models have an infinite number of solutions. An *over-identified* model has more instruments than endogenous variables. As a general rule, at least as many instruments as treatment variables should be used in order for all the causal estimates to be identifiable. The two-stage least squares method can be extended to accommodate continuous treatment variables and instruments, although it can complicate the interpretation of the causal effects. Instruments that explain little of the variation of the endogenous variable are called *weak* instruments. A weak instrument has a low correlation with the endogenous variable. The IV estimate can be severely biased if the instruments are weak, or if many instruments are used for a single endogenous variable. Adding more weak instruments may also increase the bias of 2SLS.

6.4.2 Trend-in-trend research design of observational studies

Jones (2012) and Jones and Kingery (2014) review the methods in pharmacoepidemiology to assess causality for adverse events reported in post-marketing data, particularly spontaneous reports of these events. They note that "none (of these methods) ever achieves a *definitive* determination of causality," but that "public health needs and some regulatory bodies demand that estimates of causal association be used by drug developers, drug regulators, and clinicians to assess whether (and which) AEs are causally associated with a drug product." Their list of "obstacles" to causality assessment basically amounts to a list of unmeasured confounding, together with uncertainties in "the reporter's motivation for that assessment and the impact of that inference on their actions."

Ji et al. (2017) have recently introduced a novel design called "trend-in-trend" (TT) to address unmeasured confounding in observational studies as an alternative to instrumental variables, to relax the assumptions under which a calendar time IV study is valid. Although TT is equivalent to IV that uses calendar time as an instrument "if only a single stratum is used in the trend-in-trend design," they point out:

> However, use of calendar time as an IV can be biased by any time trend in the prevalence of an unmeasured factor that affects outcome. In contrast, the trend-in-trend design is biased by such a trend only if the time trend in the unmeasured factor is correlated with the time trends in exposure across strata defined by factors associated with exposure.

They have also applied TT to Clinformatics Databases (OptumInsight, Eden Prairie, MN) to examine the association between rofecoxib and acute myocardial infarction (AMI), severe hypoglycemia, and nonvertebral bone fracture. They first identify all persons age 18 years or older in Optum who received one or more prescriptions for rofecoxib during the study period from April 1, 2000 to December 30, 2004. For each rofecoxib-exposed person episode, they ascertain the first month and the last month of their continuous enrollment episode (or episodes, for persons with multiple enrollment episodes) during the study period; a period could contribute to multiple episodes. For each rofecoxib-exposed episode, they randomly sample without replacement 9 rofecoxib-unexposed enrollment episodes with an enrollment start date on or before no more than 1 year of the rofecoxib-exposed subjects enrollment start date, and with an enrollment end date on or after the rofecoxib-exposed subjects enrollment end date. They fit a logistic regression to estimate the cumulative probability of exposure using age, sex, diagnosis of rheumatoid arthritis, and diagnosis of osteoarthritis as explanatory variables. They use a method described below to stratify the population into $K = 5$ groups. Their analysis is able to reproduce the known positive association between rofecoxib and AMI for previous pharmacoepidemiologic studies using meta-analysis, and shows rofecoxib to have no statistically significant effect on severe hypoglycemia nor on nonvertebral bone fracture.

The "cumulative probability of exposure" mentioned in the preceding paragraph is the predicted probability of exposure over the entire study period, based on variables other than exposure, outcome, and their potential effects: "In particular, suppose we observe a population in which each individual's binary exposure status over the study period is observed" and "variables that affect but are known from subject-area knowledge not to be affected by exposure, such as age, sex, geographic residence, diagnoses, etc.," leading to the aforementioned logistic regression model that uses these variables as independent variables, with the dependent variable being exposure, so that the fitted value is the estimated cumulative probability of exposure. Ji et al. (2017) also point out that "the cumulative probability of exposure is similar to the propensity score, because both predict exposure, but differs from it in that the propensity score is used to balance observed covariates across exposure groups, while the cumulative probability of exposure is used to identify strata with different time trends in exposure." They note that estimation of the cumulative probability of exposure is the first stage of a "two-stage analysis" of the data from a TT design, the second stage of which is to provide a "quantitative estimate of a causal effect." They propose two models for such estimation, assuming that the study population consists of N individuals and there are T time periods, and letting $\mathbf{X}_i^t$ denote the vector of covariates associated with individual i at time t, which represents intrinsic characteristics that might influence a particular exposure and/or outcomes. Using their notation, we describe below their models and also their approach to stratification of the population by using the quantiles of the subject's estimated cumulative probability of exposure, under the assumption of a common distribution of the $\mathbf{X}_i^t$ that "can be observed, unobserved, or partially observed." The models are of the generalized linear type, with Z_i^t and Y_i^t denoting the exposure and outcome variables for subject i at time t, and g denoting the stratum to which this subject belongs.

Subject-specific model. For completely observed $\mathbf{X}_i^t$, this is a generalized linear model, with link function h, for the expected outcomes $\mu_i^t = E\left(Y_i^t | g, Z_i^t, \mathbf{X}_i^t\right)$:

$$h(\mu_i^t) = \beta_0 + \beta_1 Z_i^t + \beta_2 t + \boldsymbol{\gamma}^T \mathbf{X}_i^t. \tag{6.15}$$

If the $\mathbf{X}_i^t$ are unobserved, then (6.15) becomes a mixed effects model, with exposure and time being the fixed effects and the covariates of the individual being the random effects. An obvious generalization also yields a random effects model if the $\mathbf{X}_i^t$ are partially observed. The coefficient β_1 for exposure has a causal interpretation at the individual level. It is also the logarithm of the odds ratio when both exposure and outcome are binary, and the function of h is logit.

Population-average model. This model does not involve $\mathbf{X}_i^t$ and is a generalized linear model, with link function h^*, for the marginal expectation $\nu_i^t = E\left(Y_i^t | g, Z_i^t\right)$ of the subject-specific model:

$$h^*(\nu_i^t) = \beta_0^* + \beta_1^* Z_i^t + \beta_2^* t + C(Z_i^t, g), \tag{6.16}$$

in which the function C represents heterogeneity across exposed and unexposed groups. It does not require knowledge of covariates or assumptions of the heterogeneity across individuals. Its coefficients are directly estimable from the aggregated data on exposure and outcome, but do not have individual causal interpretation. Ji et al. (2017) refer to Zeger et al. (1988) in which details for identity, log, probit, and logit link functions are provided and corresponding mathematical relations between $(\beta_0, \beta_1, \beta_2)$ and $(\beta_0^*, \beta_1^*, \beta_2^*)$ are listed in detail. They also show that "under plausible assumptions, the trend-in-trend method is unconfounded by measured and unmeasured factors, provided that there are no trends in the prevalence of covariates that are correlated with the prevalence of the exposure over time."

Stratification based on estimated cumulative probability of exposure. Ji et al. (2017, p. 530) say that "because the unit of analysis for the cumulative probability of exposure model is the individual, and covariates are treated as invariant, each subject will be in the same cumulative probability of exposure stratum for all observation periods." Hence the subjects can be divided into K groups, using the quantiles of the estimated cumulative probabilities of exposure to define the group boundaries.

Advantages of the TT design to address unmeasured confounding in observational studies. Concerning the TT design, Ji et al. (2017) highlight its "causal contrast," defined as the "effect of use of the exposure of interest rather than the exposure(s) (if any) that the increasing (or declining) trend in use of the exposure of interest displaced (or was displaced by)", and that it "avoids the Achilles heel of most epidemiologic studies of healthcare interventions: conflation of receiving a treatment with needing that treatment." They also say:

> Unlike cohort studies, the trend-in-trend design does not assume no unmeasured confounders, but instead examines changes in outcome occurrence as a function of changes in exposure prevalence across strata with differential time trends in exposure. Therefore, the results of a trend-in-trend study will be unconfounded unless there are unmeasured factors affecting outcome for which there are time trends in prevalence that are correlated with time trends in exposure across the strata defined by exposure trend. This could occur if there are cointerventions for which the trend in use is positively correlated with trends in use of the exposure, or alternatives for which the trend in use is negatively correlated with trends in use of the exposure. As the scenarios that would produce a confounded trend-in-trend estimate are a subset of those that would produce a confounded cohort estimate, the trend-in-trend design is more resistant to confounding. However, the trend-in-trend design is feasible only if there is a strong time trend in exposure prevalence. Similarly, the effect estimates produced using calendar period as an IV will be biased if there is any time trend in an unmeasured causal factor, whereas a trend-in-trend study will

be biased only if changes in the prevalence of such a factor are correlated with changes in exposure prevalence across cumulative probability of exposure strata.

Schneeweiss and Suissa (2012) advocate the use of study designs to address confounding and other biases in post-marketing safety studies. They consider in this connection multi-time case-control designs and case-cohort designs, which have potential bias that the TT design avoids, as pointed out in the preceding quotation from Ji et al. (2017).

6.5 Structural causal models and causal calculus

6.5.1 From structural equation models to SCMs

As pointed out by Pearl (2009a), the Structural Causal Model (SCM) that he developed in Pearl (1995, 2009b) combines features of (a) the Neyman-Rubin potential outcomes framework that we have described in Section 6.2.2, (b) structural equation models and (c) graphical models for probabilistic reasoning and causal representation. This paragraph provides some basic background on structural equation models. Structural equations were originally introduced by Wright (1921) in conjunction with the associated "path diagrams" for genetic path modeling and Pearl (2009a,b) provides causal interpretations and nonparametric extensions of these equations. He starts by considering the following example. Let X denote a disease variable and Y a certain symptom of the disease, with both variables standardized so that they have mean 0 and variance 1. A linear structural equation linking Y to X takes the form $y = \beta x + u_Y$, in which x (respectively, y) stands for the level or severity of the disease (respectively, the symptom), and u_Y is an exogenous variable, incorporating all factors other than the disease that could possibly affect Y when X is held constant. "Because algebraic equations are symmetrical objects", rewriting the above linear equation as $x = (y - u_Y)/\beta$ "might be misinterpreted to mean that the symptom influences the disease", hence Wright (1921) augmented the algebraic equation with a path diagram, "in which arrows are drawn from perceived causes to their perceived effects", with an arrow from X to Y and another arrow from u_Y to Y for the above structural equation. The path diagram may also feature another exogenous variable u_X, with an arrow from u_X to X and possibly also arrows between u_X and u_Y. The exogenous variables "represent observed or unobserved background factors that the modeler decides to keep unexplained, that is factors that influence but are not influenced by other variables (called 'endogenous') in the model."

We next describe some basic background on causal diagrams, directed acyclic graphs (DAGs), conditional independence and graphical models. We begin with DAGs. A *graph* is a collection of nodes and edges. Two nodes are *adjacent* if there is an edge between them, and the graph is *complete* if there is an edge between every pair of nodes. An edge is *directed* if it goes out of one node, called the "parent", and into the other node, called the "child", with the direction indicated by an arrow head. Otherwise, the edge is called "undirected". A *directed graph* is a graph in which all of the edges are directed. A *directed path* from node X to node Y is a sequence of directed edges connecting the nodes, called *descendants* of X on the path and X is called the *ancestor* of these descendant nodes. In the case $Y = X$, the directed path is called a "cycle". A directed graph with no cycles is called *acyclic*.

A *graphical model* (or *probabilistic graphical model*) uses a graph to express the conditional dependent structure of random vectors. Two classes of graphical representations are often used to model multivariate distributions, namely, Bayesian networks and Markov random fields. The semantic basis of Bayesian networks is the *product decomposition rule*:

$$P(y_1, \ldots, y_n) = \prod_{i=1}^{n} P(y_i | pa_i), \qquad (6.17)$$

where pa_i stands for the set of the variables that precede Y_i (called the "parents" of Y_i) in the causal diagram associated with the model. Pearl et al. (2016, p. 30) point out the importance of (6.17) in empirical estimation of the joint distribution from a data set generated by the model, reducing high-dimensional estimation to a few low-dimensional distribution estimation tasks. For example, for the chain graph $X \to Z \to Y$, (6.17) reduces to $P(X = x, Z = z, Y = y) = P(X = x)P(Z = z | X = x)P(Y = y | Z = z)$, "we can count the frequencies of each x, $(z|x)$ and $(y|z)$ and multiply" to estimate the joint distribution from a trivariate data set, instead of computing the frequency of every triple (x, z, y). Suppose that $X = 1$ (or 0) if the subject takes (or does not take) aspirin and Y is the binary outcome variable, with $Y = 1$ (or 0) representing heart disease (or no heart disease) in the chain graph $X \to Z \to Y$, where Z denotes platelet aggregation (with 1 for high and 0 for low). Without Z, one would expect X and Y to be associated because aspirin has an effect on heart disease. Since individuals with low platelet aggregation ($Z = 0$) have a lower than average risk of heart disease, their risk is lower than average regardless of whether they are treated ($X = 1$) or untreated ($X = 0$). In the subset of individuals with $Z = 0$, treatment X and outcome Y are not associated, and a similar argument can be applied to individuals in the group with $Z = 1$.

More generally, a path p in a DAG G is said to be *blocked* by a set $\mathbf{Z}$ of nodes if and only if (a) p contains a chain of nodes $A \to B \to C$ or a *fork* $A \leftarrow B \to C$ such that the middle node B is in $\mathbf{Z}$, or (b) p contains a *collider* $A \rightarrow B \leftarrow C$ such that the collision node B is not in **Z**, and no descendants of B are in **Z**. If **Z** blocks every path between two nodes X and Y, then X and Y are said to be *d-separated* conditional on **Z**. In view of the conditional independence implied by (6.17), *d*-separation of X and Y conditional on **Z** implies that X and Y are *conditionally independent* given **Z**.

Dawid (1979) provides an early discussion of the role of conditional independence of X and Y given **Z** in statistical theory. Pearl (2009a) argues that "most judgments about conditional independence emanate from our understanding of cause-effect relationships" and that "the standard decision to assume independence among certain statistical parameters and not others (in a Bayesian prior) rely on causal information", although the causal rationale for these judgments and decisions is seldom explicitly mentioned for lack of a suitable "vocabulary that differs substantially from the one Bayesian statisticians have been accustomed to articulate." He continues to mention Simpson's paradox, which will be discussed in Supplement 3 of Section 6.6, as a "classical example demonstrating the obstacle of causal vocabulary". Koller and Friedman (2009, Parts III and IV) also discuss causality and structure learning in Bayesian networks, for which they also consider utilities, decisions, and optimization in influence diagrams; see Supplement 4 of Section 6.6 for the background in influence diagrams, decision analysis, and how Bayesian networks and causal modeling have enriched structured decisions.

The Bayesian network structure has the *local Markov property* that each node X_i is conditionally independent of its "non-descendants" (which are nodes in the graph that are not descendant of X_i) given the set of parents pa_i; see (6.17). Markov random fields (MRFs) are *mixed graphs* (which consist of three types of edges: directed $\rightarrow$, bidirected $\leftrightarrow$, and undirected $-$) that satisfy *global Markov* assumptions that are defined in the next paragraph. For a mixed graph G, α is called a spouse of β (or belongs to sp(β)) if $\alpha \leftrightarrow \beta$, and α is called a *neighbor* of β (or belongs to ne(β)) if $\alpha - \beta$. A sequence of edges between α and β in G is an ordered set of edges $e_1, \ldots, e_n$ such that e_i has vertices x_{i-1} and x_i with $x_0 = \alpha$ and $x_n = \beta$; the sequence of edges is called a *path* if the vertices x_i are all distinct. A vertex α is an *ancestor* of vertex β if there is a directed path $\alpha \rightarrow \ldots \rightarrow \beta$ or if $\alpha = \beta$; it is *anterior* to β if there is an anterior path to β (i.e., on which every edge is either $\gamma \rightarrow \delta$ or $\gamma - \delta$, with δ between γ and β) from α or if $\alpha = \beta$; see Richardson and Spirtes (2002) who review previous works by Darroch, Lauritzen, and Speed (1980), Lauritzen and Wermuth (1989), Frydenberg (1990), Koster (1996, 2002), Andersson, Madigan, and Perlman (1997, 2001), and who introduce ancestral graphs that satisfy global Markov assumptions. An *ancestral graph* G is a mixed graph whose vertices α satisfy (i) pa(α)$\cup$sp(α) $= \emptyset$ if ne(α) $\neq \emptyset$, and (ii) $\alpha \notin$ ant(pa(α)$\cup$sp(α)), where pa(α) $= \{a : a \rightarrow \alpha\}$ is the set of parents of α and ant(S) $= \{\alpha : \alpha$ is anterior to β for some $\beta \in S\}$. Richardson and Spirtes (2002) point out that despite the large literature on graphical models, there are identifiability difficulties and inference issues based on limited observations, and say that their proposed class of ancestral graph Markov models "is intended to provide a partial resolution to this conundrum."

The concept of d-separation for DAGs can be extended to a mixed graph G as follows. Letting $\mathbf{X}$, $\mathbf{Y}$, $\mathbf{Z}$ be sets of nodes in G, $\mathbf{Z}$ is said to separate $\mathbf{X}$ and $\mathbf{Y}$ if between any nodes $X \in \mathbf{X}$ and $Y \in \mathbf{Y}$ there does not exist a path $X_1 - \ldots - X_k$ for which none of the X_i belongs to $\mathbf{Z}$. The global Markov assumptions associated with G are defined by the conditional independence of $\mathbf{X}$ and $\mathbf{Y}$ given $\mathbf{Z}$, for any $(\mathbf{X}, \mathbf{Y}, \mathbf{Z})$ such that $\mathbf{Z}$ separates $\mathbf{X}$ and $\mathbf{Y}$; see Koller and Friedman (2009) who also give the following characterization of a positive distribution (which does not take the value 0) P over n nodes $V_1, \ldots, V_n$ of G that satisfies the global Markov assumptions: P is a *Gibbs distribution*, i.e., it has the form

$$P(v_1, \ldots, v_n) \propto \pi_1(\mathbf{D}_1) \ldots \pi_m(\mathbf{D}_m) \tag{6.18}$$

for some complete subgraphs $\mathbf{D}_1, \ldots, \mathbf{D}_m$ and positive functions $\pi_1, \ldots, \pi_m$.

6.5.2 Symbolic causal calculus

In this section we give an introduction to causal calculus using symbolic logic, dating back to McCain and Turner (1997) and Lifschitz (1997). We then use this machinery to give Pearl's operational definition of structural causal models and subsequent generalizations by others.

Representing intervention with the $do(\cdot)$ operator. Pearl et al. (2016, pp. 55-57) use $do(x)$ to denote the case where a treatment variable X is fixed at x, distinguishing it from the case where X takes the value x naturally. As an illustration, they consider X, "a hypothetical intervention by which we administer a drug uniformly to the entire population and compare the recovery rate to what could obtain under the complementary intervention, where we prevent everyone from using the drug," and binary outcome variable Y (=1 for recovery) so that the problem of interest is to estimate the average causal effect $P(Y = 1|do(X = 1)) - P(Y = 1|do(X = 0))$, which "cannot be estimated from the data set itself without a causal (assumption)." The causal assumption can be described by a graphical model that involves another measured covariate Z (e.g., gender) such that X and Y are d-separated conditional on Z. "The proportions of males and females remain the same, before and after the intervention" and "the process by which Y responds to X and Z, $Y = f(x, z, u_Y)$, remains the same, regardless of whether X changes spontaneously or by deliberate manipulation." Moreover, Z and X are independent under this treatment assignment and therefore

$$P\left(Y = y | do(X = x)\right) = \sum_z P\left(Y = y | X = x, Z = z\right) P\left(Z = z\right), \qquad (6.19)$$

which can be consistently estimated from the data. This formula "instructs us to condition on gender, find the benefit of the drug separately for males and females, and only then average the result using the percentage of males and females in the population", but estimating $P\left(Y = 1 | X = 1\right)$ and $P\left(Y = 1 | X = 0\right)$ separately from the data and taking their differences "might falsely conclude that the drug has a negative effect overall."

Pearl (2009a, pp. 108-112) describes how the $do(\cdot)$ operator can represent interventions (treatments) in general causal graphical models for which the treatment X is fixed at level x and Z is covariate that affects the amount of treatment received. For a general response variable Y (not necessarily binary), he says that "$P\left(z, y | do(x)\right)$ describes the post-intervention distribution of variables Y and Z", from which one can assess treatment efficacy by conditioning the average treatment difference $E_M\left(Y | do(x')\right) - E_M\left(Y | do(x)\right)$ for two levels (or types) of treatment, or the risk ratio $E_M\left(Y | do(x')\right) / E_M\left(Y | do(x)\right)$, of causal model M and that "the central question in the analysis of causal effects is the question of *identification*: Can the post-intervention distribution $P\left(Y = y | do(x)\right)$ be estimated from data governed by the pre-intervention distribution $P\left(z, x, y\right)$?" He defines identifiability as follows: A quantity $Q(M)$ is identifiable given a set of assumptions (which are encoded in the causal diagram) if for any two models M_1 and M_2 satisfying these assumptions, $P_{M_1} = P_{M_2} \Rightarrow Q(M_1) = Q(M_2)$. He says: "When (identifiability) happens, Q depends on P only, and should be expressible in terms of the parameters of P." An important result using the $do(\cdot)$ operator is the refinement of the product decomposition rule (6.17) for DAGs into the following *truncated product* formula:

$$P\left(y_1, \ldots, y_n | do(x)\right) = \prod_{i | Y_i \notin \mathfrak{X}} P\left(y_i | pa_i\right), \qquad (6.20)$$

allowing multiple interventions (such as those that dictate the values of several variables simultaneously or time-varying levels of a treatment), where $P(\cdot | \cdot)$ denotes the pre-intervention conditional probability under model M and $\mathfrak{X}$ denotes the intervention set of variables whose values are already determined by $do(x)$. This formula "demonstrates how the causal assumptions embedded in M permits us to predict the post-intervention distribution from the pre-intervention distribution, which further permits us to estimate the causal effect of X on Y from non-experimental data," and in the case of time-varying confounders "coincides with Robins' (1987) G-computation formula, which was derived from a more complicated set of (counterfactual) assumptions."

Back-door criterion for variable selection. To adjust for possible confounding in non-experimental studies, the truncated product formula (6.20) suggests that one should adjust for a variable's parents, some of which "may be unmeasurable, such as genetic trait or life style" and therefore one faces the problem of selecting an "admissible set" of covariates for measurement and adjustment to estimate the treatment effect. A set S of covariates is *admissible* for estimating the causal effect of X on Y if it satisfies the *back-door criterion* that (a) no element of S is a descendant of X and (b) S blocks every path between X and Y that ends with an arrow pointing to X (called a "back-door path"); see Pearl (2009a, p. 114) who calls a path p to be "blocked" by a set S of nodes if either (i) p contains at least one arrow-emitting node that is in S, or (ii) p contains at least one collision node that is outside S and has no descendant in S, and who also explains his underlying intuition:

> The back-door paths carry spurious associations from X to Y, while the paths directed along the arrows from X to Y carry causative associations. Blocking the former paths (by conditioning on S) ensures that the measured association between X and Y is purely causative, namely, it correctly represents the target quantity: the causal effect of X on Y.

Definition of SCM and a generalization. In the structural causal model introduced by Pearl (2009b, Chapter 7), every endogenous variable is associated with a structural equation that describes its causal dependence on other variables in the system which may also include exogenous variables; the structural equation can be nonlinear or even nonparametric. Using bold capital letters to denote sets of variables and indexing the variables in $\mathbf{Y}$ by $I_{\mathbf{Y}}$ (so that the elements of $\mathbf{Y}$ are Y_i, $i \in I_{\mathbf{Y}}$), a causal model consists of a family of probability measures $\{P_{do(\mathbf{X}_I)} : I \subset I^*\}$, in which I^* is the set of indices i for which Y_i has (nonrandom) target values ξ_i under $do(\mathbf{X}_I)$ for $i \in I \subset I^*$. SCM is a causal model that also consists of a family of functions $f_j : \mathfrak{Y}_{pa(j)} \times \mathfrak{X}_{pa(j)} \to \mathfrak{Y}_j$ for $j \in I_{\mathbf{Y}}$, where $\mathfrak{X}_i$ is the set of possible values of X_i, $\mathfrak{X}_I = \prod_{i \in I} \mathfrak{X}_i$, and $\mathfrak{Y}_I$ is defined similarly. This definition of SCM, due to Bongers et al. (2016), differs slightly from Pearl's because it does not assume acyclicity that leads to the "recursiveness" and "uniqueness" axioms in Pearl (2009b, p. 231). Bongers et al. (2016) call their SCM *uniquely solvable* if the structural equations $y_i = f_j\big(\mathbf{y}_{pa(j)}, \mathbf{x}_{pa(j)}\big)$, $j \in I_{\mathbf{Y}}$, has a unique solution. Using this definition that allows cyclic SCMs, Blom and Mooij (2018) have developed *generalized structural causal models* (GSCMs) that can capture the causal semantics of equilibrium states in dynamical systems with initial conditions.

Counterfactual and potential outcomes in the SCM framework. Pearl
(2009a, pp. 119–120) says that "not all questions of causal character can
be encoded in $P\left(y|do(x)\right)$ type expressions" as causal questions of attribu-
tion (e.g., fraction of death cases due to specific exposure) or susceptibility
(e.g., fraction of healthy unexposed population who would get the disease
had they been exposed) require "a probabilistic analysis of counterfactuals (such as) Y would be y had X been x in situation $U = u$, denoted
$Y_x(u) = y$" but that remarkably "structural equation models provide the
formal interpretation and symbolic machinery for analyzing such counterfactual relationships" because of the following "key idea":

> Interpret the phrase "had X been x" as an instruction to make
> a minimal modification in the current model...replacing the equa-
> tion for X by a constant x (while keeping the rest of the model un-
> changed)... Let M be a structural model and M_x a modified version
> of M (with X replaced by x in the structural equations). Denote the
> solution for Y in the equations of M_x by $Y_{M_x}(u)$. The counterfac-
> tual $Y_x(u)$ (or the value of Y in unit u if X had been x) is given by:
> $Y_x(u) = Y_{M_x}(u)$.

Pearl (2009a, Section 4) points out that this structural definition of
counterfactuals subsumes the Neyman-Rubin potential outcome framework, in which the primitive object of analysis is $Y_x(u)$, "the value that
outcome Y would obtain in experimental unit u, had treatment X been
x." Moreover, the missing data paradigm for this framework treats U as a
random variable so that the value of the counterfactual $Y_x(u)$ "becomes a
random variable as well, denoted as Y_x." Under the assumption of condi-
tional ignorability $Y_x \perp\!\!\!\perp X | \mathbf{Z}$, introduced by Rosenbaum and Rubin (1983)
for a set of covariates $\mathbf{Z}$, and using P^* to denote the augmented probability function defined over both the observed and counterfactual variables,
the causal effect $P\left(y|do(x)\right) = P^*\left(Y_x = y\right)$ can be evaluated by

$$P^*\left(Y_x = y\right) = \sum_{\mathbf{z}} P^*\left(Y_x = y|\mathbf{z}\right) P(\mathbf{z}) = \sum_{\mathbf{z}} P^*\left(Y_x = y|x, \mathbf{z}\right) P(\mathbf{z})$$

$$= \sum_{\mathbf{z}} P^*\left(Y = y|x, \mathbf{z}\right) P(\mathbf{z}) = \sum_{\mathbf{z}} P(y|x, \mathbf{z}) P(\mathbf{z}), \qquad (6.21)$$

in which the last expression contains no counterfactual quantities. The
second equality in (6.21) follows from the conditional independence of Y_x
and X given $\mathbf{Z}$, while the third equality follows from the consistency constraint for counterfactual:

$$X = x \;\Rightarrow\; Y_x = Y, \qquad (6.22)$$

which states that the value of Y_x would take on if X were x is the actual value of Y (Robins, 1986). Pearl (2009a, pp. 115–117) says that judging whether "X is conditionally ignorable given Z" is a "formidable mental task that can be circumvented by the back-door criterion which also enables the (propensity score) analyst to search for an optimal set of covariates – namely, a set Z that minimizes measurement cost or sampling variability." He also points out that propensity score methods cannot be expected to reduce bias in case the set Z does not satisfy the back-door criterion and that "the prevailing practice of conditioning on as many pretreatment measurements as possible should be approached with great caution; some covariates may actually increase bias if included in the analysis."

Transportability via selection diagrams. Pearl and Bareinboim (2014) point out that "the generalizability of empirical findings to new environments, settings or populations, often called 'external validity', is essential in most scientific explorations" and consider in particular "transportability", defined as a "license to transfer (generalize) causal effects learned in experimental studies" from population Π to a new population Π^*. Noting that "licensing transportability requires knowledge of the mechanisms, or processes, through which population differences come about", they say:

> To this end, we will use causal diagrams augmented with a set S of "selection variables", where each member of S corresponds to a mechanism by which the two populations differ, and switching between the two populations will be represented by conditioning on different values of the S variables.

They define a *selection diagram* as follows. Let M and M^* be SCMs associated with the populations Π and Π^*, respectively, sharing a causal diagram G. The pair (M, M^*) is said to induce a selection diagram D if

(a) Every edge in G is also an edge in D, and

(b) D contains an extra edge $s_i \to v_i \in G$ whenever the selection variable $s_i \in S$ shows a discrepancy between M and M^*.

In the selection diagram, "the S variables locate the mechanisms where structural discrepancies between the two populations" occur and therefore "the absence of a selection node pointing to a variable represents the assumption that the mechanism responsible for assigning value to that variable is the same for the two variables." Combining the concepts of intervention and identifiability with *do*-calculus and the selection diagram representation of the SCMs associated with Π and Π^*, they give the following operational definition of transportability:

> Let D be a selection diagram for (Π, Π^*). Let (P, I) be the pair of observational and interventional distributions of Π, and P^* be

the observational distribution of Π^*. The causal relation $R(\Pi^*) = P^*(y|do(x), z)$ is said to be *transportable* from Π to Π^* in D if $R(\Pi^*)$ is uniquely computable from P, P^*, I in any model that induces D.

They use this definition to reduce questions of transportability to symbolic derivations in the *do*-calculus, yielding graph-based procedures for deciding, prior to observing any data, whether causal effects in Π^* can be inferred from experimental findings in Π. They also derive "transport formulas" such as

$$P^*(y|do(x)) = \sum_z P(y|do(x), z) \sum_w P(w|do(x)) P^*(z|w) \qquad (6.23)$$

for certain selection diagrams, in which the factors $P(\cdot|\cdot)$ are estimable from the experimental study and $P^*(\cdot|\cdot)$ through observational studies from Π^*.

6.6 Supplements and problems

1. *Partial identification and bounds for probability of causation.* Noting that "the credibility of (statistical) inference decreases with the strength of the assumptions maintained", Manski (2003) says in his introductory chapter:

> It is useful to distinguish combinations of data and assumptions that point-identify a population parameter of interest from ones that place the parameter within a set-valued identification region. Point identification is the fundamental necessary condition for consistent point estimation of a parameter... The classical theory of local asymptotic efficiency characterizes, through the Fisher information matrix, how attainable precision increases as more is assumed known about a population distribution. Nonparametric regression analysis shows how the attainable rate of convergence of estimates increases as more is assumed about the shape of the regression. These and other achievements provide important guidance to empirical researchers (in comparing) precision of alternative point estimates... (In) nonparametric regression with missing outcome data, empirical researchers estimating regressions commonly assume that missingness is random, in the sense that the observability of an outcome is statistically independent of its value. Yet this and other point-identifying assumptions have regularly been criticized as implausible. So I set out (in the late 1980s)

to determine what random sampling with partial observ-
ability of outcomes reveals about mean and quantile regres-
sions if nothing is known about the missingness process or
if assumptions weak enough to be widely credible are im-
posed. The findings were sharp bounds whose forms vary
with the regression of interest and with the maintained assumptions... Study of regression with missing outcome data
stimulated investigation of more general incomplete data
problems. Some sample realizations may have unobserved
outcomes, some may have unobserved covariates, and others
may be entirely missing. Sometimes interval data on outcomes or covariates are available, rather than point measurements.

He also traces "the long but sparse history" of partial identification,
dating back to 1934 when Frisch developed sharp bounds on the slope
parameter of simple linear regression when the covariate is measured
with mean-zero errors, followed by Marschak and Andrews' partial
identification approach to inference on production functions in 1944,
and by Koopmans and Reiersol's dictum in 1950 that the specification
of a model ought to be based on the underlying econometrics and assumptions with universal or almost universal acceptance but should
not be geared primarily toward point identifying the parameters.

After Manski's influential work on partial identification and credible
inference, there has been steady progress in this direction in econometrics, and Tamer (2010) gives a review of this approach, for which
the abstract says:

Identification in econometric models maps prior assumptions and the data to information about a parameter of interest. The partial identification approach to inference rec-
ognizes that this process should not result in a binary answer that consists of whether the parameter is point identified, (and instead uses the data to) characterizes the informational content of various assumptions by providing a
menu of estimates, each based on different sets of assumptions, some of which are plausible and some of which are
not. Of course, more assumptions beget more information,
so stronger conclusions can be made at the expense of more
assumptions. The partial identification approach advocates
a more fluid view of identification and hence provides the
empirical researcher with methods to help study the spectrum of information that we can harness about a parameter
of interest using a menu of assumptions... Naturally, with
finite sample sizes, this approach leads to statistical complications, as one needs to deal with characterizing sampling

uncertainty in models that do not point identify a parameter. Therefore, new methods for inference are developed. These methods construct confidence sets for partially identified parameters, and confidence regions for sets of parameters, or identifiable sets.

In particular, he reviews the new methods using subsampling for construction of the confidence regions for an identified parameter or for interval bounds. A new approach recently developed by Chen et al. (2018) makes use of MCMC to construct confidence regions for identified sets.

2. *Likelihood and Bayesian imputation methods for missing data.* Domain knowledge of why data are missing is important to handle adequately the remaining data for the objectives of the study. If values are *missing completely at random* (MCAR), the data sample is still representative of the population. A weaker form is *missing at random* (MAR), introduced by Rubin (1976) who also introduced MCAR, when missingness is not random but can be fully accounted for by variables that provide complete information. Although MAR appears to be an implausible assumption in practice, as noted in the preceding supplement by Manski (2003), the substantive application can provide insight into its reasonableness; see Little (2002). When data are MCAR or MAR, Rubin calls the response mechanism *ignorable* because the analysis can ignore the reasons for missing data, allowing the use of standard maximum likelihood; see also Heitjan and Basu (1996). When the response mechanism is nonignorable, the reasons for the missing observations need to be involved in the data analysis; see Schafer (1997) and Little and Rubin (2014). The likelihood approach involves the density $f(y|\theta)$ of the complete data and the conditional density $f(M|\mathbf{Y}, \psi)$ of the mechanism given the complete data so that the likelihood has the form

$$f\left(\mathbf{Y}_{\text{obs}}, M | \theta, \psi\right) = \int f\left(\mathbf{Y}_{\text{obs}}, \mathbf{Y}_{\text{miss}} | \theta\right) f\left(M | \mathbf{Y}_{\text{obs}}, \mathbf{Y}_{\text{miss}}, \psi\right) d\mathbf{Y}_{\text{miss}},$$

$$(6.24)$$

since $(\mathbf{Y}_{\text{obs}}, \mathbf{Y}_{\text{miss}})$ is the complete data. The Bayesian approach puts priors on (θ, ψ) and can be implemented by the Gibbs sampler, which also provides multiple imputations of missing values and which is a sampling version of the ECM (Expectation-Conditional Maximization) algorithm, yielding draws from the posterior distribution of the parameters.

For ignorable mechanisms in which the likelihood function is proportional to $f(\mathbf{Y}_{\text{obs}}|\theta)$, Rubin (1987) has worked out the Bayesian theory of multiple imputation (MI), and in particular the MI approximations to the posterior mean and the posterior variance, while Little and his coauthors have focused on making MI more robust by using penalized spline of propensity prediction (PSPP); see Little and An (2004) and Zhang and Little (2009, 2011). For *missing not at random* (MNAR) data, Bayesian imputations are much more difficult. Schafer (1999) has developed a NORM program for a relatively simple missing data mechanism, acting on multivariate normal complete data, which allows data augmentation to be used; see Pigott (2001). Giusti and Little (2011) introduce a pattern mixture (PM) model to handle income nonresponse in a sample survey with a rotating panel design. Andridge and Little (2011) and West and Little (2013) use an alternative proxy PM analysis that avoids specifying the missing data mechanism by introducing a sensitivity analysis parameter λ for which $\lambda = 0$ corresponds to the case of MAR.

3. *Simpson's paradox.* Blyth (1972) relates a paradox described by Simpson (1951) concerning the interpretation of interaction in contingency tables in the context of choosing from many possible random losses and payoffs. He describes Simpson's paradox as: "It is possible to have $P(A|B) < P(A|B')$ and have at the same time both $P(A|BC) \geq P(A|B'C)$ and $P(A|BC') \geq P(A|B'C')$", where $'$ denotes the complement of an event, even though "$P(A|B)$ is an average of $P(A|BC)$ and $P(A|BC')$ and $P(A|B')$ is an average of $P(A|B'C)$ and $P(A|B'C')$", because "these two averages (can) have different weightings". On the other hand, when the two weightings coincide, which is the case for independent B and C, the "paradoxical possibility" cannot happen. He also gives the following extension of Simpson's paradox: "Subject to the conditions $P(A|BC) \geq \gamma P(A|B'C)$ and $P(A|BC') \geq \gamma P(A|B'C')$ for some $\gamma \geq 1$, it is possible to have $P(A|B) \approx 0$ and $P(A|B') \approx 1/\gamma$."

Pearl et al. (2016, pp. 2, 3, 57) focus on Simpson's example involving "a group of sick patients given the option to try a new drug", for whom "a lower percentage recovered among those who took the drug than among those who did not" but "more men taking the drug recovered than did men were not taking the drug, and more women taking the drug recovered than did women were not taking the drug." They argue that "in order to decide whether the drug will harm or help a patient" one has to understand the causal mechanism that generates the observed results, and that segregated (by gender in this case) data are "more specific, hence more informative, than the unsegregated data." They apply (6.19) with $X = 1$ for the patient taking the drug, $Y = 1$ for the patient recovering and $Z = 1$ (or 0) for male (or female) patients to show a clear positive advantage to drug-taking from the data that show women more likely to take the drug than men. They also provide a possible explanation: "Estrogen has a negative effect on recovery, so women are less likely to recover than men, regardless of the drug."

4. *Influence diagrams, decision analysis, and Bayesian networks.* Pearl (2005) gives a review of influence diagrams, which "command a unique position in the history of graphical models" as an extension of Wright's path diagrams and informal precursors of Bayesian networks, providing "a computational tool for automated reasoning" and first developed by decision analysts in the 1970s; see Howard and Matheson (1984). He says that lacking in these early developments was causal modeling that could provide formal structure and conceptual understanding of the mystical relationships between graphs and (conditional) probabilities in these influence diagrams. Work by Pearl and others in the Artificial Intelligence community to fill this gap has greatly enhanced influence diagrams, which have become widely adopted tools for structured decision problems; see Koller and Friedman (2009, Chapters 22 and 23). An influence diagram is a DAG with three types of nodes (uncertainty node that corresponds to each uncertainty being modeled, value node that is associated with the utility function, and decision node that corresponds to each decision made) and three types of arrows that end in an uncertainty node ("conditional" type), or a value node ("functional" type), or a decision node (called "informational" type). Backward induction techniques are used for optimization in influence diagrams, and computational algorithms to evaluate the expected utilities and the value of information are used to solve the structured decision problems.

7

Safety Databases: Statistical Analysis and Pharmacovigilance

Collection and submission of safety data in different phases of clinical trials are required by regulatory agencies for drug approval and post-marketing safety evaluation. In addition, beginning in 1968, the FDA established the Adverse Event Reporting System database to collect adverse event information associated with drugs from patients, health care professionals, and other sources through a spontaneous reporting system, and these data are available online through the Freedom of Information Act. Pharmacovigilance is the pharmacological science concerning data collection, monitoring, and detection of adverse reactions of medical products after they have been licensed for use in a country. Section 7.1 gives an overview of the large variety of safety databases, ranging from preclinical data to adverse event reporting systems for drugs and vaccines and health insurance claims databases. Section 7.2 discusses statistical issues in the analysis of spontaneous adverse event report databases and Sections 7.3–7.7 describe statistical methods to address them, and Section 7.8 gives an overview of pharmacoepidemiologic approaches to the analysis of these data. Section 7.9 describes the actual experience of pre- and post-marketing studies with the combination vaccine MMRV, about which Chapter 5 has described clinical safety data when it is used in combination with PedvaxH1B®. Supplements and problems are given in Section 7.10.

7.1 Safety databases

7.1.1 Preclinical data

In biopharmaceutical development, preclinical (or nonclinical) studies are commonly performed to assess the safety (or toxicity) profiles of potential new drugs, biologics, medical devices, gene therapy solutions, and diagnostic tools. Regulatory agencies generally require preclinical safety assessment of a pharmaceutical product before marketing approval (ICH, 2008; Brock et al., 2013). Depending on the category of the potential product, different types of preclinical testing have to be conducted. Typically *in vitro* and *in vivo* tests are carried out to determine a product's inherent toxicological properties, which include

- genotoxicity: the potential of a compound to induce chromosomal aberrations or genetic damage (gene mutation) directly or indirectly,

- carcinogenicity: the tumorigenic potential of a substance in animals and to the associated risk to humans,

- reproductive and developmental toxicity: the potential toxicological effects of a compound on fertility and early embryonic development, embryo-fetal development, pre- and postnatal development, including maternal function,

- immunotoxicity: the potential of a compound to stimulate or suppress the immune system, hence impacting humoral or cell-mediated immunity,

- local toxicity: the individual toxic reactions that can be evaluated through single or repeated dose toxicity studies.

These preclinical studies are often exploratory in nature and use a variety of human organ-specific cell lines or animal species with a limited number of experimental units. We next describe the characteristics (e.g., scope, objectives, available databases) of both *in vitro* and *in vivo* toxicity tests. *In vitro* studies constitute the first step of toxicity screening tests for potential products, and are often conducted in a test tube or culture media using components of organisms such as living microorganisms or cells. In addition to determining other pharmaceutical properties such as cellular absorption, metabolism, drug-drug interactions, etc., *in vitro* assays are commonly used for early screening of product toxicity, especially human organ-specific toxicity, such that they can provide information on mechanism(s) of action as well as an early indication of the potential for some kinds of toxic effects for subsequent study design (Li, 2005; Pugsley et al., 2008; Roggen, 2011; Anadón et al., 2014). *In vitro* tests are usually less expensive, faster to run, and somewhat less predictive of toxicity in intact organisms, as compared to *in vivo* tests described below.

In general, cytotoxicity endpoints are of primary interest and consist of membrane integrity, cellular metabolite contents, lysosomal functions, cellular apoptosis, etc. For instance, liver models such as liver slices, liver cell lines, and primary hepatocytes, etc., have been widely used over the years in *in vitro* liver toxicity testing. (Soldatow et al., 2013; Bale et al., 2014). Similarly, the primary human cell culture systems include hepatocytes for hepatotoxicity, neuronal and glial cells for neurotoxicity, cardiomyocytes for cardiotoxicity, renal proximal tubule epithelial cells for nephrotoxicity, and skeletal myocytes for rhadomyolysis (Li, 2005; Bal-Price and Jennings, 2014).

It is important to recognize that results of *in vitro* studies are rarely published due to a variety of reasons, e.g., lack of public interest or lack of enthusiasm for publishing toxicology results for failed compounds, or other ongoing activities in failed compounds to preclude revealing the properties of the compound to potential competitors. Therefore, comprehensive databases for *in vitro* toxicity testing results from individual biopharmaceutical companies and/or research institutes are generally scarce (Briggs et al., 2012; Cases et al., 2014; Briggs et al., 2015). Nevertheless, some publicly accessible databases containing published or publicly available *in vitro* results are available for toxicity research and are described below.

- TOX21 (https://ntp.niehs.nih.gov/results/tox21/index. html) is a multi-agency collaborative effort among the National Toxicology Program (NTP) of the National Institute of Environmental Health Sciences (NIEHS), National Center for Advancing Translational Sciences (NCATS)/NIH Chemical Genomics Center (NCGC), National Institutes of Health (NIH), and the US Food and Drug Administration (FDA). Built upon the HTPS (high throughput screening) technology, TXO21 gives the characteristics and chemical reactivity in biochemical- and cell-based assays of more than 10,000 chemicals, drugs, and formulations. It can be used for profiling signatures of compound mechanism of toxicity and for stipulation of further in-depth toxicological testing (Casey, 2013; Attene-Ramos et al., 2015; Huang et al., 2016). Its goal is to identify chemical structure-activity relations derived through *in vitro* testing that could potentially act as predictive surrogates for *in vivo* toxicity and reduce the use of animals for *in vivo* tests and provide information directly related to human health (Casey, 2013).

- Acutoxbase (www.acutetox.org) is a data management system for *in vitro* toxicology developed by the AcuteTox project that was funded by the European Commission Directorate General for Research for the prediction of human acute oral toxicity. It consists of six basic sections: (i) *in vitro* experiments, (ii) *in vivo* animal data, (iii) human poisoning cases, (iv) *in vitro* biokinetic data, (v) chemicals and (vi) data reporting (Kinsner-Ovaskainen et al., 2009).

- TOXNET (https://toxnet.nlm.nih.gov/) is a cluster of databases covering toxicology, hazardous chemicals, environmental health, and related areas, and is managed by the Toxicology and Environmental Health Information Program of the National Library of Medicine, which provides free access to and easy searching of these special databases (Wexler, 2001).

- ToxML (http://www.leadscope.com/toxml.php) is a structurally searchable database, built upon a public data standard ToxML, using

FDA's administrative toxicity records that include a large variety of chemical-structural classes for substances used as human drugs. It consists of four frameworks that are compiled into a single database: bacterial mutagenesis, *in vitro* chromosome aberration, *in vitro* mammalian mutagenesis, and *in vivo* micronucleus (Arvidson, 2008).

- AltTox (`www.alttox.org`) is a database dedicated to advancing non-animal methods of toxicity testing. With the goal of improving the health of humans, animals, and the environment, it is designed for the exchange of technical and policy information on *in vitro* and *in silico* methods of toxicity testing (Kavlock et al., 2007).

It should be pointed out that although *in vitro* screening assays can provide some mechanistic insights on human-specific toxicity, a major drawback of *in vitro* systems is the lack of whole-body pharmacokinetics and toxicokinetics processes in carrying out toxicity assessment of pharmaceutical compounds (Li, 2005; Anadón et al., 2014). Even with the independent discrete multiple organ co-culture systems where cells from different organs as physically separated cultures are co-cultured and hence inter-connected by an overlying medium (Annaert and Brouwer, 2005), it is still challenging to model the multiple organ interactions *in vivo* and to evaluate the organ-specific effect of a compound and its metabolites. After *in vitro* screening assays, a compound usually goes through *in vivo* toxicity tests for further development. Specifically, results of *in vivo* toxicology studies should (a) establish a safe starting dose for further clinical development, (b) provide information to design a drug treatment regimen that would generate desired therapeutic effects, e.g., the least toxicity and maximum efficacy, (c) assess target organ specific toxicity and its reversibility after treatment termination, and (d) provide insights into biomarkers for possible treatment enrichment and clinical monitoring in subsequent development activities among humans. *In vivo* animal studies are conducted in two species, i.e., rodent (rat, mouse) and non-rodent (dog, nonhuman primate). Other species (e.g., rabbits, ferrets, hamsters, mini-pigs) may be used for special studies (e.g., vaccine studies). Although test results for most *in vivo* experiments are not publicly available, there have been collaborative efforts in the biopharmaceutical industry and among research institutes to develop publicly accessible databases of *in vivo* test results. An example is eTOX (`http://www.etoxproject.eu/project.html`) "integrating bioinformatics and chemoinformatics approaches for the development of expert systems allowing the *in silico* prediction of toxicities." It provides published and unpublished test results from 13 biopharmaceutical companies and more than 11 research institutes, covering five species - rat, dog, guinea pig, mouse, rabbit; see Briggs et al. (2012), Cases et al. (2014), Briggs et al. (2015), Karp et al. (2015). It should be pointed out that most *in vitro* and *in vivo* databases are in the format of summaries, hence the information on experimental units is usually unavailable.

7.1.2 Clinical trial data

Safety data are routinely collected during clinical trials of medical products. The objectives and safety endpoints of the clinical studies may differ from one phase to another, but the trials data are typically incorporated into the Case Report Form (CRF, which is a paper or electronic form) and the CRF is usually initially stored in the sponsor's database with the Clinical Data Interchange Standards Consortium (CDISC) format, details of which can be found in www.cdisc.org. During the conduct of a clinical trial, the adverse events experienced by the study subjects are recorded in the CRF. Besides patient demographic variables and baseline characteristics that relate to a particular disease indication, the CRF usually includes the following information on each adverse event: starting and ending dates, grade or severity, temporal relationship with therapy (before, during, or after therapy), treatment associated with the adverse event, whether the event is a SAE, and outcome of the adverse event. In addition to the clinical manifestation of adverse outcomes, vital signs (e.g., body temperature, heart rate, and blood pressure), electrocardiogram (ECG), and laboratory testing results (hematology, biochemistry, and urinalysis) are also recorded in the CRF. Upon completion of a clinical study, the sponsor or investigator is required to upload, within a certain period of time, at least the following information (except for patient confidential information, e.g., patient identification number) to a publicly accessible clinical trial registry database:

- summaries of protocols: the purpose of the study, the disease or condition and medical product under study, trial phase, study design, recruitment status, inclusion and exclusion criteria, study site(s), and contact information,

- summaries of study results: description of study participants, number enrolled, overall outcomes of the study, summary of adverse events experienced by participants.

There are many clinical trial registry databases, some at the national level and some at the international level. The most widely used clinical trial registry databases are ClinicalTrials.gov of the US National Library of Medicine, the International Clinical Trials Registry Platform (ICTRP) maintained by the WHO (http://www.who.int/ictrp/en/).

7.1.3 FDA Adverse Event Reporting System (FAERS)

After regulatory approval and subsequent marketing of a medical product, regulatory agencies and manufacturers continue collecting safety data on patients who use the product and experience adverse events. These data are reported by consumers, health care providers, and product manufactures in an Individual Case Safety Report (ICSR) that contains the following information (ICH, 2001):

- Administrative and Identification Information: Sender's information, type of report (spontaneous report, report from clinical trial, other), seriousness, dates received and transmitted, case identification number, receiver of case safety report.

- Information on the case: patient characteristics (age, gender, height, weight), medical history and concurrent medications, adverse event duration and outcomes, laboratory test results, drug information (identification, batch and lot numbers, manufacturer, authorization number, route of administration, dates of administration), narrative case summary including clinical course, therapeutic measures, and sender's comments.

The post-marketing ICSR data are entered into a spontaneous adverse event reporting system (SAERS). Different countries maintain their own SAERS; the most comprehensive SAERS database is the US FDA Adverse Events Reporting System (FAERS) for post-marketing safety surveillance of all approved drugs and therapeutic biologics. Originally labeled Spontaneous Reporting System (SRS) since its inception in 1967, FAERS contains over seven million reports of adverse events up to 2012 and is updated quarterly, representing all spontaneous reports submitted directly to the FDA. Reports submitted by manufacturers are categorized into 15-day reports, serious periodic reports, and non-serious periodic reports for new molecular entity products within the first 3 years following FDA approval (FDA, 2014a). Note that individual pharmaceutical companies also maintain their own database containing the ICSRs of patients who use the company's products. Though much smaller in comparison with FAERS, the company's database provides more database information for safety signal detection for the company's products (Lehman et al., 2007). FAERS is commonly used by the FDA not only to monitor for new adverse events and medical errors that might be associated with the use of post-licensure products, but also to evaluate the manufacturer's compliance to reporting regulations and responding to outside requests for information (Almenoff et al., 2005; FDA, 2014a). Adverse events reported to FAERS are coded using the Medical Dictionary for Regulatory Activities (MedDRA).

7.1.4 Vaccine Adverse Event Reporting System and Vaccine Safety Datalink

The Vaccine Adverse Event Reporting System (VAERS) (`http://vaers.hhs.gov/index/about/index`) is a national vaccine post-marketing safety surveillance program co-managed by the FDA and the Centers for Disease Control and Prevention (CDC). It was established in 1990 in response to the requirement by the National Childhood Vaccine Injury Act (NCVIA) that health professionals and vaccine manufacturers report adverse events (possible side effects) that occur after the administration of vaccines licensed for use in the United States (Chen, 1994; Singleton et al., 1999; Iskander et al., 2004; CDC, 2012). In addition to vaccinee's characteristics (which include the birth weight and the number of siblings for children of age 5 and younger), the VAERS report form also contains the following information:

- Description of adverse events(s) (symptoms, signs, time course) and treatment,

- Whether the adverse events are serious, and the outcome of the adverse events,

- Dates and times of vaccination and adverse event onset,

- Names, manufacturers, lot numbers, route of administration, and dosages of the vaccines,

- Vaccination sites and purchase information,

- Pre-existing physician-diagnosed allergies, birth defects, medical conditions,

- Adverse event history following previous vaccination.

VAERS has been used in numerous studies with data mining and signal detection methods to establish the association of the occurrence of adverse events with the administration of vaccines. For example, analysis of VAERS data suggested a potential connection of Guillain-Barre's syndrome with the meningococcal conjugate vaccine, Menactra (Chen et al., 1994; Iskander et al., 2004; Souayah et al., 2012), which prompts a further investigation on this association (https://vaers.hhs.gov/about/index).

The Vaccine Safety Datalink (VSD) was established in 1990 jointly by the Immunization Safety Office of the US CDC and 4 (currently expanded to 9) health maintenance organizations (HMOs). The primary purpose of VSD is to monitor vaccine safety and conduct studies about rare and serious adverse events following immunization. It uses a prospectively collected, computerized medical record linkage system of subjects enrolled in the participating HMOs for the vaccine safety studies based on safety concerns raised from literature or excessive reports of adverse events to VAERS. Information collected in VSD consist of data from emergency departments, hospital and laboratory data, and outpatient data, together with potential confounding covariates. It allows for estimation of background rates of various conditions of interest and for rare adverse events. In addition to addressing vaccine safety issues, the database is also used to evaluate cost-effectiveness (Chen et al., 1997; DeStefano, 2001).

7.1.5 VigiBase

VigiBase, an international drug safety database developed in 1968, is maintained by the WHO's Uppsala Monitoring Centre (UMC). It is one of the largest and most diversified spontaneous reporting databases with over 100 countries contributing to the WHO Medicines Safety Programme. All ICSRs reported to this database use the medical terminologies WHO-ART, ICD, MeddRA, and the vocabularies WHO-DD and -DDE. The database is continually updated with incoming ICSRs. Although individual nations are recommended to send their updated ICSRs quarterly, some countries do so more frequently (Lindquist, 2008). In comparison with other spontaneous reporting databases, the inconsistency of reporting regulations and data quality across the member countries is its drawback.

7.1.6 Medicare, Medicaid, and health insurance claims databases

As part of the US Sentinel Initiative for monitoring drug safety, the SafeRx project was launched in 2008 collaboratively by the US FDA and the Center for Medicare and Medicaid Services (CMS) to develop methods for near-real time safety surveillance of medical products and to facilitate pharmacoepidemiologic studies for Medicare and Medicaid recipients (FDA, 2008b, 2010b; Racoosin et al., 2012). The CMS database contains comprehensive diagnostic and treatment information of those who join the Medicare and Medicaid programs. The collected information also includes demographic characteristics, prescription (including drugs prescribed, quantity dispensed, days supplied, prescriber information, payment), fee for services (FFS) (including inpatient hospital care, outpatient institutional care, and doctor visits, co-morbidities, procedures, occurrence of laboratory tests, physician information, payments). The FFS claims data are updated on a weekly basis; see Hartzema et al. (2011), Racoosin et al. (2012), and Robb et al. (2012) and references therein.

Similar to the US national CMS claims database, health insurance claims databases are electronic, longitudinal, and comprise information of policy holder's demographic characteristics, FFS, and prescription. The major difference between health insurance claims databases and the CMS is the composition of patient's age, with the former covering a wide age range, and the latter only those who meet the age requirements for eligibility. Examples of such health insurance claims databases that have been used for medical product safety research and signal detection are those maintained by Kaiser-Permanente (Chen et al., 2009), i3® (Dore et al., 2009), and GE health care database (DuMouchel et al., 2013). Caution should be exercised in interpreting the results derived from individual claims databases as different insurance programs may cover different populations (Lanes and de Luise, 2006).

7.1.7 Adverse event reporting database for medical devices

The US FDA collects medical device reports (MDRs) of suspected device related deaths, serious injuries, and malfunctions through its MedWatch program, and uses these reports to monitor device performance, detect potential device-related safety issues, and evaluate the benefit-risk profile of these products. As of August 14, 2015, it requires manufacturers and importers to submit mandatory MDRs to the FDA in an electronic format that the FDA can process, review, and archive (FDA, 2014b). It also encourages health professionals, care-givers, patients, and product customers who find problems related to medical devices to submit reports through the FDA through the MedWatch program. All voluntary and mandatory adverse event reports are entered into the Manufacturer and User Facility Device Experience (MAUDE) database, which has been used for reviewing the adverse event reports and detecting device-related safety signals (Gurtcheff, 2008; Levinson, 2006).

7.2 Statistical issues in the analysis of spontaneous AE reporting databases

Although FAERS, VAERS, and VigiBase have been recognized as useful tools for signal detection and data mining, it is important to realize their limitations and the statistical issues in their analysis (Almenoff et al., 2005; Rodriguez et al., 2001; Bailey et al., 2010; Chakravarty, 2010). Reporting of adverse events from the viewpoint of care is voluntary in the US, and some adverse events may never be reported to the FDA by health professionals and consumers, hence under-reporting can be serious. On the other hand, there may also be duplicate reporting because health professionals and consumers may report adverse events to both the FDA and the product manufacturer, and the latter is required to send the report to the FDA upon receiving the reports. In addition, the adverse event report rates vary from year to year, and over different regions where habits and regulations differ substantially. There are also changes in drug names and medical terminology during the fifty years of data accumulation. The database had over 300,000 "verbatim" drug names, which include generic and trade names, and after years of effort have been reduced to much fewer ingredient names. Since spontaneous reporting is not governed by research protocols, it is difficult to assess if the reported adverse reaction is caused by the product.

Bate et al. (2014, pp. 331-354) point out potential biases in the statistical analysis related to (a) the spontaneous reporting of drug-event pairs, (b) the reporting database structure, and (c) the trends in reporting and under-reporting. Concerning (a), they say:

> The drugs mentioned are usually mostly responsible for the event(s). However, a drug will not be suspected only on the basis of its pharmacological properties or safety profile. The time sequence between drug exposure and event occurrence will also be crucial... This leads to numerous SDRs (signals of disproportionate reporting) in which a drug is found associated with an event because it is indicated in patients with comorbidities that increase the risk of that event. This *indication bias* is related to the preferential... Similarly, the *co-prescription bias* may generate spurious SDRs, associating an event with drugs that do not intrinsically increase the risk of the event, but are frequently co-prescribed with drugs that really do.

Concerning (b), they note:

> In epidemiology, a traditional 2×2 contingency table opposes exposed to non-exposed, and cases to control. In spontaneous reporting databases, all information concerns patients receiving drugs and having suspected adverse reactions... The 2×2 contingency tables that underlie DAs thus oppose patients exposed to a drug to patients exposed to other drugs, and patients with a specific event to patients with another event. ... This bias is called the "masking effect" or the "event competition bias", and may mask SDRs for any drugs with a specific and highly reported event, which has an important weight in the drug's overall reporting.

They point out concerning (c) the following:

> Underreporting varies, especially in the case of media attention for a given drug-event association. This can lead to trends in reporting: an event can be more reported (or less underreported) with a given drug, though its occurrence remains constant. ... This has been designated as the "notoriety bias"... and is related to the classical detection bias in epidemiology.

West et al. (2014) point out validity concerns when using these data to arrive at safety conclusions from statistical analysis. As an analogy, they note that "physicians rely on patient-supplied information on past drug use and illness to assist with the diagnosis of current disease", and that patients' poor recall of past illnesses and medication use can "compromise a physician's ability to diagnose and/or prescribe successfully." Acri and Gross (2014) describe pharmacoepidemiologic studies of medication adherence, which show the patients not taking medication as prescribed, "resulting in more than $100 billion of avoidable hospitalizations" in the serious cases and in causing adverse events that are reported to the databases without accounting for non-compliance. Seidling and Bates (2014) also review pharmacoepidemilogic studies of medication errors "in the process of ordering, dispensing, or administering a drug." The methods used in these studies include "manual or automatic screening of claims data, administrative databases, medical records, electronic health records, incident reports mostly by providers in hospitals, patient (self-reporting) approaches," and there has been "no single approach that is considered the gold standard for detecting medication errors." The review concludes that "medication errors happen with considerable frequency during therapy" but that their incidence and severity cannot be quantified by the approaches used that do not have consistent use of definitions and classifications of medication errors.

DuMouchel (1999) discusses statistical modeling issues with the spontaneous reporting databases. He points out that a major statistical difficulty was in "the search for 'interestingly large' counts in a large frequency table, having millions of cells, most of which have an observed frequency of 0 or 1." According to the discussion by O'Neill and Szarfman (1999) on this paper, which was related to a project in response to the FDA's goal "to screen all the drug-event combinations for possible further investigation," the SRS (Spontaneous Reporting System) database of the FDA provides statistical challenges to "both describe the database in a big picture manner and to be able to proceed from this big picture down to the particulars in a logical manner that would facilitate medical understanding and insight into the drug-event associations in the database." DuMouchel presents this big picture in terms of counts N_{ijk} of the number of reports involving drug i (having 1398 levels) and event j (having 952 levels), and with $952 \times 1398 = 1,330,896$ cells that are further stratified into 18 groups by report date (with 6 first-year periods) and gender (with 3 classes: male, female, unreported). The database shows that multiple reports are often received for the same patient-event from the same or different sources and that the N_{ijk} "must be carefully interpreted as reporting rates are not occurrence rates," and because of "differential reporting of adverse events by drug." The last point is called "dilution bias" by Ahmed et al. (2015), who say:

> Drugs that have been on the market for a long time will be mentioned in many more reports than will more recently marketed drugs. The drugs with longer tenure will be less prone to generate disproportionality signals... This class of antidepressant drugs

(SSRIs, or selective serotonin reuptake inhibitors) was presented (in the UK) as causing suicides during a TV program. A transient peak of reports of suicide cases involving SSRIs was observed after the program was broadcast.

7.3   Reporting ratios and disproportionality analysis of safety database

In his seminal work on search for "unusually frequent drug-event combinations" from the SRS database that has many limitations as discussed above, DuMouchel (1999) asks: "Can drug-event combinations of potential interest be identified from internal evidence (SRS) alone? How can a rate be defined without a denominator?" To overcome this difficulty without resorting to external measures of exposure, he introduces the *baseline frequencies* E_{ij}, which is the expected number of reports under some independence assumption in the reporting of a specific drug and event. Letting $n_{ij} = \sum_k N_{ijk}$, $n_{i.} = \sum_j n_{ij}$, and $n_{.j} = \sum_i n_{ij}$, note that $n_{i.} - n_{ij}$ (respectively, $n - n_{ij}$) is the number of all other events than j for drug i (respectively, all drugs) in the spontaneous reports, where n is the total number of reports (Table 7.1). The *proportional reporting ratio* (PRR$_{ij}$) is defined by n_{ij}/E_{ij}, where

$$E_{ij} = n_{.j}\frac{n_{i.} - n_{ij}}{n - n_{ij}}, \tag{7.1}$$

which basically assumes independence of event j and all other events for reports on drug i. The *relative risk* (RR$_{ij}$) is defined by RR$_{ij} = n_{ij}/\widetilde{E}_{ij}$, where

$$\widetilde{E}_{ij} = \frac{(n_{i.} - n_{ij})(n_{.j} - n_{ij})}{n - n_{i.} - n_{.j} + n_{ij}}, \tag{7.2}$$

whose denominator is the number of reports on all other drugs than i and all other events than j. Note that

$$\text{PRR}_{ij} = \frac{n_{ij}/n_{.j}}{(n_{i.} - n_{ij})/(n - n_{ij})} \tag{7.3}$$

measures the disproportionality in rates of the target event j to all other events for exposure to drug i in the 2×2 contingency table (Table 7.1). In view of the independence hypothesis underlying (7.1), a higher value of PRR signals a stronger association between the adverse event and the drug. A closely related alternative for the 2×2 table is the *reporting odds ratio*

$$\text{ROR}_{ij} = \frac{n_{ij}}{\widetilde{E}_{ij}} = \frac{n_{ij}/(n_{i.} - n_{ij})}{(n_{.j} - n_{ij})/(n - n_{i.} - n_{.j} + n_{ij})} \tag{7.4}$$

TABLE 7.1 Summary table for a target drug with a target event from a spontaneous reporting database.

Target drug	Target event	All other events	Total
Yes	n_{ij}	$n_{i.} - n_{ij}$	$n_{i.}$
No	$n_{.j} - n_{ij}$	$n - n_{i.} - n_{.j} + n_{ij}$	$n - n_{i.}$
Total	$n_{.j}$	$n - n_{.j}$	n

of the exposed group (receiving target dose i) to the non-exposed group for the target adverse event j. DuMouchel (1999) also considers other baseline models and χ^2-tests for $(n_{ij} - E_{ij})/E_{ij}$, but points out that while statistical significance should not be taken seriously because of multiplicity issues and other issues with SRS data, the test statistics or associated P-values "might be a useful measure for ranking the degree of association" of drug i and event j over different (i, j) pairs. Note that n_{ij}/E_{ij}, which will be called the "standardized rate" for event j and drug i, is within the purview of "standardization" discussed in Section 6.3.1.

7.4 Empirical Bayes approach to safety signal detection

Assuming the count n_{ij} to be Poisson with mean μ_{ij}, DuMouchel (1999) introduces an empirical Bayes approach to the challenging high-dimensional problem of estimating the ratios $\lambda_{ij} = \mu_{ij}/E_{ij}$ (or $\mu_{ij}/\hat{E}_{ij}$). Disproportionality analysis (DA) combined with empirical Bayes estimation has become a widely used method for other databases beyond the SRS database considered in DuMouchel's seminal paper, in which he points out that the empirical Bayes approach tries "to achieve the interpretability of the relative risk measures but also to adjust properly for the sampling variation." In particular, DuMouchel et al. (2013) have applied it to 5 real healthcare databases and 6 simulated databases to evaluate its performance for safety signaling and have found that it "did not discriminate true positives from true negatives using healthcare data as they seem to do using spontaneous report data", unlike its good performance for spontaneous report databases. They say: "One possible explanation for why DA methods work well for spontaneous report databases is that a spontaneous report of a suspected drug-adverse event association has the benefit of a focused interpretation by the reporter, whereas the data in a healthcare database, being collected for a different purpose such as insurance billing, may tend to be subject to many more random sources of noise and bias."

DuMouchel's empirical Bayes approach assumes a common prior distribution on λ_{ij} so that the posterior distribution of λ_{ij} given n_{ij} can be used to rank the cell counts via $\text{rank}(i,j) = E[\log_2(\lambda_{ij}) \mid n_{ij}]$, where $\log_2$ stands for logarithm to base 2. "Empirical Bayes" refers to his use of the observed counts to estimate by maximum likelihood the hyperparameters of the prior distribution, which he assumes to be a mixture of two gamma distributions, with shape and scale parameters α_i and β_i ($i = 1, 2$) and prior probability π of choosing the $\text{Gamma}(\alpha_1, \beta_1)$ distribution. He argues that using $E[\log_2(\lambda_{ij}) \mid n_{ij}]$ has the effect of taking the geometric mean $\text{EBGM}_{ij} = 2^{E[\log_2(\lambda_{ij}) \mid n_{ij}]}$, which has an information-theoretic interpretation as "the number of bits of information connecting row i and column j in the table of frequencies". He assumes the following model for all (i,j) pairs:

$$\begin{cases} n_{ij} \sim \text{Poisson}(\mu_{ij}), \\ \lambda_{ij} \;(= \mu_{ij}/E_{ij}) \sim P\,\text{Gamma}(\alpha_1, \beta_1) + (1-P)\,\text{Gamma}(\alpha_2, \beta_2). \end{cases} \tag{7.5}$$

He also explains the rationale behind this Bayesian model, saying:

> We assume that the majority of the cells (e.g., $1 - P = 2/3$ of them) have values of λ clustered at or below the null hypothesis value of $\lambda = 1$. A corresponding gamma distribution with parameters $\alpha_2 = 2$, $\beta_2 = 4$ (with mean = 0.5 and standard deviation = 0.35) is suggested (as starting values for α_2 and β_2) for this component. The remaining P (e.g., $P = 1/3$) of the cells (for which $\lambda > 1$) are hypothesized to have a λ-distribution with very high variance and a somewhat higher mean, with suggested parameters (starting values) $\alpha_1 = 0.2$, $\beta_2 = 0.1$, having mean = 2 and standard deviation = 4.5.

The reason why he only considers one-sided departures of the null hypothesis $\lambda = 1$ is that "if (the relative risk $\text{RR}_{ij} =) n_{ij}/\tilde{E}_{ij} = 1,000$, then cell (i,j) occurred 1,000 times as frequently as the baseline frequency predicts," hence only exceedances of λ_{ij} over 1 flag safety concerns as the goal of data mining the SRS database "is to screen all drug-event combinations for possible further investigation." He points out that the relative risk measure RR_{ij} "has the great advantage of being easy to interpret " but that "its biggest disadvantage is the extreme sampling variability of RR when the baseline and observed frequencies ($\tilde{E}_{ij}$ and n_{ij}, respectively) are small." O'Neill and Szarfman (1999) provide the following important insights into E_{ij} or $\tilde{E}_{ij}$ and the SRS database of the FDA, which also explain the major difference between the empirical Bayes methods here and those in Chapter 5 for clinical trial data:

> Most of the literature on signal detection methods for adverse

events attempts in some way to create a control group for a comparison, either of a drug with itself in prior time intervals, or with other drugs and events, or with external data sources of relative drug usage and exposure. Currently, there is no external control group, nor independent external measure of patient exposure for all drugs available (in the SRS database). DuMouchel's model attempts to deal with this by taking all the frequency count data in the entire table into account by using as controls all other drugs and all other events... This may be considered analogous to the data set up for a case-control design, where the odds ratio, the difference of proportions, or other measures of association in a four-cell table may be used for testing the independence of row and column (for Drug A and Drug B, with the reports for each drug categorized into events for ADR1 and ADR2). DuMouchel's approach generalizes this paradigm by including all other drugs and all other adverse events as the controls, and by introducing the Bayesian modeling of the distribution of the ratios of observed counts to the expected counts for all cells in the total table under the assumption (null hypothesis) of independence of rows and columns.

Let $\theta = (\alpha_1, \beta_1, \alpha_2, \beta_2, P)$ be the hyperparameter vector of the mixture Gamma prior distribution of the Poisson counts n_{ij}. Because the Gamma distributions are a conjugate family of prior distributions for Poisson data, the posterior distribution of λ_{ij} given $n_{ij} = N$ and $E_{ij} = E$ (which, in view of (7.1), involves other $n_{i,\tilde{j}}$ and $n_{\tilde{i},j}$ values through $n_{i.}$ and $n_{.j}$) is the following mixture of Gamma distributions:

$$P_N \, \text{Gamma}(\alpha_1 + N, \beta_1 + E) + (1 - P_N) \, \text{Gamma}(\alpha_2 + N, \beta_2 + E), \quad (7.6)$$

$$P_N = \frac{P f(N; \alpha_1, \beta_1/E)}{P f(N; \alpha_1, \beta_1/E) + (1 - P) f(N; \alpha_2, \beta_2/E)}, \quad (7.7)$$

where $f(\cdot; a, b)$ is the density function of a negative binomial distribution:

$$f(N; a, b) = \left(\frac{1}{1+b} \right)^N \left(\frac{b}{1+b} \right)^\alpha \frac{\Gamma(\alpha + N)}{N! \Gamma(\alpha)}, \quad (7.8)$$

which is the marginal density of counts in a Gamma mixture of Poisson distributions. Noting that $P f(\cdot; \alpha_1, \beta_1/E) + (1 - P) f(\cdot; \alpha_2, \beta_2/E)$ is the marginal density of the observed counts n_{ij} over all (i, j) pairs, DuMouchel (1999) proposes to estimate the hyperparameter vector θ by maximizing the likelihood function

$$L(\theta) = \prod_{i,j} \left\{ P f(n_{ij}; \alpha_1, \beta_1/E_{ij}) + (1 - P) f(n_{ij}; \alpha_2, \beta_2/E_{ij}) \right\}, \quad (7.9)$$

saying: "The maximization involves an iterative search in the five-dimensional parameter space, where each iteration involves computing $\log(L(\theta))$ and its first and second derivatives," which are sums of several million terms. However, using the starting values suggested in our quotation below (7.5), he reports that "in testing runs using several datasets, the maximization typically takes between 5 and 15 iterations" to converge.

DuMouchel's empirical Bayes estimate of λ_{ij} has been referred to as the Multi-item Gamma-Poisson Shrinker (MGPS), following a paper by DuMouchel and Pregibon (2001) that uses the method for the "market basket problem" of screening for "multi-item associations" in a database of transactions, and the paper by Szarfman et al. (2002) on the use of the method to "efficiently signal higher-than-expected combinations of drugs and events" in the FDA's spontaneous reports database. It is also called the "Gamma-Poisson Shrinker" in the R implementation by Canida and Ihrie (2017). CDER (Center for Drug Evaluation and Research) of the FDA published a memorandum in August 2006 on data mining of AERS spontaneous reporting database by using MGPS. Concerning the question about the opportunities provided by MGPS, it says that MGPS provides "a large collection of positive and negative controls, reminders of what other experts know that serve to assess biologic plausibility of results, clues to complex safety issues quickly," and "signals important information that might be missed if the question is not asked, aids in predicting future trends or behaviors (e.g., of drugs in the same class), and enables decision-makers to make proactive, knowledge driven decisions" (Szarfman and Levine, 2006). It points out the limitations of AERS, including reporting bias, potential for confounding due to multiple drugs being prescribed to individual patients, lack of exposure or background rate, and being a "passive reporting system" in which reports to companies from patients or healthcare providers are voluntarily submitted. It also points out the limitations of data mining that "cannot prove or refute causal associations between drugs and events" and that only "identifies adjusted disproportionality of drug-event reporting patterns" in AERS. The CDER's memorandum notes that MGPS "does not estimate incidence or prevalence" and "does not adjust for polypharmacy," using "no dosage and formulation information." Hence, "to further study the adverse-event risk, the signals generated by MGPS can be evaluated by individual case review and compared with various analyses from other sources (e.g. clinical trials, general practice databases, literature reports)." It also reports some results of the MGPS analysis of the FDA's spontaneous reports database, "which currently has over 2.9 million such reports," presenting the results only on 16 drugs and only "for drug-PT pairs for severe adverse events where $EBGM_{ij} \geq 2$ and $n_{ij} \geq 2$ for at least one year." PTs (Preferred Terms) that are most likely related to the indications being treated were excluded. Recall that $EMBG_{ij}$ refers to the empirical Bayes geometric mean estimate of λ_{ij} and is used to rank the λ_{ij} pairs; see the first paragraph of this section. As pointed out by DuMouchel (1999, p. 202), graphical techniques have also been developed by Ana Szarfman and colleagues at the FDA "for interpreting and sorting through" thousands of potentially interesting interactions among millions of counts in applying MGPS-EBGM to the analysis of these data. These graphical techniques are "an essential part of the overall project," since "the results are much more convincing when one can show with a graph or two how consistent the discovered patterns are, and the graphics themselves are potent discovery tools." The presentation of the results in the aforementioned FDA memorandum in August 2006 clearly demonstrates the power of these graphical tools.

A subsequent enhancement of MGPS is the regression-adjusted GPS algorithm (RGPS) introduced by DuMouchel and Harpaz (2012), published in a November 2012 white paper by Oracle Health Sciences, which says:

> The main methodology for coping with the fact that spontaneous reports mention multiple drugs per report is logistic regression or its variants. A regression model attempts to compute the probability that a given AE will be mentioned in a report based on the set of drugs mentioned in the report as well as the before-mentioned report covariates such as age, sex, or report year... (Logistic regression) can have the unexpected disadvantage of implicitly assuming that multiple drugs affect risk multiplicatively, whereas an additive effects model or some other model may fit the observed event frequencies much better... We denote one such extension, implemented within (the Oracle Health Sciences software) Empirical Signal, as extended logistic regression (ELR)... By combining ideas from ELR and MGPS, RGPS aims to achieve the best of both methods.

7.5 Bayesian signal detection from AE databases

Gould (2007) notes that DuMouchel's use of a common P for the gamma mixture prior for λ_{ij} over all drug-event pairs (i, j) has certain disadvantages although it facilitates maximum likelihood estimation of P in the empirical Bayes approach. He proposes to allow P to vary with (i, j), similar to the prior (5.9) that he also uses for signal detection from clinical trials data. Using i to label the drug-event pairs, $i = 1, \ldots, m$, his prior distribution is the gamma mixture

$$\lambda_i \sim (1 - \gamma_i)\text{Gamma}(a_0, b_0) + \gamma_i \text{Gamma}(a_1, b_1), \qquad (7.10)$$

in which a_0, b_0, a_1 and b_1 are specified hyperparameters, with (a_0, b_0) for the null distribution of no association between the drug and the event, and (a_1, b_1) for the gamma component in which there is association. The γ_i is assumed to have a Bernoulli distribution whose parameter follows a beta distribution; see Section 5.4.2 and Supplement 3 in Section 5.5. Gould (2007) uses this hierarchical Bayesian model to identify drug-event pairs with small posterior probabilities of γ_i for further investigation. His simulation studies show that it has (a) good performance in terms of sensitivity and specificity and (b) better performance than DuMouchel's MGPS-EBGM method and the Bayesian Confidence Propagation Neural Network (BCPNN) of Bate et al. (1998), which we describe below.

Consider the cell counts n_{ij} in the $I \times J$ table of an AE (adverse event) database for drug-AE pairs (i, j). Assume $n_{ij}|p_{ij} \sim \text{Binomial}(n_{..}, p_{ij})$ with $p_{ij} \sim \text{Beta}(\alpha_{ij}, \beta_{ij})$, in which $\alpha_{ij} = 1$ and $\beta_{ij} = [E(p_{i.}|n_{i.}) + E(p_{.j}|n_{.j})]^{-1} - 1$. Then, for the marginal row and marginal column totals in the $I \times J$ table under the assumption of independence, $n_{i.}|p_{i.} \sim \text{Binomial}(n_{..}, p_{i.})$ with $p_{i.} \sim \text{Beta}(1, 1)$, and $n_{.j}|p_{.j} \sim \text{Binomial}(n_{..}, p_{.j})$ with $p_{.j} \sim \text{Beta}(1, 1)$, where p_{ij}, $p_{i.}$, and $p_{.j}$ denote the probabilities of the occurrence of cell counts. Bate et al. (1998) define the information component for cell (i, j) to be $\text{IC}_{ij} = \log_2 [p_{ij}/(p_{i.}p_{.j})]$, which leads to the estimate

$$\widehat{\text{IC}}_{ij} = \log_2 \left[\frac{(n_{ij} + 1)(n_{..} + 2)^2}{(n_{ij} + 1)(n_{..} + 2)^2 + n_{..}(n_{i.} + 1)(n_{.j} + 1)} \right] \tag{7.11}$$

with variance estimate

$$\hat{\sigma}_{ij}^2 = \frac{1}{(\log 2)^2} \left[\frac{n_{..} - n_{ij} + \gamma - 1}{(n_{ij} + 1)(n_{..} + \gamma + 1)} \right.$$
$$\left. + \frac{n_{..} - n_{i.} + 1}{(n_{i.} + 1)(n_{..} + 3)} + \frac{n_{..} - n_{.j} + 1}{(n_{.j} + 1)(n_{..} + 3)} \right], \tag{7.12}$$

where $\gamma = \frac{(n_{..}+2)^2}{(n_{i.}+1)(n_{.j}+1)}$, as suggested by Heckerman (1997). This leads to $\widehat{\text{IC}}_{ij} \pm z_{1-\alpha/2}\hat{\sigma}_{ij}$ as an approximate $100(1-\alpha)\%$ confidence interval for IC_{ij}; see also Huang et al. (2011). The AE database used by Bate et al. (1998) is the WHO database in Section 7.1.5, which they say "is held by Uppsala Monitoring Centre and now contains nearly two million reports of ADRs (Adverse Drug Reactions)." The neural network in BCPNN provides "the computational power to consider all links and the ability to highlight potential signals", which is "extremely advantageous as most reports in the databases contain some empty fields." The information component IC_{ij} is "the strength of the association between two variables (indicator variables of taking drug i and experiencing AE j) and is the logarithmic form of the factor relating the prior and posterior probabilities (hence propagation)." The IC is "only calculated on a finite number of reports (and is therefore) merely an estimate of the real IC", hence a confidence interval for the real IC is needed.

7.6 Likelihood ratio test-based approach and other signal detection methods for ADR monitoring

7.6.1 LR test-based approach to QSD

In their overview of quantitative signal detection (QSD) for monitoring adverse drug reactions (ADRs), Bate et al. (2014) point out that from a public health and epidemiological perspective, signals of potential harmful effects of medical products arise from analysis of large amounts of data from spontaneous reporting systems (SRS), observational studies, and clinical trials. They say that QSD "implies a prior statistical analysis attesting that the observed value (of proportions, odds, incidence rate, or severity of AE) is outside what would be expected." They point out that disproportionality analyses (DAs) of spontaneous reporting databases usually result in signals of disproportionate reporting (SDRs) that differ from safety signals, as "a safety signal does not always imply a corresponding SDR and the existence of an SDR is not sufficient to constitute a safety signal." They further note that applications of DAs to spontaneous reporting databases may suffer from potential biases that may impact signal detection from DAs. For example, if a drug is prescribed to prevent the reported event or to treat a disease predisposing to this event, this may lead to *indication bias* in which the drug is found to be associated with the event because it is being given to "patients with comorbidities that increase the risk of that event." On the other hand, if a drug is contraindicated in a high-risk population, then other drugs without the contraindication could be found associated with such events. Another potential bias, called *co-prescription bias*, may incur when a drug is frequently co-prescribed with other drugs and spurious SDRs may be generated with this drug which in fact does not intrinsically increase the risk of the event. Moreover, if a high proportion of an event is reported for a drug and a lower proportion of the same event is reported for all other drugs, then the ability to detect SDRs not involving the event would be limited, which is called "*event competition bias*" or "masking effect." Bate et al. (2014) also discuss biases related to the variability of reporting rates, in which an event may be more likely reported with a given drug (e.g., due to the media focusing on the event), even though its occurrence remains constant.

Huang et al. (2011) note that "identifying the safety signals in large databases such as FAERS is important for public health" and propose a frequentist test-based approach using large spontaneous adverse event reporting databases and clinical trial databases, as an alternative to Du-Mouchel's (1999) empirical Bayes MGPS approach. Using the FAERS database as an illustrative example, they propose to summarize the data in a two-dimensional table with AE as the row variable and drug as the column variable. Let I denote the total number of AEs, J the total number of drugs, and the cell count n_{ij} the number of reports on the ith AE and jth drug. Let $n_{i\cdot}$ and $n_{\cdot j}$ be the marginal totals for the ith AE and jth drug, respectively. Huang et al. (2011) transform the $I \times J$ table into many 2×2 tables so that for drug j there are potentially I tables, each associated with a particular AE. They assume that $n_{ij} \sim \text{Poisson}(n_{i\cdot}p_i)$, where p_i is the reporting rate of the jth drug for the ith AE, and $n_{\cdot j} - n_{ij} \sim \text{Poisson}((n_{\cdot\cdot} - n_{i\cdot})q_i)$, where q_i is the reporting rate of all the other AEs combined (after excluding the ith AE). They consider the null hypothesis $H_0 : p_i = q_i$ for all i, and the one-sided alternative $H_a : p_i > q_i$ for at least one i. The likelihood ratio test (LRT) statistic is

$$\text{LR}_{ij} = \frac{(n_{ij}/n_{i\cdot})^{n_{ij}} [(n_{\cdot j} - n_{ij})/(n_{\cdot\cdot} - n_{i\cdot})]^{n_{\cdot j} - n_{ij}}}{(n_{\cdot j}/n_{\cdot\cdot})^{n_{\cdot j}}}$$

$$= \left(\frac{n_{ij}}{E_{ij}}\right)^{n_{ij}} \left(\frac{n_{\cdot j} - n_{ij}}{n_{\cdot j} - E_{ij}}\right)^{n_{\cdot j} - n_{ij}}, \tag{7.13}$$

where $E_{ij} = n_{i\cdot}n_{\cdot j}/n_{\cdot\cdot}$ is the expected value of n_{ij} under H_0. The likelihood ratio test rejects H_0 if $\max_{1 \leq i \leq I} \text{LR}_{ij}$ exceeds some threshold.

Huang et al. (2011) use FDR (false discovery rate) control to determine the threshold. They therefore apply a step-down procedure involving the p-values associated with the likelihood ratio statistics. They note that under $H_0, n_{1j}, \ldots, n_{Ij}$ are conditionally independent given $(n_{1\cdot}, \ldots, n_{I\cdot})$, with $n_{ij} \sim \text{Poisson}(n_{i\cdot}p_0)$, where p_0 is the common value of p_i under H_0, and therefore

$$(n_{1j}, \ldots, n_{Ij})|(n_{1\cdot}, \ldots, n_{I\cdot}; n_{\cdot j}) \sim \text{Multinomial}\left(n_{\cdot j}; \frac{n_{1\cdot}}{n_{\cdot\cdot}}, \ldots, \frac{n_{I\cdot}}{n_{\cdot\cdot}}\right). \tag{7.14}$$

In view of (7.14), they use simulation from the multinomial distribution to determine the p-value of the maximum likelihood ratio (MLR), leading to the following step-down procedure to signal AEs associated with the jth drug, with FDR control at $\alpha = 0.05$:

We rank the likelihood ratio test statistic values for the observed dataset from the largest to the smallest one. After the AE associated with MLR is identified as the signal when its p-value is less than 0.05 (so that) we have rejected H_0, we move to the AE with the second largest value of the likelihood ratio test statistic (i.e., ranked 2nd), determine its p-value from the empirical null distribution of MLR values obtained using Monte Carlo simulation, and if this p-value is smaller than 0.05, we declare the corresponding AE as a signal and move to the next AE associated with the third largest value of the likelihood ratio test statistic, and so on.

This differs from the step-down procedure in Section 5.3 because it does not use adjusted p-values, hence the claims in Huang et al. (2011, p. 1233) that the procedure controls FDR at level α needs justification. This actually follows from the general theory of test-based variable selection of Lai et al. (2018b) for generalized linear models. By making the use of the closed testing principle, they show that the procedure actually controls the FWER at level $\alpha + o(1)$ as $n_{..} \to \infty$.

7.6.2 Tree-based scan statistics

A scan statistic, introduced by Naus (1965a) for studying the maximum cluster of points on a line, has been widely used for identifying clusters of a one-dimensional, and later multi-dimensional, point process and applied to drug safety signals; see Wallenstein et al. (1994), Glaz et al. (2001), Turnbull et al. (1989), Kulldorff (1997), Kulldorff et al. (1998), Kulldorff et al. (2003), Yih et al. (2011), and Kulldorff et al. (2013). Here we first describe the one-dimensional scan statistic that involves the distribution of a random variable X which takes values in $(0, 1]$ and can be parameterized as follows. Partitioning the interval $(0, 1]$ into subintervals, each of length d, the density function of X is

$$
f(x) = \begin{cases} a, & \text{for } b \leq x \leq b + d \\ (1 - ad)/(1 - d) & \text{for } 0 \leq x < b \text{ or } b + d < x \leq 1, \end{cases} \tag{7.15}
$$

in which a and b are unknown parameters. Suppose $X_1, \ldots, X_N$ are i.i.d observations and have the same distribution as X. To test the null hypothesis $H_0 : a = 1$ (which corresponds to the case of uniform X) against the alternative hypothesis $H_1 : 1 < a \leq 1/d$ (which corresponds to X being stochastically larger than uniform), Naus (1965a) uses a generalized likelihood ratio (GLR) test statistic

$$
\Lambda(X_1, \ldots, X_N) = \frac{\sup_{\Theta_1} \prod_{i=1}^{N} f(X_i)}{\sup_{\Theta_0} \prod_{i=1}^{N} f(X_i)}, \tag{7.16}
$$

where Θ_0 and Θ_1 denote the parameter spaces corresponding to H_0 and H_1, respectively. Under H_1, the density function of X_i is a piecewise constant function with 3 pieces and the largest value in the middle piece. Let n be the number of observations in the middle piece. Since the denominator of (7.16) is a constant, (7.16) can be written as $\Lambda = \sup_{\Theta_1} a^n \left[(1 - ad)/(1 - d)\right]^{N-n}$, which reduces to

$$
\left(\frac{n}{N}\right)^n \left(\frac{N - n}{N}\right)^{N-n} \left(\frac{1}{d}\right)^n \left(\frac{1}{1 - d}\right)^{N-n} \tag{7.17}
$$

for known d, and to

$$
\sup_{0 < d < n/N} \left(\frac{n}{N}\right)^n \left(\frac{N - n}{N}\right)^{N-n} \left(\frac{1}{d}\right)^n \left(\frac{1}{1 - d}\right)^{N-n} \tag{7.18}
$$

for unknown d. In the context of scan statistics for a one-dimensional point process, $N = \sup_{0 < x < 1-d} n_d(x)$, where $n_d(x)$ denotes the number of points X_i falling in the scanning window $(x, x + d\,]$, and the scan statistic is used to test the null hypothesis of constant intensity.

For a multidimensional scan statistic, the scanning window may be a rectangle, circle, triangle, sphere, cylinder, etc. (Naus, 1965b; Turnbull et al., 1989; Kulldorff, 1997), and the preceding Poisson point process with constant intensity has been extended to more general multivariate point process models, including non-homogenous Poisson processes (Naus, 1965b; Wallenstein et al., 1994; Kulldorff, 1997; Glaz et al., 2001). This has led Kulldorff (1997) and Kulldorff et al. (1998) to extend scan statistics to a tree, for which "all the data are in the leaves" of the tree and "the scanning window is defined by a cut, which can be made on any branch of the tree" so that "the cut defines a branch of the tree whose leaves may contain excess events." They first consider "simple cuts" and illustrate them in application to occupational silicosis surveillance using the National Center for Health Statistics Multiple Cause of Death Database, for which "each leaf corresponds to a specific occupation" and the tree-based scan statistic considers "all possible cuts, on any branch" and calculates, for each cut, "the total number of deaths and the total number of silicosis deaths for all the leaves defined by that cut." Letting c_i denote the observed number of silicosis deaths and n_i denote the total number of deaths in leaf (occupation) i, they assume that $c_i|n_i \sim \text{Poisson}(\lambda_i n_i)$, where λ_i is the probability that a death in leaf i is due to silicosis. They justify the Poisson approximation for rare diseases and let $C = \sum_{i=1}^{I} c_i$ and $N = \sum_{i=1}^{I} n_i$ (summing over the I leaves) so that conditional on $(C, n_1, \ldots, n_I)$, $(c_1, \ldots, c_I)$ has a multinomial distribution and therefore the likelihood function is

$$L(\lambda_1, \ldots, \lambda_I) = \prod_{i=1}^{I} \left(\frac{n_i \lambda_i}{\sum_{j=1}^{I} n_j \lambda_i} \right)^{c_i}. \tag{7.19}$$

They consider testing the null hypothesis H_0 of no occupational difference in silicosis mortality rate (i.e., the λ_i are equal for all leaves i) against the composite alternative hypothesis H_G that there is a group G of occupations for which $\lambda_i = \lambda_G$ for all $i \in G$ while $\lambda_j = \lambda^* < \lambda_G$ for $j \notin G$ for unspecified parameters λ^* and λ_G. Letting $c_G = \sum_{i \in G} c_i$ and $n_G = \sum_{i \in G} n_i$, they show that the GLR statistic for testing H_0 versus H_G has the form

$$R_G = \frac{\sup\{L(\lambda_1, \ldots, \lambda_I) : \lambda_i = \lambda_G \text{ for } i \in G, \lambda_j = \lambda^* \text{ for } j \in G, \lambda_G > \lambda^*\}}{\sup\{L(\lambda_1, \ldots, \lambda_I) : \lambda_1 = \ldots = \lambda_I\}}$$
$$= \left(\frac{N}{C}\right)^C \left(\frac{c_G}{n_G}\right)^{c_G} \left(\frac{C - c_G}{N - n_G}\right)^{C - c_G} \text{ or } 1, \tag{7.20}$$

according to whether c_G/n_G (which is the MLE of λ_G) exceeds the MLE

$(C - c_G)/(N - n_G)$ of λ^* or not. Maximizing over G and taking logarithms then leads to their log-likelihood ratio statistic

$$\ell = \max_G \left\{ c_G \log\left(\frac{c_g}{n_g}\right) + (C - c_G)\left(\frac{C - c_g}{N - n_G}\right) \right\} I \left(\frac{c_G}{n_G} > \frac{C - c_G}{N - n_G}\right),$$
(7.21)

in which $I(\cdot)$ is the indicator function and each possible cut on the tree corresponds to a particular group G of occupations. The MLE of the common λ_i under H_0 is C/N. They implement the GLR tests by using Monte Carlo simulations to calculate the null distribution of (7.21) assuming C/N as the common λ_i, which is tantamount to a bootstrap test of H_0.

They extend the preceding tree-based scan statistic for simple cuts to "combinatorial cuts", which they explain as follows:

> Suppose we have four branches A, B, C, and D, originating from the same node. Rather than only considering the simple cuts, which would correspond to [A], [B], [C], and [D], one could consider all possible combinations of the four branches, giving the additional cuts [A, B], [A, C], [A, D], [B, C], [B, D], [C, D], [A, B, C], [A, B, D], [A, C, D], and [B, C, D]... For (an occupational) example, there are three simple cuts: farmers, cowboys, and hunters (at a node). If we used combinatorial cuts for that node, we would also evaluate (additional) sets of combined data: farmers + cowboys, cowboys + hunters, farmers + hunters, and farmers + cowboys + hunters.

They also consider "ordinal cuts", which they illustrate as follows:

> Take, for example, teachers of kindergartens, elementary schools, high schools, and colleges. This is an ordered list defined by the age of the students, and while it may make sense to combine neighbors on that ordered list, it makes less sense to combine kindergarten teachers together with college teachers without including the other two... Note that the simple cuts are a subset of the ordinal cuts, which is a subset of the combinatorial cuts.

Their Section 6.3 says that "an important practical consideration is whether to use a tree with only simple cuts, or whether to use combinatorial and ordinal cuts as well." Their Section 6.4 says:

> Another important potential application of (tree-based scan statistic) is in pharmacovigilance, where the goal is to find unexpected adverse drug effects that are too rare to find during preapproval phase III clinical trials. This could be done in a hospital or HMO setting, where the number of people receiving each drug is known, and where the emergence of serious side effects is closely followed. The tree-based independent variable would consist of all the administrated drugs, and closely related drugs would be near each

other on the tree. The method can also be turned around, creating a hierarchical tree for the dependent variable, with closely related side effects close to each other on the tree. Using proportional incidence of adverse effects, the tree-based scan statistic could also be used for data from the FDA's spontaneous reporting system.

Their Section 5 also briefly discusses extension of the tree-based scan statistic to multiple trees, saying:

From a mathematical perspective, it is trivial to generalize the above defined method to incorporate two or more trees, as long as the collection of leaves is the same. After the first tree has been scanned, simply continue with the second one, and so on, until all cuts on all trees have been evaluated. The cut with the maximum likelihood is then taken over all the trees, so that there is still only one most likely cut. In this way, the multiple testing is taken care of for all cuts on all trees simultaneously.

Kulldorff et al. (2013) have applied the tree-based scan statistic, adjusting for age, sex, and health plan, to assess the safety of selected antifungal and diabetes drugs from the electronic health records database of approximately 3.4 million members in nice health plans in the HMO Research Network Center for Education and Research on Therapeutics from 1999 through 2003. They "identify drug exposures from the pharmacy dispensing file, which includes generic and brand drug names, dispensing dates, national drug code for drug product dispensed, units dispensed, and days supplied" and use the "diagnosis file (which) contains ICD-9-CM codes for all diagnosis, dates of diagnosis, and an impatient/outpatient indicator." After removing "diagnoses unlikely to be drug-related acute AEs", they group the remaining ICD-9 diagnosis codes using MLCCS (Multi-Level Clinical Classification Software), which "is a hierarchical system with four levels' in which the top level identifies 18 body systems and each of them can have up to three sublevels. Their finding is that "several previously known AEs were detected while the total number of signals was modest." Brown et al. (2013) also apply DuMouchel's empirical Bayes method (EBGM described in Section 7.4) to these data and compare with the findings of the tree-based scan statistics, which they call TreeScan, for two antifungal and two diabetes drugs. They say that "TreeScan identified 71 signals, 49 at the highest threshold (with multiple testing adjusted p-value of < 0.001) and 22 at the medium threshold ($0.001 < p$-value < 0.05)" and that EBGM "identified 48 signals", of which the high threshold ones were also high-threshold TreeScan signals. Supplement 3 in Section 7.10 describes a recent extension of TreeScan to "tree–temporal scan statistics" for post-licensure monitoring of vaccines.

7.6.3 Ontological reasoning approach

Using the structural and terminological properties of MedDRA terms, ontological reasoning in which semantically linked adverse events are grouped to improve the performance of signal detection in spontaneous reporting systems provides an approach to describing clinical similarity of certain adverse events. As discussed in Chapter 1, adverse events are coded using adverse event dictionaries such as MedDRA, which do not take into account signal detection. To improve signal detection performance, Henegar et al. (2004) develop a formal ontology of adverse drug reactions and data mining tools that use descriptive representations of MedDRA terms to "group medically related case reports". Signal detection using ontological reasoning proceeds in two steps. The first step is terminological preprocessing, which performs simple reasoning by "subsumption with the formal ontology or within the classic MedDRA taxonomical hierarchy." For example, the drug-event pairs associated with "hepatitis_NOS" are grouped with pairs associated with the "subsumed concepts," such as "hepatitis_toxic" and "hepatitis_fulminant." The second step is signal detection using a hierarchical Bayesian approach that groups similar drug-event pairs at various levels of the formal ontology to determine posterior probabilities of the AEs after taking the drug. Henegar et al. (2004) show that this ontological reasoning approach improves the performance of signal detection by increasing the sensitivity without decreasing the specificity of signal detection. They also acknowledge that the "huge workload involved in the knowledge engineering step" limits the use of this ontological reasoning approach for signal detection.

7.6.4 Deep learning for pharmacovigilance

Traditional data mining and statistical modeling approaches to identifying drug-event pairs to detect safety signals (Schuemie et al., 2012; Patadia et al., 2015; Pacurariu et al., 2015) face many challenges because of insufficient knowledge on the pathophysiological mechanisms of the occurrence of adverse events, heterogeneity, temporal dependency, sparsity of signals, and high-dimensional covariates. To address these challenges, machine learning approaches have been increasingly used in pharmacovigilance. Bisgin et al. (2011) apply an unsupervised learning technique called "topic modeling" to FDA-approved drug labels with the goal of uncovering "topics" that group drugs with similar safety and therapeutic labels for detecting "potential adverse events that might have arisen from specific medications via topics." Using the FAERS data to build profiles of adverse events based on the side effects of drugs known to be associated with the events, Tatonetti et al. (2011) divide the FAERS data into two separate sets: reports listing exactly one drug and reports listing exactly two drugs, develop predictive models using supervised machine learning methods based on the first dataset, and validate the models for adverse event prediction using the second dataset. This approach helps identify drug-drug interactions in adverse event reports and provides an option for detecting hidden interactions by "using side effect profiles to infer the presence of unreported adverse events." Other applications of machine learning approaches to signaling adverse drug reactions have been provided by Du et al. (2017), Munsaka (2017), and Gao et al. (2017).

More recently, deep learning networks (see Section 2.1.3) have been advocated as effective predictive models for detection of adverse drug reactions using complex databases (e.g., EHRs) and social media (e.g., Twitter posts). Miotto et al. (2017) give a review of the opportunities and challenges of deep learning, such as Google DeepMind which differs from traditional machine learning in "how representations are learned from the raw data". Deep learning has great potential because of its "superior performance, end-to-end learning scheme with integrated feature learning, capability of handling complex and multi-modality data." Realizing the value of social media in pharmacovigilance and infeasibility of human review of the data, Cocos et al. (2017) use recurrent neural networks with word-embedding vectors (such as ADR membership tags in an input sequence) to detect ADRs from Twitter posts. Shickel et al. (2017) and Huynh et al. (2016) have also given additional applications of deep learning to safety signal detection.

7.7   Meta-analysis of multiple safety studies

Meta-analysis refers to statistical analysis methods that are applied to combine results from multiple studies to derive an overall conclusion on a common problem across these studies. For example, suppose that there are I two-arm randomized trials, each of which contains summary information such as d_{ij} patients having the AE of interest among a total of n_{ij} subjects in the jth treatment group of the ith trial, with $j = 0$ (or 1) for the control (or treatment). Let $\hat{\pi}_{ij} = d_{ij}/n_{ij}$ denote the response rate and $n_i = n_{i0} + n_{i1}$ the total sample size in the ith trial, $i = 1, \ldots, I$. Regarding $\hat{\pi}_{ij}$ as the sample estimate of the population rate π_{ij}, one can define the treatment effect θ_i as the risk difference $\pi_{i1} - \pi_{i0}$, or risk ratio π_{i1}/π_{i0}, or log odds ratio $\text{logit}(\pi_{i1}) - \text{logit}(\pi_{i0})$, where $\text{logit}(p) = \log(p/(1-p))$. Combining these treatment effects from the I studies using meta-analysis methods yields an overall conclusion on the treatment effect. There is extensive literature on statistical methodologies for meta-analysis in biomedical research and practice (Petitti, 2000; Olkin and Saner, 2001; Van Houwelingen et al., 2002; Haidich, 2010; Whitehead, 2002; CIOMS, 2016). Meta-analysis can be particularly useful in safety analysis because

- many interventional studies, especially clinical trials, are designed for the evaluation of efficacy and hence do not have much statistical power to detect clinically important safety events, and pre-defined inclusion and exclusion criteria for patient recruitment also make it difficult to generalize drug-event associations to a general population;

- evidence on rare events can be aggregated through scientific synthesis of multiple studies as rare events may not even be observed in a single study;

- evidence of drug-event relationship can be quantified and estimated more precisely with more data from multiple sources;

- inconsistent or inconclusive results can be further addressed and elucidated with increased sample size from multiple studies.

To achieve these goals, meta-analysis should carefully select the studies to be included. Whereas studies with identical or similar designs and inclusion-exclusion criteria are ideal to be combined for meta-analysis, care should be taken when combining studies with different designs and indications because the differences may be confounding factors for the problem of interest (Brookhart et al., 2010; Higgin et al., 2003). In addition, selecting published results for meta-analysis may introduce selection bias as unpublished studies are excluded from the analysis (Greco et al., 2013).

Ioannidis (2016) has given the following warning on "massive production of unnecessary, misleading, and conflicted systematic reviews and meta-analysis":

> Instead of promoting evidence-based medicine and health care, these instruments often serve mostly as easily produced publishable units or marketing tools. Suboptimal systematic reviews and meta-analyses can be harmful given the major prestige and influence these types of studies have acquired. The publication of systematic reviews and meta-analyses should be realigned to remove biases and vested interests and to integrate them better with the primary production of evidence.

On the other hand, he also says: "Systematic reviews and meta-analysis are indispensable components in the chain of scientific information and key tools for evidence-based medicine...it is irrational not to systematically review what is already known before deciding to perform any new study. Moreover, once a new study is completed, it is useful to update the cumulative evidence." He launched the Meta-Research Innovation Center at Stanford (METRICS) in 2014 to delve into how to best address bias, study design, data sharing, peer review, registration of studies, and reproducibility issues of meta-analysis. Berlin et al. (2012, 2014) give overviews of the use of meta-analysis in pharmacoepidemiology and in the evaluation of adverse events in clinical trials, respectively. The former focuses on non-experimental studies and the latter on clinical trials. We summarize below basic methods for meta-analysis not only in pharmacovigilance but also in the statistics and epidemiology literature for more general biomedical applications.

7.7.1   Fixed and random effects models for meta-analysis

Under the fixed effects model, individual studies estimate the same treatment effect θ which is unknown and the observed differences in treatment effect $\hat{\theta}_i$ are attributable to random sampling error. The overall treatment effect can be estimated by the weighted average

$$\hat{\theta} = \frac{\sum_{i=1}^{I} \omega_i \hat{\theta}_i}{\sum_{k=1}^{I} \omega_i}, \tag{7.22}$$

where ω_i represents the weight assigned to the ith study for which $\hat{\theta}_i$ is the estimate of θ. As noted by Deeks and Higgins (2010) and Schwarzer et al. (2015), one needs to first choose an appropriate treatment effect measure suitable for the study objective and available data (e.g., whether risk difference or percent risk increase should be used) and then to find its estimate $\hat{\theta}_i$. There is also an issue of how the weights should be chosen, which we next discuss.

Inverse-variance, Mantel-Haenszel, and Peto methods of weighting

A widely used method to combine multiple studies is the inverse-variance approach with the overall treatment effect estimate $\hat{\theta}$ given by (7.22) in which $\omega_i = 1/\text{Var}(\hat{\theta}_i)$. With this weighting, $\sum_{i=1}^{I} \omega_i(\hat{\theta}_i - \hat{\theta})^2$ has an approximately χ^2_{I-1} distribution under the null hypothesis of homogeneity across studies. Another commonly used method to combine the odds ratios from I studies in the case of binary outcomes was introduced by Mantel and Haenszel (1959) and uses weights that yield the corresponding Mantel-Haenszel estimate. The weight assigned to the results of the ith study is $\omega_i = b_i c_i / n_i$, where b_i, c_i, and n_i are the frequencies of the ith study in Table 7.2. Since the odds ratio is $y_i = \left(\frac{a_i}{c_i}\right) / \left(\frac{b_i}{d_i}\right) = \frac{a_i d_i}{b_i c_i}$, the Mantel-Haenszel (overall) odds ratio can be expressed as follows:

$$\frac{\sum_{i=1}^{I} a_i d_i}{\sum_{i=1}^{I} b_i c_i} = \frac{\sum_{i=1}^{I} \omega_i y_i}{\sum_{i=1}^{I} \omega_i}, \tag{7.23}$$

where $\omega_i = b_i c_i$. The Mantel-Haenszel test for the null hypothesis (of no treatment effect across the I studies) $H_0 : p_{i1} = p_{i2}$ for $i = 1, \ldots, I$ uses the Mantel-Haenszel statistic

$$\text{MH} = \frac{\sum_{i=1}^{I} (a_i - E_{0,i})}{\sqrt{\sum_{i=1}^{I} V_{0,i}}}, \tag{7.24}$$

where p_{i1} (respectively, p_{i2}) is the probability of event occurrence in treatment (respectively, control), $E_{0,i} = \frac{n_{1i}m_{1i}}{n_i}$ is the mean of a_i, and $V_{0,i} = \frac{n_{1i}n_{2i}m_{1i}m_{2i}}{n_i^2(n_i-1)}$ is the variance of a_i conditional on $(n_{1i}, n_{2i}, m_{1i}, m_{2i})$, which has a limiting standard normal distribution under H_0.

TABLE 7.2 Contingency table of adverse events for the ith study.

Group	With adverse events	Without adverse events	Total
Treatment	a_i	b_i	n_{1i}
Control	c_i	d_i	n_{2i}
Total	m_{1i}	m_{2i}	n_i

For the case of rare events in binary outcomes, the Peto method for weighting odds ratios from multiple studies is "currently the estimation methods of choice," as noted by Brockhaus et al. (2014). This method, which was introduced in the Statistical Appendix of Yusuf et al. (1985), yields the Peto odds ratio

$$\text{POR} = \exp \left(\frac{\sum_{i=1}^{I} (a_i - E_{0,i})}{\sum_{i=1}^{I} V_{0,i}} \right). \tag{7.25}$$

This corresponds to weighting $y_i = (a_i - E_{0,i})/V_{0,i}$ by its inverse variance $\omega_i = 1/V_{0,i}^{-1} = V_{0,i}$ to obtain the log-odds ratio estimator $\left(\sum_{i=1}^{I} \omega_i y_i \right) / \left(\sum_{i=1}^{I} \omega_i \right)$. Although such weighting is a special case of (7.22) for the log odds ratio, exponentiation in (7.25) gives a biased estimate of the overall odds ratio because of Jensen's inequality for strictly convex function $\exp(\cdot)$, as Brockhaus et al. (2014) have demonstrated in their simulation studies and in the case of $n_{1i} \neq n_{2i}$ and $I(= i) = 1$. They therefore argue that the Peto odds ratio should be viewed as "a new overall effect measure" instead of an overall odds ratio.

Extended Peto method for time-to-event data

Deeks et al. (2008) point out that for time-to-event data, the overall hazard ratio across the I studies can be estimated by pooling the hazard ratios from individual studies using the inverse-variance method as described above. Alternatively, one can divide the follow-up time into K

subintervals, and calculate the expected number of events for the jth treatment group in each subinterval for individual studies under the null hypothesis of no treatment effect on the time-to-event outcome. Let n_{ijk} denote the number of patients at risk right before the kth subinterval and d_{ijk} the number of patients experiencing the AE during the kth subinterval for the jth treatment group in the ith trial, $i = 1, \ldots, I$, $j = 0, 1$ and $k = 1, \ldots, K$. Let

$$\bar{d}_{i1k} = E(d_{i1k}) = n_{i1k} \times \frac{d_{i \cdot k}}{n_{i \cdot k}} \tag{7.26}$$

be the expected number of events for treatment in the kth subinterval of the ith trial, where $d_{i \cdot k} = d_{i1k} + d_{i0k}$ and $n_{i \cdot k} = n_{i1k} + n_{i0k}$. Note that conditional on n_{i1k} and $d_{i \cdot k}$, d_{i1k} has a hypergeometric distribution with variance

$$V_{ik} = \frac{d_{i \cdot k}(n_{i \cdot k} - d_{i \cdot k})}{n_{i \cdot k} - 1} \cdot \frac{n_{i1k}}{n_{i \cdot k}} \cdot \left(1 - \frac{n_{i1k}}{n_{i \cdot k}} \right). \tag{7.27}$$

Therefore, using the same argument as in (7.25) for the Peto odds ratio, Deeks et al. (2008) propose to estimate hazard ratio for the ith study by

$$\hat{\lambda}_i = \exp \left(\frac{\sum_{k=1}^{K} d_{i1k} - \sum_{k=1}^{K} \bar{d}_{i1k}}{\sum_{k=1}^{K} V_{ik}} \right), \tag{7.28}$$

and use $\omega_i = \sum_{k=1}^{K} V_{ik}$ to weight this hazard ratio, thereby giving a Peto-type overall hazard ratio

$$\hat{\lambda}_{\text{Peto}} = \exp \left(\frac{\sum_{i=1}^{I} \omega_i \log(\hat{\lambda}_i)}{\sum_{i=1}^{I} \omega_i} \right). \tag{7.29}$$

Generalized linear models with fixed effects

Borenstein et al. (2009) estimate the treatment effect on a response variable across multiple studies via a generalized linear model in which individual studies are treated as a fixed factor i

$$g(y_{ij}) = \beta_0 + \beta_i + \tilde{\beta} I(j = 1) \tag{7.30}$$

where $g(\cdot)$ is a suitable link function, β_0 denotes the regression intercept, β_i and $\tilde{\beta}$ are the regression slopes for the ith study and the study treatment group ($j = 0$ for control and $j = 1$ for treatment), respectively. Model (7.30) assumes that there is no interaction between treatment group and individual studies. Depending on the type of response variable y_{ij}, the link function $g(\cdot)$ can be a log link for count data (Poisson regression) or logit link for proportion data (logistic regression).

Random effects model of DerSimonian and Laird

DerSimonian and Laird (1986, abbreviated by DSL) note that the main difficulty in meta-analysis of clinical studies "stems from the sometimes diverse nature of the studies, both in terms of design and methods employed" as "some are carefully controlled randomized experiments while others are less well controlled" and have "different sample sizes and patient populations." For meta-analysis of these clinical studies, they introduce a random effects model to address the issues of (a) assignment of weights that "reflect the relative value of the information provided in a study" and (b) how to combine evidence from "incommensurable studies to answer the same question." The DSL model assumes that "the numbers of patients with the (adverse) event in the (treatment and control) groups are independent binomial random variables with associated probabilities p_{T_i} and p_{C_i}" for $i = 1, \ldots, I$ and that

$$\theta_i = \mu + \delta_i, \tag{7.31}$$

where "θ_i is the true treatment effect in the ith study, μ is the mean effect for a population of possible treatment evaluation, and δ_i is the ith study's effect from the population mean" with $E(\delta_i) = 0$ and $\text{Var}(\delta_i) = \sigma^2$. DSL describes three commonly used specifications of θ_i: risk difference $p_{T_i} - p_{C_i}$, relative risk p_{T_i}/p_{C_i} and relative odds $\left(\frac{p_{T_i}}{1-p_{T_i}}\right) / \left(\frac{p_{C_i}}{1-p_{C_i}}\right)$, and argues for using the risk difference because "besides relevance of the measure and statistical efficiency, it is also desirable to choose a measure that is nearly constant over studies, so that the effect of heterogeneity can be minimized."

Let Y_i be the effect size and s_i^2 its sampling variance of the ith study. Then $E(Y_i) = \mu$ and $\text{Var}(Y_i) = \sigma^2 + s_i^2$, hence μ can be estimated by

$$\hat{\mu}_\sigma = \frac{\sum_{i=1}^{I} w_i(\sigma^2) Y_i}{\sum_{i=1}^{I} w_i(\sigma^2)}, \text{ where } w_i(\sigma^2) = (\sigma^2 + s_i^2)^{-1}. \tag{7.32}$$

The null hypothesis $H_0 : \sigma^2 = 0$ of constancy of treatment effect across the I studies can be tested by using Cochran's test statistic

$$Q = \sum_{i=1}^{I} w_i(Y_i - \hat{\mu}_0)^2, \text{ where } w_i = 1/s_i^2. \tag{7.33}$$

Then Q is approximately χ_{I-1}^2 under the null hypothesis. In particular, if Y_i is the difference of proportions $\hat{p}_{T_i} - \hat{p}_{C_i}$, then

$$s_i^2 = \hat{p}_{T_i}(1 - \hat{p}_{T_i})/n_{T_i} + \hat{p}_{C_i}(1 - \hat{p}_{C_i})/n_{C_i}, \tag{7.34}$$

where n_{T_i} and n_{C_i} are the sample sizes of the treatment and control groups, respectively, in the ith study. For $\sigma^2 \neq 0$, DSL uses the method of moments (MOM), maximum likelihood (ML), and restricted maximum likelihood (REML) to estimate σ^2. MOM estimates σ^2 by equating $Q_\sigma = \sum_{i=1}^I w_i(\sigma^2)(Y_i - \hat{\mu}_\sigma)^2$ to its expected value $E(Q_\sigma) = \sigma^2 \left\{ \sum_{i=1}^I w_i(\sigma^2) - \sum_{i=1}^I w_i^2(\sigma^2)/\left[\sum_{i=1}^I w_i(\sigma^2)\right] \right\} + I - 1$, which leads to the estimating equation

$$\sigma^2 = \max \left\{ 0, \frac{Q_\sigma - (I-1)}{\sum_{i=1}^I w_i(\sigma^2) - \sum_{i=1}^I w_i^2(\sigma^2)/\left[\sum_{i=1}^I w_i(\sigma^2)\right]} \right\}. \quad (7.35)$$

DSL carries out empirical studies of using these methods to estimate σ^2 and finds that MOM "is an attractive procedure because of the comparability of its estimates with those of maximum likelihood methods and because of its relative simplicity."

Robust refinement and repurposing DSL for Big Data

Three decades after the publication of DSL, DerSimonian and Laird (2015) review subsequent developments related to their random effects model for meta-analysis: "According to the Web of Science Core Collection, the paper has over twelve thousand citations to date. Moreover, the popularity does not seem to be subsiding in that more than 50% of those citations occurred in the last few years with more than two thousand in the year 2014 alone... In the later years (2010–2014), citations in general internal medicine and public health related topics (during 1986–2009) are replaced by additional citations in oncology and science & technology research related topics." To explain the popularity of DSL, they note that it "requires simple data summaries from each study that are generally readily available" and that it is "simple and easy to implement' and "can be useful in identifying sources of heterogeneity." They point out in the modern Big Data era, "it is natural to consider analyzing data summaries, rather than to consider pooling the data from different studies into one mega-sized database" in conducting meta-analysis of I studies, when I is relatively small compared to the magnitude of data collected from each individual study, and use Genome Wide Association Studies (GWAS) to illustrate their discussion of repurposing the DSL approach to meta-analysis of these studies to locate genetic variants that are causal for a complex disease.

DerSimonian and Laird (2015) also review several simulation studies comparing MOM with "more sophisticated yet computer intensive methods", which have concluded that MOM "remains adequate in most scenarios and there is little to gain from using more computationally intensive techniques." They also refer to the literature on confidence intervals for σ^2

but point out that "using an estimate of σ^2 as a measure of heterogeneity is unsatisfactory as it depends heavily on the scale of measurement and has no absolute interpretation." They propose to use the measure of heterogeneity $\mathcal{H}^2 = Q_\sigma/(I-1)$ or $\mathcal{I}^2 = \sigma^2/(\sigma^2 + s^2)$ proposed by Higgins and Thompson (2002) and to construct confidence intervals of $\mathcal{H}^2$ or $\mathcal{I}^2$, where s^2 is the mean of the s_i^2 in the random effects model. Letting $\hat{w}_i = w_i(\hat{\sigma}^2)$ and $\hat{\mu} = \mu_{\hat{\sigma}}$, where $\hat{\sigma}^2$ is the MOM estimate of σ^2 defined by the estimating equation (7.35), they note that "when the focus is on testing (or confidence interval estimation), several simulation studies have highlighted limitations" of the DSL method that "ignores variability in the weights $\hat{w}_i$", resulting in anticonservative tests (or confidence intervals) when I is small "and/or the sample sizes of each study are small, or highly unequal." They propose a robust estimate of $\mathrm{Var}(Y_i) = \sigma^2 + s_i^2 = 1/w_i(\sigma^2)$ that replaces $\hat{w}_i^{-1}$ by the residual $(Y_i - \hat{\mu})^2$. The robust estimate is

$$\frac{\sum_{i=1}^{2} \hat{w}_i (Y_i - \hat{\mu})^2}{\left(\sum_{i=1}^{I} \hat{w}_i\right)(I-1)}, \tag{7.36}$$

which "reduces to the model-based estimate, apart from a factor of" $I/(I-1)$, and which "gives valid confidence intervals and tests under a wide range of assumptions."

7.7.2 Meta-analysis of rare events

Let y_{ij} denote the number of events in the jth treatment group of the ith study, and assume that $y_{ij} \sim \mathrm{Binomial}(n_{ij}, p_{ij})$, $j = 0, 1$ and $i = 1, \ldots, I$. There are statistical challenges in analyzing rare adverse events with low incidence rates or low counts both for individual studies and for their meta-analysis, for which large-sample approximations are not valid and risk ratios or odds ratios are not even defined when cells have zero count; see Sweeting et al. (2004). To address these challenges, Bhaumik et al. (2012) use the random effects model

$$\log\left(\frac{p_{ij}}{1 - p_{ij}}\right) = \mu + \theta I(j = 1) + \epsilon_i \quad \text{and} \quad \epsilon_i \sim N(0, \sigma^2), \tag{7.37}$$

in which σ^2 represents the heterogeneity parameter. Adding a positive constant a to the observed frequencies, one obtains an estimate of the treatment effect for the ith study

$$\hat{\theta}_i(a) = \log\left(\frac{y_{i1} + a}{n_{i1} - y_{i1} + a}\right) - \log\left(\frac{y_{i0} + a}{n_{i0} - y_{i0} + a}\right), \tag{7.38}$$

which gives an unbiased estimate $\hat{\theta} = I^{-1} \sum_{i=1}^{I} \hat{\theta}_i(1/2)$ of θ_i when $a = 1/2$. To estimate σ^2, Bhaumik et al. (2012) use the DSL estimating equation

(7.35) with $Y_i = \hat{\theta}_i \left(\frac{1}{2}\right)$ and $s_i^2 = [n_{i1}\hat{p}_{i1}(1 - \hat{p}_{i1})]^{-1} + [n_{i0}\hat{p}_{i0}(1 - \hat{p}_{i0})]^{-1}$, where $\hat{p}_{ij} = (y_{ij} + 1/2) / (n_{ij} + 1)$.

Cai et al. (2010) use a likelihood-based approach with Poisson random effects for the baseline (corresponding to the control group) event rates that can vary from study to study, but a constant relative risk of treatment to control across studies. Specifically, letting $X_{ij} = 1$ for the treatment group $j = 1$, and $X_{ij} = 0$ for the control group $j = 0$, they assume that the observed number of y_{ij} of adverse events among the n_{ij} subjects in study i and treatment group j follows a Poisson distribution with mean $n_{ij}\lambda_{ij}$, where

$$\lambda_{ij} = \xi_i \exp(\tau X_{ij}), \tag{7.39}$$

in which ξ_i represents the baseline event rate for the ith study and e^τ is the constant relative risk across studies. They say: "the obvious approach of assuming a normal distribution on $\log(\xi_i)$ results in a non-closed form likelihood", which entails computationally intensive methods; see Tian et al. (2009) who assume a fixed-effects framework and use an exact method for inference on a parameter of interest without using continuity correction for cell frequencies. Cai et al. (2010) assume instead $\xi_i \sim \text{Gamma}(\alpha, \beta)$, resulting in a closed-form Poisson-gamma mixture distribution. The likelihood function of parameters of interest, namely, (α, β, τ), is given by

$$L(\alpha, \beta, \tau) = \prod_{i=1}^{I} \frac{(n_{i0})^{y_{i0}}}{y_{i0}!} \frac{[n_{i1}e^\tau]^{y_{i1}}}{y_{i1}!} \frac{\Gamma(y_{i\cdot} + \alpha)\beta^\alpha}{\Gamma(\alpha)\,[\beta + n_{i0} + n_{i1}e^\tau]^{y_{i\cdot}+\alpha}}, \tag{7.40}$$

where $y_{i\cdot} = y_{i0} + y_{i1}$. The MLE of the parameter vector (α, β, τ) can be obtained through nonlinear numerical maximization in most computing software. They say that the method was applied to meta-analysis of "48 comparative trials involving rosiglitazone, a type 2 diabetes drug, with respect to its possible cardiovascular toxicity" that had been considered by Nissen and Wolski (2007). Although the DSL could have been used, "this method may not work well in the context of rare events where it is likely for several of the studies being combined to have no events at all," as in the case of rosiglitazone for which "25 of the 48 studies include no deaths and 10 studies have no cardiac events." Whereas "Nissen and Wolski took the conventional approach of omitting studies with zero events from their fixed effects odds ratio analysis," Cai et al. (2010) cite simulation studies by Tian et al. (2009) showing that "standard MH and Peto's methods may lead to invalid or inefficient inference about the treatment difference when studies with zero events are deleted or artificially imputed". This motivated their development and application of (7.39), which was used by Brumback et al. (2000) to "assess the impact of chorionic villus sampling on the occurrence of rare limb defects using data from a series of 29 studies." They use likelihood-based methods to construct confidence intervals for τ and also carry out comparative studies with other methods, including a more general random effects model for $\tau_i \sim N(\mu, \sigma^2)$ that is independent of ξ_i (see the fully Bayesian model in Supplement 4 of Section 7.10 and the following "conditional model"). Conditional on $y_{i\cdot}$, y_{i1} is binomially distributed as $y_{i1} \sim \text{Binomial}(y_{i\cdot}, p_i)$, where $p_i = \exp(\tau_i)/[w_i + \exp(\tau_i)]$ and $w_i = n_{i1}/n_{i0}$ is the ratio of sample sizes. The conditional model can be used to model the random effects for τ_i via $p_i \sim \text{Beta}(\psi\gamma, \psi w_i)$, giving a Beta-Binomial model with

$$E(p_i) = \mu_i = \frac{\gamma}{w_i + \gamma}, \text{Var}(p_i) = \frac{\mu_i(1 - \mu_i)}{\psi(\gamma + w_i) + 1}. \quad (7.41)$$

The MLE's of α, β, γ can easily be obtained by maximizing the likelihood function because of the convenient conjugate relationship of the binomial-beta distributions. The evidence of overall treatment effect on the rare event is characterized through the estimated value of γ exceeding 1.

7.7.3 Network meta-analysis

Meta-analysis to combine evidence from multiple comparative clinical trials, each of which contains the same set of treatment and control therapies, yields *direct treatment comparisons*. On the other hand, healthcare professionals, policy makers, and patients are often interested in evidence synthesis via *simultaneous indirect comparisons* of a wide array of therapies that are investigated across various studies for a given medical condition using network meta-analysis methodologies. Dias et al. (2018) describe network meta-analysis as "an essential component of health technology assessment (HTA) routinely used in submissions not only to reimbursement agencies...but also, increasingly, to similar organizations worldwide, including the Canadian Agency for Drugs and Technologies in Health, and the US Agency for Healthcare Research and Quality." They use the following simple example to illustrate the basic idea. Let $\hat{\theta}_{AB}^{dir}$ denote the treatment effect difference estimated from a randomized clinical trial comparing treatments A and B, and let $\hat{\theta}_{AC}^{dir}$ be the treatment effect difference estimated from another trial comparing treatments A and C. An *indirect* estimate of the treatment effect difference between treatment B and treatment C, denoted by $\hat{\theta}_{BC}^{ind}$, is the difference $\hat{\theta}_{BC}^{ind} = \hat{\theta}_{AC}^{dir} - \hat{\theta}_{AB}^{dir}$, which has variance $\text{Var}(\hat{\theta}_{BC}^{ind}) = \text{Var}(\hat{\theta}_{AC}^{dir}) + \text{Var}(\hat{\theta}_{AB}^{dir})$. Dias et al. (2018) extend this idea to three sets of trials on AB, BC, and AC that yield the direct estimate $\hat{\theta}_{BC}^{dir}$ and indirect estimate $\hat{\theta}_{BC}^{ind}$, by using inverse-variance weighting to combine the direct and indirect estimates via

$$\hat{\theta}_{BC}^{pooled} = \frac{w_{BC}^{dir} \, \hat{\theta}_{BC}^{dir} + w_{BC}^{ind} \, \hat{\theta}_{BC}^{ind}}{w_{BC}^{dir} + w_{BC}^{ind}}, \quad (7.42)$$

where $w_{BC}^{dir} = 1/\text{Var}(\hat{\theta}_{AC}^{dir})$ and $w_{BC}^{ind} = 1/\left[\text{Var}(\hat{\theta}_{AB}^{dir}) + \text{Var}(\hat{\theta}_{AC}^{ind})\right]$. The mean treatment effect difference between A and C can be estimated by $\hat{\theta}_{AB}^{pooled}$ and $\hat{\theta}_{AC}^{pooled}$ from the same three sets of trials.

Cipriani et al. (2013) argue that "a valid indirect comparison (such as AB) requires that the sets of AC and BC studies are similar in their distributions of effect modifiers" and illustrate by using two sets of studies, with one set of studies on AC including patients with severe condition and another set of studies on BC including patients with moderate condition, which could result in invalid indirect comparison of AB if severity of the condition is a treatment effect modifier. Baker and Kramer (2002) graphically demonstrate different ways of "transitive fallacy" that can arise due to changes in unobserved or unadjusted variables across randomized trials and point out that "even with large sample sizes, combining results from a randomized trial on BC with results from another randomized trial on AB will not guarantee correct inference about AC" if the transitivity assumption is violated. *Transitivity* (or similarity) requires the distribution of patients or study characteristics that are treatment effect modifiers to be sufficiently similar across different sets of randomized trials for inclusion in indirect comparisons. Lack of transitivity in these studies can lead to significant *inconsistency* (or *incoherence*) measure $(\hat{\theta}_{BC}^{dir} - \hat{\theta}_{BC}^{ind})/[\text{Var}(\hat{\theta}_{BC}^{dir}) + \text{Var}(\hat{\theta}_{BC}^{ind})]^{1/2}$, which is approximately normal under the null hypothesis of consistency. Similar tests can be carried out for $\hat{\theta}_{AB}^{dir} - \hat{\theta}_{AB}^{ind}$ and $\hat{\theta}_{AC}^{dir} - \hat{\theta}_{AC}^{ind}$; see Bucher et al. (1997) for additional background.

Jones et al. (2011) give a general regression-based framework of fixed and random effects models for network meta-analysis, in which a generalized linear model (GLM) is assumed for binary data with log-linear link function. Specifically, suppose that r_{ij} events are observed among n_{ij} subjects in treatment group j of study i and that $r_{ij} \sim \text{Binomial}(n_{ij}, \pi_{ij})$, where π_{ij} is the probability for a subject in the jth treatment group of the ith study to have the event, $i = 1, \ldots, I$ and $j = 1, \ldots, J$. They consider a fixed effects model of the form

$$\text{logit}(\pi_{ij}) = \log\left(\frac{\pi_{ij}}{1 - \pi_{ij}}\right) = a + s_i + t_j, \qquad (7.43)$$

where a is an intercept representing the effect of the reference group across all studies, s_i is the ith study effect and t_j is the jth treatment effect. Jones et al. (2011) apply (7.43) to an example involving 26 studies, of which (a) the first two contain three-arm comparisons of treatments A, B, and C, (b) the next seven are two-arm studies for direct comparisons of treatments A and C, and (c) the last seventeen are two-arm studies for direct comparisons of treatments B and C. Fitting the model (7.43) gives the pooled estimate $\hat{\theta}_{AB}^{pooled}$ as there is no significant evidence of inconsistency between the direct and indirect estimates. The random effects model assumes that the treatment effects vary from study to study and has the form

$$\text{logit}(\pi_{ij}) = a + s_i + t_j + \varepsilon_{ij}, \qquad (7.44)$$

in which ε_{ij} are independent normal random effects for the ith study.

7.8 Pharmacoepidemiologic approaches

7.8.1 Information content differences among safety databases and from web-based epidemiologic studies

Gould (2015a) points out that different medical product safety databases, including spontaneous reporting databases, insurance claims databases, and various EHR databases provide sources of information for identifying potential toxicities or AE risks of the medical products, but "are subject to deficiencies that limit the interpretability of analyses based on (these) data." In particular, he says:

> Claims databases do not ordinarily provide information about AEs as such (nor about prescribed or unprescribed over-the-counter medications or unfilled prescriptions), so that the recurrence of an AE reflecting possible product-related harm must be inferred from information about physician visits, diagnosis codes, medical indications, or dispensed medications that the database provides... Claims usually will be reasonably accurate for drugs and vaccines because filling is often made for the particular therapy dispensed, but the same may not be true for medical devices. EHR databases in principle capture patient records within a healthcare system, including records of results of laboratory tests, vital signs measurements, diagnoses, medications, and so on, so that a longitudinal picture of patient experience can be obtained... as long as the patient stays in the healthcare system. EHR databases provide an opportunity to study the temporal pattern of occurrence of AEs... However, only whether a medicine was prescribed generally is recorded, not whether it was taken as prescribed. Also, information about the occurrence of potential AEs generally needs to be inferred from the record whereas the occurrence of an AE as such has been recorded because EHR databases are designed for patient care management, not for detection of harm.

Hence different databases have different types of information on the AEs experienced.

Section 7.8.3 introduces the Observational Medical Outcomes Partnership (OMOP), established in 2008, to study how information from different observational databases (claims and EHR) can be combined and used for pharmacovigilance. The OMOP Research Lab has been recently named the Innovation in Medical Evidence Development and Surveillance (IMEDS) Lab (http://imeds.reaganudall.org/). In addition, Observational Health Data Sciences and Informatics (OHDSI) has been established as a multi-stakeholder, interdisciplinary collaborative to carry out large-scale analytics of observational health data and provide open-source software. The FDA launched the Sentinel Initiative in 2008 to track the safety of drugs, and its "Mini Sentinel" program analyzes claims data from more than 100 million patients as of 2014 (http://www.mini-sentinel.org/). The European Adverse Drug Reaction project supplements spontaneous report systems for detecting AEs by EHR data using epidemiological, text mining, and computational techniques (http://www.euadr-project.org).

Gould (2015a, p.356) points out that "a growing body of internet-based information that includes patient inquiries about health-related issues presents some potentially useful avenues for early detection of potential drug toxicities." He refers to epidemiologic methods of using electronic information from the internet for detection and surveillance as "infoepidemiology" and finds medical discussion boards potentially useful for identifying drug toxicity. In particular, he refers to a project by White et al. (2013) to evaluate potential interactions between the antidepressant paroxetine and the lipid-lowering product pravastatin with respect to the occurrence of hyperglycemia, using search logs of millions of consenting web users during 2010. He points out that these internet data, analyzed using text mining approaches, "may be useful for identifying late-onset AEs that would be difficult to detect using spontaneous reporting systems or even observational databases.

7.8.2   Case-control and self-controlled case series (SCCS)

Case-control studies start with the selection of a set of subjects with an adverse event as the cases and another set of subjects without the event as controls, and then trace back their history of exposure to a medical product. The controls are often selected separately to match with each of the cases based on their characteristics (e.g., age, gender, birthplace, etc.), so that potential risk factors (except for the exposure to the product) between each case and its matched controls are as close as possible and inference can be made with improved efficiency. If the matched controls are selected from a pre-specified cohort among those in the cohort who have not developed the adverse event by the time of event occurrence in the cases, then the design is called a nested case-control design (Ernster, 1994), which is particularly useful for studies of biologic precursors of adverse outcomes. However, it is important to realize some of its critical statistical challenges and limitations. First, unlike prospective or retrospective cohort design where incidence rates of adverse events can be calculated, case-control studies can provide the likelihood of an adverse event for the cases relative to that of controls but the incidence rate can not be estimated (Ernster, 1994; Lao et al., 2016). Second, in addition to the precise definition of cases (such as stages, severity of an event), controls have to be selected with great care to avoid potential selection bias (Strom, 2006). Third, like any other retrospective studies, recall bias may exist because information on exposure to risk factors is collected retrospectively. Fourth, no temporal relationship of any risk factors with an event can be concluded since subjects are only cross-classified as cases and controls with or without risk factors and no temporal sequences are necessarily recorded.

Case series studies are studies of the past history (including medical history, family history, history of exposure to the product of interest) of patients who have experienced the target adverse event, and inference can be made based on medical and scientific judgment of the relationship of the event with the product exposure. They are used to decide whether or not an adverse event is an adverse drug reaction and are the most widely used tool by physicians to evaluate clinical safety (Chakra et al., 2010). When a fixed, pre-specified time period is identified and exposure or non-exposure to a product is determined during that time period for each case, then one can estimate the relative incidence of the rate of event during exposure time period to the rate of event during non-exposure time period. This is often called the self-controlled case series (SCCS) design (Wilson and Hawken, 2013), and was originally developed to investigate the association between a vaccine and an adverse event (Farrington, 1995; Farrington et al., 1996). In the SCCS design, the observational period following each exposure for each case is divided into a risk period (number of days immediately following each exposure) and a control period (the remaining observational period). Let n be the number of patients in an observational study of an adverse event E (case) and exposure to drug D. The occurrence of E identifies an index date of the case, with an observation period for the case being a prespecified period of time (e.g., 180 days) preceding the index date. The index date for a control (not experiencing E) that is matched to the case by characteristics such as age and gender is usually the same as for the control for whom the same observation period is also used. Let n_{DE} (respectively, $n_{\bar{D}E}$) denote the number of cases (respectively, controls) in the study sample who are exposed (respectively, not exposed) to drug D. Then $n\bar{D}E = n - n_{DE}$ (respectively, $n_{D\bar{E}} = n - n_{\bar{D}E}$) is the number of exposed cases (respectively, non-exposed controls) in the study sample. A commonly used statistic to compare event rates between exposed and non-exposed groups is the odds ratio $(n_{DE}n_{\bar{D}\bar{E}})/(n_{\bar{D}E}n_{D\bar{E}})$. Among the limitations of the SCCS design are event-unaffected probability of exposure, requirement of variability in the time or age of the event, and no incidence rate estimates (Whitaker et al., 2006).

SCCS can be viewed as a cohort crossover study, a particular application of which uses pharmacy prescription histories in large databases for detection of drug adverse reactions by the following rationale: If a drug causes an adverse reaction on a patient, then another drug or class of drugs is usually prescribed to the patient to treat the adverse condition following the prescription of the previous drug, hence the unusual frequency of particular prescription sequences such as drug A → drug B can reveal adverse outcomes caused by drug A (referred to as an *index drug*) "whose side-effect is the indication for the prescription" of drug B (referred to as an *outcome drug*); see Hallas (1996), who calls the cohort crossover analysis in this kind of applications a *prescription sequence symmetry analysis* (PSSA), and Supplement 6 in Section 7.10 for further details of PSSA. Suchard et al. (2013) have also introduced a refinement of SCCS. They consider J drugs (instead of a single drug) and a fixed observation period of T days during which each subject may be exposed to one or more of the drugs. Let y_{it} be the number of AEs experienced by subject i on day t and $x_{ijt} = 1$ or 0 according to whether subject i is exposed to drug j on day t or not. Assuming that y_{it} is Poisson with parameter $\exp(\beta_0 + \sum_{j=1}^{J} \beta_j x_{ijt})$, where β_0 is the exposure-free event rate and β_j is the event rate after exposure to drug j, they use likelihood inference on the event rates $\beta_0, \beta_1, ..., \beta_J$. When J is large, one has a high-dimensional Poisson regression problem, and Simpson (2013) introduces regularization to avoid overfitting and numerical instability.

7.8.3 OMOP and systematic pharmacovigilance

As noted by Stang et al. (2014), the Observational Medical Outcomes Partnership (OMOP) was established as a public-private partnership between the FDA, the Foundation for the National Institutes of Health (FNIH), the Pharmaceutical Research and Manufacturers Association, academic, and owners of healthcare claims data or EHR data; it was subsequently transitioned from FNIH to the Reagan-Udall Foundation for the FDA. The OMOP has three principal objectives:

(a) Develop methods and capabilities for transforming observational data from disparate sources that include both central (housed in the OMOP research lab) and distributed (housed by collaborators that own the data) databases to standards-based "common data" and for analyzing the data.

(b) Evaluate the performance of the analytic methods for estimating from the observational data the association between the medical products and the health outcomes.

(c) Provide resources for the broader research community to advance the science of safety surveillance.

Stang et al. (2014) point out that in contrast to spontaneous reports, the claims data and EHR data have the advantage of "representing a defined population with known denominators and potentially more robust medication and outcome information" for the development of a systematic process to identify associations between medical products and outcomes. Concerning objective (a), they describe a Common Data Model (CDM) to accommodate data from various sources, incorporating standard terminology and standard definitions of drug exposure and outcomes. They also list and summarize 14 analytic approaches provided by a "community of methods developers" for estimating "the strength of association between exposure to medical products and the occurrence of health outcomes of interest." Some of the listed analytic methods have been described in other parts of this chapter. Concerning objective (b), they say:

> Before assessing the performance of an analytic method, it was necessary to establish a set of gold standards against which each method could be tested. This entailed identifying a set of health outcomes known to be associated with specific drugs or drug classes (e.g., warfarin and bleeding) against which the performance of databases, statistical methods, and health outcome definitions could be assessed empirically. We performed systematic literature reviews to develop a spectrum of definitions of 10 health outcomes of interest..., paired with 10 drugs/drug classes for which there was evidence from other students and product information of an association. These became our "positive controls" (e.g., drug-outcome pairs where the drug is believed to cause the outcome) and our set of "negative controls" (e.g., drug-outcome pairs where we could find no evidence of an association for which any method should not produce an association).

For (c), they refer to the OMOP website (`http://omop.org`), where "all processes, procedures, techniques, and results are posted" and "technical reports, presentations, and papers are also available." Ryan et al. (2012) and Madigan et al. (2014) point out that different procedures and techniques applied to the OMOP data from the same observational study can lead to different conclusions about the adverse event risks of the intervention.

7.8.4 Postmarketing pharmacoepidemiologic studies: Examples from biologic therapies

Acquavella et al. (2014) point out some fundamental differences, "from a drug safety and risk management perspective," between biologic therapies, which are medicines derived from living cells using recombinant DNA technology, and the more traditional small-molecule therapies that have been the main focus of the drug safety literature. Even in the preclinical phase, they note the following main differences:

- Selection of species for toxicology and pharmacology studies: For small molecules, it is typical to study rodent and nonrodent species. For biologic therapies, targets may not be expressed in rodents, and therefore toxicology studies are often conducted in one species — nonhuman primates (e.g., monkeys).

- Duration of therapeutic action: In comparison with small molecules for which there is a more direct relationship between PK and PD, monoclonal antibodies and other biologic therapies generally have a longer half-life and lag time for a PD effect.

- Observed toxicities: Whereas "off-target" toxic effects are of concern to small-molecule therapies, the toxicities of biologic therapies are typically extensions of the desired pharmacologic effects and the toxicology profiles may be unrevealing, with no adverse events in nonclinical toxicology studies.

Acquavella et al. (2014) note that "large clinical trials (for both biologics and nonbiologics) provide an estimate of frequency of common drug-related adverse effects or adverse reactions" and that "rare adverse effects are detected when sufficient numbers of subjects have been exposed to the therapeutic of interests" in postmarketing pharmacovigilance. They discuss the role of pharmacoepidemiologic studies in pharmacovigilance, using four biologic therapies as illustrative examples. Two of them, Prolia and XGEVA, "have only recently been approved" and "the development of a pharmacoepidemiologic study of prespecified adverse events of interest was an important part of the regulatory approved negotiations." The other two, Epogen and Enbrel had been approved and marketed prior to the FDA Amendment Act of 2007 when the agency acquired authority to mandate postmarketing studies, and pharmacoepidemiologic studies were subsequently designed to examine certain potential safety concerns of the agency.

Osteoporosis is a chronic disease characterized by low bone mass and predisposes those effected, particularly postmenopausal women over age 50, to increased bone fracture risk. Several pharmacologic agents are available for the prevention and/or treatment of the disease, and the newest among them, denosumab, is a monoclonal antibody used to block the RANK ligand, thereby decreasing bone resorption and increasing bone mass and strength. Prolia (denosumab 60 mg administered every 6 months) was approved by other countries for treatment of postmenopausal osteoporosis (PMO) in women at high risk for bone fracture. During review of the marketing application by Amgen, the FDA raised potential safety concerns based on mechanism of action, clinical trial evidence, and findings from studies of other anti-resorptive agents. A comprehensive postmarketing risk analytics and management plan was proactively developed by Amgen with input from the FDA for the approval of Prolia. It incorporates a large prospective pharmacoepidemiologic study involving a 10-year open cohort of more than 20 million women, and a list of specified AEs of interest including osteonecrosis of the jaw, fracture healing, complications, hypocalcemia serious dermatological AEs leading to ER visit on hospitalization, and acute pancreatitis. Incidence rates of these AEs are to be compared between women exposed to Prolia and those exposed to the currently commonly used bisphosphonate treatments. Stang et al. (2014) give an overview of the study design issues that were considered in this pharmacoepidemiologic study "of unprecedented size and scope," in addition to the external landscape into which Prolia was introduced. In particular, since prevention of osteoporosis, a large proportion of Prolia users may have been previously treated with bisphosphonates. They point out that "when comparing event incidence in Prolia versus bisphosphonate users, one must account for such previous exposure, which may confound the risk of on-study events." The 10-year study duration poses additional challenges that need to be addressed, including "changes over time in physician prescription patterns, treatment landscape, and patient case-mix in addition to complexities due to approvals in new countries and for new indications," which may also require interim reevaluation and modifications of the study plan.

XGEVA (denosumab 120 mg SQ Q4W) is another Amgen drug to prevent skeletal-related events (SREs) in patients with bone metastases from solid tumors. Prior to its approval, intravenous bisphosphonates were the only approved treatment to prevent SREs in these patients. There are important differences between PMO and advanced cancer patients that resulted in different study designs for the XGEVA and Prolia postmarketing pharmacoepidemiologic studies, as noted by Acquavella et al. (2014). Incidence of ONG and serious infections is much higher among cancer patients than among PMO patients. Moreover, cancer patients with bone metastases have short life expectancy, precluding outcomes with extended induction-latent periods. They describe the postmarketing program for XGEVA as multi-faceted, including continued assessment of patients in clinical trials, follow-up of spontaneous reports of AEs and physicians' understanding of recommendations related to ONG prevention provided in the denosumab prescribing information, and a trinational Nordic prospective study of cancer patients treated with XGEVA or the standard of care (intravenous zoledronic acid). The Nordic study also involves collaboration with dental researchers at centers where virtually all suspected cases of ONG would be evaluated to establish a trinational database of known ONG cases for linkage with the treatment cohorts in the prospective study.

Epogen and Enbrel are also Amgen drugs. Epogen (epoetin alfa, or EPO) received FDA approval in 1989 and has been widely used by nephrologists for the treatment of anemia in patients with chronic kidney disease (CKD). Patients with late-stage CKD, particularly those receiving dialysis, do not produce enough erythropoietin and become severely anemic. EPO is a biologic administered intravenously or subcutaneously to raise and maintain hemoglobin (Hb) levels to a desired level. Results from randomized controlled trials published in 1998 and 2006 raised safety concerns that higher doses used to achieve higher target levels might have elevated risk of cardiovascular events and mortality. Although the safety concerns were then incorporated into product labeling, it was unclear whether these risks were applicable to current clinical practice. In 2004, two non-interventional database studies using Medicare hemodialysis data showed an association between higher average monthly EPO doses and elevated mortality, but the studies had limitations in design and analysis. This led Amgen to "initiate a multifaceted pharmacoepidemiologic program to investigate whether higher EPO doses in clinical practice increase the risk of mortality in dialysis patients" in 2005, as described by Acquavella et al. (2014) who also summarize the analytic techniques including instrumental variables, marginal structural models, multilevel modeling, and split-sample design to address time-dependent confounding and confounding-by-indication and the findings to date.

The biotechnology company Immunex, acquired by Amgen in 2002, received FDA approval of its biologic Enbrel (etanercept) in 1998 to treat rheumatoid arthritis (RA), ankylosing spondylitis (AS), juvenile idiopathic arthritis (JIA), psoriatic arthritis (PsA), and plaque psoriasis (Ps). Immunex committed to a 3-year follow-up of Enbrel-treated RA patients enrolled in open-labeled extension studies. Subsequently, Amgen extended the follow-up to 10 years. These data were used later in conjunction with data from EU registries to evaluate the potential association of Enbrel with lymphoma in adult RA patients, showing that the incidence of lymphoma in this patient population did not increase over time with increasing exposure to Enbrel (Gibofsky et al., 2011). In 1999, a phase IV clinical trial was initiated to evaluate the safety of Enbrel in children with systematic-onset JIA. Patient recruitment was slow, perhaps because of potential assignment to placebo, and the FDA later released Amgen from this commitment. The FDA then required the establishment of a prospective observational study of pregnancy outcomes among Enbrel users. In 2012, the FDA issued a postmarketing requirement to assess systematically spontaneous reports of malignancies in pediatric and young adult patients for a period of 10 years. Acquavella et al. (2014) say:

> The key learnings from these studies, in addition to the contextualization of the label changes as a result of spontaneous report analyses, include (1) the difficulty in recruiting children for a randomized, placebo-controlled clinical trial when a commercial product is available, (2) the difficulty in recruiting for a pregnancy registry in general, especially when the study calls for a comparison cohort,

and (3) the value of large administrative databases to serve as an external source of information regarding drug exposure and safety outcomes to complement routine pharmacovigilance and data from controlled clinical trials.

7.9 Pre- and Post-marketing studies of MMRV vaccination

This section describes how safety signals generated from multiple post-marketing observational studies have led to changes in recommendations from the ACIP (Advisory Committee on Immunization Practice) of the CDC regarding administration of the combination MMRV vaccine in MMRW (Morbidity and Mortality Weekly Report) 2008 (Vol. 57, pp. 258-260). The MMRV vaccine has been described in Chapter 5, where it is used in combination with another vaccine Pedvax H1B®. We first give here some background on pre-licensure clinical trials of MMRV and then describe several pivotal postmarketing observational studies that led to the ACIP recommendation in 2008.

7.9.1 Pre-licensure clinical trials

As pointed out in the review paper by a research team from Merck & Co., Inc., Kenilworth, NJ, USA, Kaiser Permanente, Primary Physicians Research, Boston Medical Center, and Marshfield Clinic (Kuter et al., 2006), two vaccines M-M-R®II and VARIVAX® produced by Merck & Co., Inc., Kenilworth, NJ, USA, have been licensed in the US and in other countries since 1979 and 1995, respectively, and "have been shown to be generally tolerated, immunogenic," and "highly effective in reducing the incidence of measles, mumps, rubella, and varicella." Both the American Academy of Pediatrics and ACIP "have indicated that combination vaccines are generally preferred over monovalent vaccines or concomitant administration vaccines at different injection sites on the same day" because they "include fewer injections for children," facilitate vaccine delivery, have significant savings in time and administrative duties, and "the potential to increase coverage rates through simultaneous administration of multiple antigens at one visit," leading Merck & Co., Inc., Kenilworth, NJ, USA, to develop the MMRV (ProQuad®). Kuter et al. (2006) say:

> The primary objective of the clinical development program for ProQuad® was to demonstrate that a single dose of ProQuad® was as immunogenic and generally well tolerated in healthy children, 12 to 23 months of age, as the standard practice of concomitant

administration of M-M-R®II and VARIVAX® at separate injection sites. Additional objectives of the clinical development program for ProQuad® were to assess the safety and immunogenicity of a 2-dose regimen of ProQuad® and to evaluate if ProQuad® could be used in place of M-M-R®II in children 4 to 6 years of age.

They describe five clinical trials in the clinical development program. Because results from earlier studies showed that the seroconversion rates and geometric mean titers (GMTs) to varicella-zoster virus (VZV) afforded by MMRV were lower than those after M-M-RII and VARIVAX® administered concomitantly but at separate injection sites, MMRV was reformulated with a higher potency of VZV to yield ProQuad®. Hence the first two trials were randomized trials to determine whether the higher potency of the VZV component, and at which dose level, of ProQuad® plus placebo could overcome the decrease in VZV antibody response rates and GMTs and elicit a similar response as concomitant administration of M-M-R®II and VARIVAX®. The results demonstrated the immunological comparability in the selected dose. The third trial was to assess the manufacturing consistency and persistency of antibody, and the fourth trial was to determine if ProQuad® could be administered concomitantly with COMVAX® (an H1B vaccine produced by Merck & Co., Inc., Kenilworth, NJ, USA) and TRIPEDIA® (a ATaP vaccine produced by Sanofi-Connaught) without impairing the immune response to any of the components of vaccines. The first trial was to determine whether ProQuad® could be used in place of M-M-R®II as a second dose in healthy 4- to 6-year old children who had been previously administered a primary dose of M-M-R®II and VARIVAX®. Kuter et al. (2006, p. 208) describe the statistical methods they use to analyze the combined data of the five trials concerning immunogenicity and safety. In particular, "logistic regression models were used for post-hoc evaluation of the relationship of fever (elevated temperatures $\geq 102.0°F$...and postvaccination measles antibody titer, and for the relationship of measles-like rashes and postvaccination measles antibody titer" and the explanatory variables in these models included "the natural logarithm of the postvaccination measles, mumps, rubella, and varicella antibody titers, the VZV potency, race, gender, and age (in months)" and "various interactions were also considered," using the usual backward stepwise test-based variable elimination method "based on a 0.05 (nominal) significant level" to select variables for the final model.

The safety results reported by Shinefield et al. (2006) for the second trial, Lieberman et al. (2006) for the third trial, and Reisinger et al. (2006) for the fifth trial basically show that MMRV was well-tolerated during the 42 days after vaccination and that the overall incidence of adverse experiences was comparable between recipients of MMRV and MMR+V. In particular, Shinefield et al. (2006) report that "only 1 serious adverse experience, a febrile seizure 8 days after the primary dose of MMRV (middle potency), was considered to be vaccine-related," while Lieberman et al.

(2006) report that "five of the 6 vaccine-related serious adverse experiences were febrile seizure." The MMRV vaccine received licensure in the US in 2005 and was recommended in 2006 by ACIP that stated a preference for its use over separate MMR and Varicella vaccines. The results of the safety analysis of the combined data from the five trials by Kuter et al. (2006) show no statistically significant difference between the rate of febrile seizures during the 42 days post vaccination in recipients of ProQuad® and that in recipients of M-M-R®II and VARIVAX®. The authors, however, point out that "the studies were not powered to detect significant differences in the rate of febrile seizures between the 2 vaccination groups." On the other hand, "the rate of vaccine-related measles-like rash was significantly higher in recipients of ProQuad® than in recipients of M-M-R®II and VARIVAX, but they remained low in both vaccination groups." Concerning the results of logistic regression mentioned in the preceding paragraph, they "showed that the level of the postvaccination measles antibody titer was positively associated with the rate of fever and the rate of measles-like rashes," as "the rate of fever and the height of the measles antibody titers increased with increasing VZV potency, but plateaued across the varicella virus dose range required for adequate immunogenicity of ProQuad®." Moreover, "the level of postvaccination rubella antibody titer was negatively associated with both fever and measles-like rashes," and race and age were also significant predictors of fever and measles-like rashes, with higher rates in Caucasians and in older children.

7.9.2 Post-licensure observational safety studies and reversal of ACIP recommendation

Section 7.1.4 introduced the Vaccine Safety Datalink (VSD), which developed a RCA (Rapid Cycle Analysis) system for monitoring potential associations between specific vaccines and prespecified adverse events. Beginning in 2007, a research group from VSD used the RCA system to monitor weekly 6 specific outcomes (seizures, thrombocytopenia, encephalitis/menigitis, ataxia, allergic reactions, and arthritis) during 42 days after vaccination in children aged 12 to 23 months; see Klein et al. (2010). Two authors of their paper together with representatives of CDC wrote the *Update: Recommendations from ACIP regarding administration of MMRV* in MMWR 2008 (CDC, 2008), saying that VSD "detected a signal of increased risk for seizures of any etiology among children aged 12-23 months after administration of MMRV vaccine compared with administration of MMR vaccine (many children also received varicella vaccine)." The *Update* also noted that in earlier studies the associations between MMR and increased risk for febrile seizures 1 to 2 weeks after vaccination (Griffin et al., 1991; Farrington et al., 1995; Barlow et al., 2001; Vestergaard et al., 2004) and that because of this CDC and Merck & Co.,

Inc., Kenilworth, NJ, USA, had initiated postlicensure studies "to better understand the risk for febrile seizures that might be associated with MMRV vaccination." It went on to report the following:

> Once the signal was detected, a VSD study was initiated that evaluated the risk for febrile seizures 7–10 days after vaccination among 43,353 children aged 12–23 months who received MMRV vaccine and 314,599 children aged 12–23 months who received MMR vaccine and varicella vaccine administered at the same visit. Medical records were reviewed to validate the diagnosis, and a multivariate logistic regression was used to adjust for age and influenza season. The preliminary results indicated a rate of febrile seizure of nine per 10,000 vaccinations among MMRV vaccine recipients compared with four per 10,000 vaccinations among MMR vaccine and varicella vaccine recipients... At the ACIP meeting (on February 27, 2008), representatives from Merck & Co., Inc., Kenilworth, NJ, USA, presented interim results of an ongoing postlicensure study being conducted among children aged 12–60 months (99% of the children were aged 12–23 months)... The interim analysis found a 2.3 times (CI = 0.6–9.0) higher relative risk for confirmed febrile seizures 5–12 days after MMRV vaccination (14,263 children; rate = five per 10,000 vaccinations) when compared with a historic control group of children (matched on age, sex, and date of vaccination) vaccinated with MMR vaccine and varicella vaccine at the same visit (14,263 children; rate = two per 10,000 vaccinations). Although the relative risk was not statistically significant, it was similar to the adjusted odds ratio reported by the VSD study for the 7–10 days after vaccination...The results (by Merck & Co., Inc., Kenilworth, NJ, USA) are considered interim; approximately half of the final sample size needed to investigate the risk for febrile seizures was available for this analysis...Availability of MMRV vaccine currently is limited in the United States because of manufacturing constraints unrelated to vaccine safety or efficacy. MMRV vaccine is not expected to be widely available before 2009; however, some clinics might have MMRV vaccine in stock.

The *Update* then reports that ACIP considered the preceding preliminary results from the VSD and studies by Merck & Co., Inc., Kenilworth, NJ, USA, the limited supply of MMRV vaccine, and alternative options for vaccination against measles, mumps, rubella, and varicella, and voted to change the preference recommendation for MMRV to not expressing such preference, modifying the preference language to read as follows: "ACIP does not express a preference for use of MMRV vaccine over separate injections of equivalent component vaccines (i.e., MMR vaccine and varicella vaccine)." The *Update* also reports a recommendation by ACIP to establish a work group for "in-depth evaluation of the findings regarding the increased risk of febrile seizures after the first dose of MMRV vaccine to present consideration of future policy options."

Nicola Klein and Katherine Yih are the two authors of Klein et al. (2010) who coauthored the *Update* with the representatives of CDC. Chapter 8 will review Klein et al. (2010) and subsequent developments of sequential monitoring of prespecified adverse events following vaccination using VSD surveillance systems for different vaccines. Here we describe another observational safety study of febrile seizures following the first dose of MMRV vaccination in a managed care setting, namely Kaiser Permanente Southern California (KPSC), by a group working at Merck & Co., Inc., Kenilworth, NJ, USA, and KPSC. Jacobsen et al. (2009) say:

> To augment the extant safety information, this observational safety study was undertaken as part of a post-licensure commitment to several health agencies to assess the short-term safety of MMRV. The goal was to follow a cohort of at least 25,000 children ages 12-60 months, who were administered a first dose of MMRV in the course of ordinary practice for the occurrence of febrile convulsion within 5-12 days following vaccination, as well as 0-4-day and 0-30-day windows, and compare this experience to a matched cohort of children who received the MMR and V vaccines given separately at the same visit and to their experience in a pre- and post-vaccination self-comparison period.

The comparison in the last sentence above consists of (1) a primary historical cohort vaccinated with MMR+V concomitantly in the period of November 2003–January 2006 immediately preceding the routine use of MMRV at KPSC, (b) two self-comparison periods for recipients of MMRV– a pre-vaccination self-comparison period defined by the period from 60 to 30 days prior to vaccination with MMRV and a post-vaccination self-comparison period defined by the period from 60 to 90 days following vaccination. Children in the historical comparison cohort were matched without replacement, using the optimal matching software by Bergstralh et al. (1996), to children vaccinated with MMRV on the basis of age, sex, and vaccination calendar day and month.

The interim analysis of this study is the one that the *Update* in MMWR 2008 (CDC, 2008) refers to as being presented by "representatives from Merck & Co., Inc., Kenilworth, NJ, USA" at the ACIP meeting. Jacobsen et al. (2009, p. 4568) say: "An independent, external safety review committee was convened to periodically monitor the safety data emerging from the study." The final analysis results are presented in cumulative incidence curves depicting the time to confirmed febrile convulsion and to pre-adjudicated convulsion diagnosis following vaccination among children vaccinated with MMRV ($n = 31,298$) and MMR+V ($n=31,298$). For the background of cumulative incidence curves, see Section 4.6.1. The issue of "confirmed" versus "pre-adjudicated" febrile convulsion shows the complexity of and care needed for observational adverse outcome data, as pointed out in Section 3.2 of Jacobsen et al. (2009):

> Of the 370 potential convulsion events, 138 cases had a claims record or visit outside the KPSC system, while 232 cases were seen within the KPSC system, as a first encounter or in follow-up to a previous encounter (Table 2). In total, 121 of the 370 potential cases were excluded for the reasons listed in Table 2 (no outside record obtained, no convulsion related visit but history of convulsion, etc.)

The cumulative incidence curve for the MMRV group lies about that of the MMR+V group for the 30-day period after vaccination, in their Figure 1, the left panel of which shows confirmed febrile convulsion and the right panel pre-adjudicated convulsion. The curves in either panel show "a modest difference in days 5-12 following vaccination" but "come close to joining by day 30." Their Table 3 gives 95% confidence intervals for relative risk and for risk difference, over the time period 0-4 days, 5-12 days, 13-30 days, and 0-30 days, of febrile convulsion (confirmed or pre-adjudicated), showing significant differences between MMRV and MMR+V for confirmed febrile convulsion in the 5-12-day period. Moreover, "the number of confirmed febrile convulsion observed in the pre-vaccination self-comparison period and in the post-vaccination self-comparison period was smaller than in either the MMRV or the primary comparison cohort." Their Table 4 provides additional information about concomitant vaccines for comparison between the MMRV and the historical cohorts, showing the MMRV cohort to more likely receive hepatitis A and pneumococcal conjugate vaccines the same day.

7.10 Supplements and Problems

1. *Limitations of Spontaneous Reporting Systems.* Spontaneous Reporting Systems (SRSs) have been widely used as data sources for disproportionality analysis of adverse drug reactions in safety signal detection. In addition to statistical issues and constraints on their analyses discussed in Section 7.2, DuMouchel (2007) has also summarizes the following limitations:

   (a) No standardized protocol: There is no research protocol governing the reporting of adverse events to an SRS, leading to inconsistency in reporting practice by healthcare providers, patients, and manufacturers.

(b) Varying reporting rates: The reporting rate can vary from drug to drug and from one AE to another AE; even for the same drug and/or the same AE, it can vary from year to year. The reporting rate can be heavily influenced by advertisements, social media, and government policy.

(c) Inconsistent terminologies: Although the names of drugs and AEs have been standardized using standard dictionaries, many SRSs have a long history with many off-marketed products included in the databases, and AE terminologies evolves over time, leading to inconsistency in AE terminologies and product inclusion.

(d) Duplicate reporting: The same AE that occurred on the same patient may be reported multiple times by different reporters (e.g., 100,000 duplicate reports removed from 3 million reports) and undetected duplicates can produce severe bias in the estimation of drug-event association.

(e) A drug-event pair association detected by disproportionality analysis of an SRS database may or may not provide a safety signal; by no means can a causal relationship be concluded from such analysis.

2. *Exercise.* Huang et al. (2011) conducted simulation studies to compare the performance characteristics of PRR, LRT defined in Sections 7.3 and 7.6.1, and BCPNN in Section 7.5. Perform simulation studies with different sample sizes to compare PRR, LRT, BCPNN, and MGPS (Section 7.4) in terms of sensitivity, specificity, power, FDR, and positive FDR of Storey (2003); see Supplement 2 in Section 5.5 for details.

3. *Tree-temporal scan statistics.* The tree-based scan statistics described in Section 7.6.2 have been extended to longitudinal data from the self-controlled case series studies in Section 7.8.2. They have been applied to post-licensure monitoring of adverse events for the Gardasil vaccine by Yih et al. (2015, 2018) and for the meningococcal conjugate vaccine Menactra® by Li et al. (2018) who give the following description of the "tree-temporal scan data mining method" in the VSD project to monitor adverse events for the vaccine following its approval by the FDA in January 2005 when the ACIP (see Section 7.9) recommended it be given routinely to pre-adolescents aged 11 to 12 years, with a booster dose at age 16. The project involves 6 VSD sites, uses the MLCCS ICD-9 diagnosis codes and "defines risk windows as any possible combinations of (time) intervals that start 1 to 21 days after vaccination and end 2 to 42 days later, with a minimum window length of 2 days and a maximum window of 28 days", excluding day 0 from the analysis "in order to remove the diagnoses that are often recorded by the health care provider on the (day of vaccination) to note pre-existing

conditions." The comparison window in the self-controlled case series study comprises "those remaining days within the 1 to 56 follow-up period but outside the risk window", as illustrated in Figure 1 of Li et al. (2018). The tree-temporal scan statistic is a "generalized log likelihood ratio (LLR)" statistic of the form that resembles (7.21):

$$\text{LLR} = \left\{ c\log\left(\frac{c}{u}\right) + (N-c)\log\left(\frac{N-c}{N-u}\right) \right\} I(C > u) \qquad (7.45)$$

for a specific AE, where c is the number of observed cases in the risk window for that AE, N is the total number of cases in the follow-up period summed over all AEs, and u is the expected number of cases (under the null hypothesis) given by $u = n(z/N)$, in which z is the number of cases in the risk interval summed over all AEs and n is the number of observed cases for that AE. The test statistic LLR is calculated for each possible risk interval, and the p-value of the maximum LLR among all possible LLRs is computed by Monte Carlo simulations; see the second paragraph of Section 2.5 of Li et al. (2018) for details. Section 3 of that paper presents the results of applying this method to identify adverse events from the electronic health records of the enrolled participants in the VSD project, who had received Menactra® vaccination during the period January 2005 to December 2014.

4. *Bayesian meta-analysis.* Bayesian methods, analogous to random effect models, provide a unified framework for synthesizing evidence from multiple yet similar studies, allowing for incorporation of prior knowledge on the parameter of interest and its uncertainty both at study level and between studies. In addition to offering predictive probability for future observations based solely on existing observed information, Bayesian meta-analysis is particularly useful in analyzing rare event data.

Following the structural framework in Berry (2000), let y_{ij} denote the observed counts for the jth group in the ith study, and

$$y_{i0} \sim \text{Poisson}(\lambda_i T_{i0}) \quad \text{and} \quad y_{i1} \sim \text{Poisson}(\rho_i \lambda_i T_{i1}), \qquad (7.46)$$

where λ_i is the hazard rate for the control group ($j = 0$) and ρ_i the relative risk of the treatment to the control in the ith study. Under the exchangeability assumption of the λ_i's and ρ_i's, one assigns independent prior probability distributions to λ_i and ρ_i

$$\lambda_i \sim LN(\mu, \sigma^2) \quad \text{and} \quad \rho_i \sim LN(\tau, \delta^2),$$

where $LN(\cdot)$ represents the log-normal distribution, and μ, σ^2, τ, and δ^2 are hyperparameters relating to the first-stage priors. The next stage priors are given by

$$\mu \sim N(\mu_0, \eta^2), \quad \sigma^2 \sim IG(\alpha, \beta),$$
$$\tau \sim N(\tau_0, \delta_0^2), \quad \delta^2 \sim IG(p, q),$$

where $IG(\cdot)$ stands for inverse-gamma distribution. The above model structure provides flexibility in modeling the hazard rates in both treatment and control groups, as well as the hazard ratio of treatment over control. Hence, the parameters ρ_i and τ are more relevant in this set-up. The hyperparameters $(\mu_0, \eta^2, \alpha, \beta)$ and $(\tau_0, \delta_0^2, p, q)$ can either be given fixed values (e.g., based on expert's opinions), or be estimated from the data.

For binary data such as adverse event counts among a given number of subjects in treatment and control groups of each study, let X_{ij} denote the number of observed events among n_{ij} subjects in the jth treatment group of the ith study. Then, it follows that

$$X_{ij} \sim \text{Binomial}(n_{ij}, \pi_{ij}), \qquad (7.47)$$

where π_{ij} is the probability of event occurrence for the jth treatment group of the ith study, $j = 0, 1$ and $i = 1, \ldots, I$. Berry (2000) uses the logit model of π_{ij}

$$\log\left(\frac{\pi_{ij}}{1 - \pi_{ij}}\right) = \begin{cases} \theta_i, & \text{for } j = 0, \\ \theta_i + \rho_i & \text{for } j = 1, \end{cases} \qquad (7.48)$$

where θ_i is the log odds for the event probability in the control group and ρ_i is the log odds ratio for the event probability in the treatment group relative to that in the control group, $i = 1, \ldots, I$. The prior distributions for the parameter θ_i is given a conditionally independent normal

$$\theta_i \sim \text{Normal}(\mu_\theta, \sigma_\theta^2). \qquad (7.49)$$

Similarly, the prior distribution for the parameter ρ_i is given a conditionally independent normal

$$\rho_i \sim \text{Normal}(\mu_\rho, \sigma_\rho^2). \qquad (7.50)$$

As in the above Bayesian meta-analysis with Poisson likelihood, one can assign the next stage priors for the hyperparameters $(\mu_\theta, \sigma_\theta^2, \mu_\rho, \sigma_\rho^2)$ or give arbitrary values based on prior experience.

5. *Meta-analysis using individual patient data (IPD).* Although meta-analysis is traditionally conducted using summary data from individual studies, it may be advantageous to perform meta-analyses using individual patient data, as pointed out by CIOMS (2016). Combining all IPD in a meta-analysis can (a) map all data to a common set of terminology, (b) estimate treatment effects in subgroups of particular interest (e.g., elderly patients), (c) perform stratified analysis according to pre-defined stratum variables, (d) use composite variables

to define adverse outcomes (e.g., weight gain may include obesity, increased appetite, etc.), (e) adjust for confounding factors (e.g., comorbidities, concomitant medications, etc.), and (f) analyze time-to-event data. There are two different approaches to meta-analysis using IPD, namely, one-stage and two-stage approaches (Simmonds et al., 2005). In the one-stage approach, the individual patient data are analyzed in a fixed or random effects model with hierarchical structure that incorporates variations and/or clustering of individual patients within studies (Riley et al., 2010), while in the two-stage approach, the data are summarized for each of individual studies and meta-analysis is performed in the traditional way with summary information. More detailed discussions on the comparison and choice of one-stage or two-stage approaches are given by Whitehead (2002), Higgins and Green (2011), CIOMS (2016), and Burke et al. (2017).

6. *Prescription sequence symmetry analysis.* The concept of prescription sequence analysis was introduced by Petri et al. (1988), but Hallas (1996) renamed it by adding "symmetry" before analysis in PSSA. Wahab et al. (2013) extended the (single) index drug to a class of structurally related index drugs that may cause a group of pathophysiologically related adverse drug reactions followed by the prescription of outcome drugs to treat the adverse reactions. A key measure in PSSA is the crude sequence ratio CSR $= (n_{A\to B})/(n_{B\to A})$, in which drug A is the index drug (which is suspected to cause an ADR under investigation), drug B is used to treat the ADR, and $n_{A\to B}$ (respectively, $n_{B\to A}$) denotes the number of patients who are prescribed drug B after (respectively, before) the index drug. As "an estimate of the incidence rate ratio of the outcome in the exposed period versus that of the non-exposed period", it may be affected by the prescribing trend which can lead to bias. Hence Hallas (1996) proposes to use a null-effect sequence ratio NSR $= p/(1-p)$ as an alternative estimate, in which the estimated probability of a B $\to$ A sequence is estimated by

$$p = \sum_{i=1}^{u} \left(\frac{B_i}{B_0}\right) \times \frac{\sum_{j=i+1}^{u} A_j}{A_0}, \qquad (7.51)$$

where u is the last day of the study window, $A_0 = \sum_{i=1}^{u} A_i$, $B_0 = \sum_{i=1}^{u} B_i$, A_i is the number of patients receiving the index drug and B_i is the number of patients receiving the outcome drug on day i. Tsiropoulos et al. (2009) modify (7.51) by placing a restriction k on the length of the exposure window so that p is replaced by

$$\tilde{p} = \frac{\sum_{i=1}^{u} \left[A_i \left(\sum_{j=i+1}^{i+k} B_j\right)\right]}{A_0 \left(\sum_{j=i-k}^{i-1} B_j + \sum_{j=i+1}^{i+k} B_j\right)}, \qquad (7.52)$$

in which $B_0 = 0$. Hallas (1996) points out that the advantages of PSSA include its ease of implementation, visual representation and robustness to unmeasured confounders because it uses self-controlled designs that includes only those patients who experience the ADR of interest and/or have exposure to the index and outcome drugs. In their simulation studies, Wahab et al. (2013) find that the PSSA method shows high specificity and moderate sensitivity when applied to adverse events identified from 120 clinical trials over 19 drugs. They show that as a complementary tool to traditional pharmacovigilance methods, PSSA can detect detect additional safety signals from administrative data sources. It has become one of the routine signal detection methods for the Asian Pharmacoepidemiology Network to support pharmacoepidemiologic research among several Asian countries (Pratt et al., 2015). On the other hand, there are some challenging issues that include false positive rates with multiple index drugs, selection of the study period, and confounding by indication or by contraindication; see Hallas (1996, Table 4), E. C. Lai et al. (2017) and Takeuchi et al. (2018) for more discussions.

8

Sequential Methods for Safety Surveillance

Timely detection of adverse health events in conjunction with public health policies to rectify the situation or prevent repeated occurrences is beneficial to the affected individuals and society. This involves systematic collection, analysis, and interpretation of large amounts of outcome-specific data by national health programs in different countries and international networks; see Sonesson and Bock (2003, pp.5–6) who also point out that there are many situations in which the sequentially accumulated data can be used prospectively to quickly detect an increased incidence of a disease so that timely rectifying actions can be taken. They note that while much of the research on statistical surveillance originated from engineering applications, "the context of public health surveillance implies specific problems that are not generally present in the case of industrial production control." These include problems of seasonal effects and reporting delays, inherent differences among diseases (such as chronic versus infections), monitoring not only cases of disease but also risk factors. Kulldorff (2011) points out that when surveillance is carried out repeatedly over time, "sequential statistical methods should be used". He distinguishes between sequential testing methods "to quickly detect (an AE) problem that has been there from the beginning of the analysis", and sequential detection methods "to monitor a process for a sudden shift or unknown shift that occurs at some unknown time," which are commonly used in an industrial setting to quickly detect a suddenly malfunctioning manufacturing process." After a comprehensive overview of sequential testing methods for pharmacovigilance in Section 8.1, we focus on a number of statistical issues and recent developments to address them in Sections 8.2 and 8.3. The supplements and problems in Section 8.4 provide additional details for sequential testing and detection.

8.1 Sequential testing for safety surveillance

Bartroff et al. (2013) have given a comprehensive review of sequential testing for efficacy, in which the null hypothesis assumes that the new treatment is no better than the control, and only rejection of the null hypothesis would result in regulatory approval of the new treatment. The approval allows beneficial claims of the drug or vaccine in its labeling; this explains why the null hypothesis H_0 takes the form that there is no such benefit so that rejection of H_0 provides enough evidence to support the claim. For safety testing, the manufacturer of the medical product does not usually make a claim about its safety but is required by the regulatory agency, which does not take the position that it is unsafe, to collect data about potential adverse events. Pre-licensure randomized clinical trials for a new drug or vaccine have to first establish that it is efficacious and group sequential tests for efficacy are often used. If the efficacy bar is passed, the next stage is to test for safety, which involves a very large sample size because adverse events are rare. Therefore the regulatory position is to presume potential safety concerns of the drug or vaccine unless proven otherwise in a large randomized trial. This position implicitly assumes that there is further post-marketing evaluation since acceptance of the null hypothesis does not have a prescribed probability guarantee that it is indeed true, i.e., that the drug or vaccine is indeed safe.

8.1.1 SPRT and CMaxSPRT

The subject called *sequential analysis*, which also includes sequential design of experiments, was born in response to demands for more efficient testing of anti-aircraft gunnery during World War II, which led to Wald's development of the sequential probability ratio test (SPRT); see Wald (1945, 1947). Let $X_1, X_2, \ldots$ be i.i.d. random variables with a common density function f. To test $H_0 : f = f_0$ versus $H_1 : f = f_1$, the SPRT based on a sample $X_1, \ldots, X_n$ of fixed size n rejects H_0 if

$$N = \inf \{n \geq 1 : L_n \notin (A, B)\} \tag{8.1}$$

where $L_n = \prod_{i=1}^{n} [f_1(X_i)/f_0(X_i)]$ denotes the likelihood ratio statistic and $0 < A < 1 < B$ are the stopping boundaries that are determined such that $P_0 \{L_n \geq A\} \leq \alpha$ and $P_1 \{L_n \geq B\} \leq \beta$. Wald (1945) developed simple formulas for α and β in terms of A and B, from which he could solve for A and B when α and β are given. These formulas are corollaries of the likelihood ratio identity and therefore apply to more general settings than the i.i.d. case. In fact, L_n in (8.1) can be defined for general, not necessarily independent X_i. For this general framework, if $P_i (N < \infty) =$

1 for $i = 0, 1$, we can use the likelihood ratio identity to obtain

$$P_0 \left(L_N \geq B \right) \leq B^{-1} P_1 \left(L_N \geq B \right), \quad P_1 \left(L_N \leq A \right) \leq A P_0 \left(L_N \leq A \right), \quad (8.2)$$

and $\leq$ can be replaced by $=$ in (8.2) if L_N falls on either boundary exactly. Ignoring overshoots, (8.2) can be treated as approximate equalities to solve the error probabilities $\alpha = P_0 \left(L_N \geq B \right)$ and $\beta = P_1 \left(L_N \leq A \right)$, yielding

$$\alpha \approx \frac{1 - A}{B - A}, \quad \beta \approx A \cdot \frac{B - 1}{B - A}. \quad (8.3)$$

Writing (8.3) as equations of (A, B) in terms of α and β yields the explicit solutions for the stopping boundaries:

$$A \approx \frac{\beta}{1 - \alpha}, \quad B \approx \frac{1 - \beta}{\alpha}. \quad (8.4)$$

Within a decade after Wald's introduction of the SPRT, it was recognized that sequential hypothesis testing might provide a useful tool in clinical trials to test the efficacy of new medical treatments; see Bartholomay (1957) in particular. Supplement 1 in Section 8.4 gives an overview of likelihood ratio identities and the theory of sequential testing of composite hypotheses, using sequential generalized likelihood ratio (GLR) statistics in lieu of the likelihood ratio statistics L_n.

Davis et al. (2005) applied Wald's SPRT to a dataset of the Centers for Disease Control and Prevention (CDC) Vaccine Safety Datalink (VSD) for surveillance of vaccine safety. The motivation of this application was driven by the need for detecting serious adverse events (e.g., intussusception in the rotavirus vaccine case) as soon as possible after the introduction of a new vaccine using the CDC's dynamic VSD database. With rhesus-rotavirus vaccine as an example, Davis et al. (2005) first defined the time frame of nearly five years, and then segmented the chronological data into weekly cohorts of vaccinated children. The data were further partitioned into a baseline period before and a surveillance period after the introduction of the rotavirus vaccine, and risk-adjustment methods (Steiner et al., 2000) were also used to account for age, calendar time, season, and gender. Applying the SPRT to test the pre-specified null hypothesis of no risk increase against the alternative hypothesis of 10-fold increase (an effect size considered to be of public health importance) of intussusception risk among vaccinated children, Davis et al. (2005) were able to reject the null hypothesis in 10 weeks after introduction of the rotavirus vaccine. They also detected decreased risk of some adverse events associated with the changeover of DTPw (diphtheria, tetanus, and whole cell pertussis) to DTPa (diphtheria, tetanus, and acellular pertussis) vaccine by a similar application of the SPRT.

Kulldorff et al. (2011) study the performance of applying the SPRT to vaccine safety surveillance as in Davis et al. (2005), by "using a historical time series of health insurance claims data from the CDC-sponsored VSD project." They say:

> With these data, we mimic a prospective weekly surveillance system for evaluating whether there is increased risk of either fever or neurological symptoms within 28 days after Pediarix vaccination. Manufactured by GlaxoSmithKline, Pediarix is a combination vaccine that with a single injection protects children from five different diseases: diphtheria, tetanus, whooping cough, hepatitis B, and polio... Let C_t be the random variable representing the number of adverse events within D days following a vaccination (or drug prescription) that was given during the time period $[0, t]$, and let c_t be the corresponding observed number of adverse events. Note that time is defined in terms of the time of the vaccination rather than the time of the adverse event and that, hence, we actually do not know the value of ct until time $t + D$. Under the null hypothesis (H_0), C_t follows a Poisson distribution with mean μ_t, where μ_t is a known function reflecting the population at risk. In our setting, μ_t reflects the number of people who received the drug/vaccine during the time interval $[0, t]$ and a baseline risk for those individuals, adjusting for age and gender.

To carry out the SPRT, one has to specify a simple alternative hypothesis, which Kulldorff et al. (2011) choose to be $\gamma\mu_t$ for the mean of the Poisson distribution of C_t, where $\gamma > 1$ is a prescribed constant representing an increased relative risk, yielding the log-likelihood ratio

$$\text{LLR}_t = \log\left(\left[(\gamma\mu_t)^{C_t} e^{\gamma\mu_t}\right] / \left[(\mu_t)^{C_t} e^{\mu_t}\right]\right) = (1 - \gamma)\mu_t + C_t \log\gamma. \quad (8.5)$$

To address the question whether there is an increased risk during the 4 weeks following Pediarix vaccination, they apply the SPRT (with $\alpha = 0.05$ and $\beta = 0.2$) to the aforementioned VSD dataset, first with $\gamma = 2$ and then with $\gamma = 1.2$. For $\gamma = 2$, it terminated after 13 weeks and rejected H_0. Hence choosing values of γ that are too high for the data may lead to the SPRT to terminate in favor of H_0 than H_1. This has led Kulldorff et al. (2011) to let the data choose γ in the MaxSPRT to test the simple null hypothesis $H_0 : \gamma = 1$ versus the composite alternative hypothesis $H_1 : \gamma > 1$. For the Poisson model, MaxSPRT replaces (8.5) by the test statistic

$$S_t = \sup_{\gamma>1}\left\{(1 - \gamma)\mu_t + C_t \log\gamma\right\}$$
$$= \left\{(\mu_t - C_t) + C_t \log(C_t/\mu_t)\right\} I_{\{C_t \geq \mu_t\}}, \quad (8.6)$$

and rejects H_0 at time $\tau = \inf\{\tau \leq T : S_t \geq a\}$, where T is the maximum duration of surveillance, accepting H_0 if $S_t < a$ for all $t \leq T$. The choice of the threshold a by using Lambert's W-function associated with (8.6) and

Poisson probabilities; see Kulldorff et al. (2011, pp. 65–67). Supplement 1 in Section 8.4 provides an alternative approach to MaxSPRT and its historical background that predated MaxSPRT.

In the SPRT and its refinement MaxSPRT, the number of adverse events of the surveillance group is considered to be random while the cumulative person-time or the cumulative number of vaccinations is considered to be fixed. Hence the expected number of adverse events under the null is assumed to be a known function of the cumulative person-time and some potential confounders such as age, sex, and site. Noting that there are usually no reliable estimates of this function in practice, Li and Kulldorff (2010) propose to condition instead on the number of adverse events in the historical data and that in the surveillance group, and to regard the cumulative person-time taken to observe the given number of adverse events as a random variable, leading to their "conditional MaxSPRT," which they denote by CMaxSPRT. Specifically, let c and Q denote the total number of adverse events and the total person-time in the historical data, respectively, and let T_k denote the cumulative person-time since the beginning of the surveillance until the kth adverse event. Here c and k are fixed numbers while Q and T_k are random. To fix the ideas, assume that the number of events over the cumulative person-time in the historical cohort and that in the surveillance group are homogeneous Poisson processes with the event rates denoted by λ_h and λ_v, respectively. Instead of working with the Poisson process, Li and Kulldorff (2010) work with the exponential inter-arrival times, or the "inter-event person-times" as they call them, like what we have presented in Section 4.2.2. Thus, the cumulative person-time T_k in the surveillance group since the beginning of the surveillance until the kth event is a sum of k i.i.d. random variables from the exponential distribution with rate λ_v, and therefore has a gamma distribution with shape parameter k and scale $1/\lambda_v$. Right after the kth adverse event in the surveillance group, the likelihood function is

$$L_k = \lambda_h^c e^{-\lambda_h Q} \lambda_v^k e^{-\lambda_v T_k} = \lambda_h^c \lambda_v^k e^{-(\lambda_h Q + \lambda_v T_k)}.$$

The null hypothesis $\lambda_h = \lambda_v$ is composite as the common value is unknown. Therefore the logarithm of the ratio of the maximized likelihood of the composite null to the composite alternative hypotheses is

$$U_k = \log \left(\frac{\max_{\lambda_v \geq \lambda_h} e^{-\lambda_h Q - \lambda_v T_k} \lambda_h^c \lambda_v^k}{\max_\lambda e^{-\lambda(Q+T_k)} \lambda^{c+k}} \right)$$

$$= I_{\{k/c > T_k/Q\}} \log \left(\frac{e^{-c}(c/Q)^c e^{-k}(k/T_k)^k}{e^{-(k+c)}[(c+k)/(Q+T_k)]^{c+k}} \right). \tag{8.7}$$

Li and Kulldorff (2010) note that (a) conditional on c, the only random part of U_k is the ratio T_k/Q, and (b) under the composite null hypothesis $H_0 : \lambda_h = \lambda_v = \lambda$ with unknown λ, the conditional distribution of T_k/Q given c does not depend on λ. Hence under H_0, the joint distribution of

$(U_1, \ldots, U_k)$ depends only on c and k. The CMaxSPRT specifies a maximum number K of adverse events from the surveillance group. If K is reached, the test stops; this serves as a truncation bound for CMaxSPRT. The test is based on the conditional distribution of $(U_1, \ldots, U_K)$ given the total number c of adverse events in the historical data, which does not depend on the unknown value of λ_h and λ_v under the null hypothesis and can be determined by Monte Carlo simulations. Tables of critical values are given in Li and Kulldorff (2010) for $\alpha = 0.05$ and different values of c and K.

8.1.2 Adjustments for confounding and risk factors

Li and Kulldorff (2010, Sect. 4.5) note that the assumption of homogeneous Poisson arrivals with event rates λ_h and λ_v over the historical and surveillance cohorts may be overly restrictive in view of population heterogeneity; for example, men and women may have different event rates. To adjust for confounding, they propose to stratify the entire population into several subgroups that are likely to have different risks for adverse events and assign different weights to the person-time from different subgroups; the weights are chosen "using either subject-matter expertise and/or published results from previous studies."

Although Wald's SPRT approach has been employed in many applied fields (e.g., process control) and in the design and analysis of clinical experiments almost right after its inception, its application in monitoring human health concerns including surveillance of medical product safety based on observational data has not taken place until fairly recently. Among the earliest applications in adverse event monitoring, Spiegelhalter et al. (2003) applied risk-adjusted SPRT to three longitudinal data sets for retrospective analyses of adverse clinical outcomes after cardiac surgery. They note that "the SPRT is the most powerful method for discriminating between two hypotheses, and was recommended well over 40 years ago (in the 1950s) in a medical context for clinical trials and clinical experiments," citing Armitage (1954) and Bartholomay (1957), but introduce adjustments for risk factors following Steiner et al. (2000) to monitor sequentially adverse events in cardiac surgery for pediatric and adult patients. They point out the need for such sequential monitoring systems to detect excess deaths after cardiac surgery, and for incorporating risk adjustments in these systems because the adverse events involve both patients and cardiac surgeons. In particular, they say: "The medical context does, however, add an additional complexity (over sequential analysis developed for sampling inspection of military supplies in the Second World War) in the need to adjust for case-mix in an attempt to avoid clinicians or trusts being unfairly penalized for treating high-risk patients," an example of which is monitoring the mortality rates for open-heart surgery on children under 1 year of age in Bristol Royal Infirmary between 1984 and

1995 relative to other medical centers in Britain. The risk adjustment in this case is as follows; they use ln to denote natural logarithm (to base e), which we denote by log instead.

> Given that the pre-operative risk is p, a doubling in the odds on death is optimally detected by adding the score $-\ln(1+p)$ to the running score total if the patient survives, and $0.69 - \ln(1+p)$ if the patient dies. The value 0.69 is equal to $\ln(2)$. ... To adjust for risk, we can allow the value of p to depend on individual patient risk factors such as age, sex, and diabetes status.

Such risk adjustment actually dates back to Steiner et al. (2000) who used risk-adjusted CUSUM charts for monitoring surgical outcomes whereby the chart "signals if sufficient evidence has accumulated that there has been a change in surgical failure rate." As noted in Supplement 1 in Section 8.4, there is a close connection between the SPRT and the likelihood ratio CUSUM rule, and this connection can be used to relate the risk-adjusted score described above to risk-adjusted log-likelihood ratio statistic of Steiner et al. (2000) who describe the score as follows:

> In most surgical contexts the risk of mortality estimated pre-operatively will vary considerably from patient to patient. An adjustment for prior risk is therefore appropriate to ensure that mortality rates that appear unusual and arise from differences in patient mix are not incorrectly attributed to the surgeon... The surgical risk varies for each patient depending on risk factors present. We define $p_t(\theta) = g(\theta, \mathbf{x}_t)$, where $\mathbf{x}_t = (x_{t1}, x_{t2}, \ldots, x_{tp})^T$ is a $p \times 1$ vector reflecting the risk factors for patient t... Since each patient has a different baseline risk level we define the hypotheses H_0 and H_A based on an odds ratio. Let R_0 and R_A represent the odds ratio under null and alternate hypotheses, respectively. To detect increases we set $R_A > R_0$. The choice of R_A is similar to defining the minimal clinically important effect in a clinical trial. If the estimated risk p_t is based on the current conditions, we may set $R_0 = 1$.

Spiegelhalter et al. (2003) assume $R_0 = 1$ so that the odds of failure under H_0 is $p_t/(1 - p_t)$, whereas under H_A the odds of failure is $R_A p_t/(1 - p_t)$, which corresponds to the probability π_t of failure equal to $R_A p_t/(1 - p_t + R_A p_t)$. The log-likelihood ratio statistic is

$$\sum_t \left\{ y_t \log\left(\frac{\pi_t}{p_t}\right) + (1 - y_t) \log\left(\frac{1 - \pi_t}{1 - p_t}\right) \right\}, \tag{8.8}$$

and therefore the log-likelihood score for patient t is

$$W_t = \begin{cases} \log\left(\frac{R_A}{1 - p_t + R_A p_t}\right), & \text{if } y_t = 1 \\ \log\left(\frac{1}{1 - p_t + R_A p_t}\right), & \text{if } y_t = 0. \end{cases} \tag{8.9}$$

"Doubling in the odds on death" for the alternative hypothesis assumed by Spiegelhalter et al. (2003) is tantamount to taking $R_A = 2$, for which $-\log(1 - p_t + R_A p_t) = -\log(1 + p_t)$ and $\log(R_A) = \log(2)$. Putting this into (8.9) yields the risk-adjusted SPRT of Spiegelhalter et al. (2003); this is also the background of the risk-adjusted CUSUM chart of Steiner et al. (2000) and the risk-adjusted CMaxPSRT of Li and Kulldorff (2010, Section 4.5).

8.2 Group sequential methods, frequency of analysis and other design considerations

8.2.1 Continuous versus group sequential monitoring for post-market safety surveillance

The preceding sections in this chapter are concerned with sequential methods for continuous post-marketing sequential safety surveillance. However, there have been discussions on whether continuous sequential or group sequential monitoring schemes should be used in post-marketing observational studies for safety surveillance. Silva and Kulldorff (2015) investigate the performance characteristics of continuous and group sequential analyses of post-marketing safety data in terms of statistical power, expected sample size (time to signal), and maximum sample size using the MaxSPRT procedure, and show that "continuous sequential analysis performs better than group sequential analysis and that more frequent group sequential analyses perform better than less frequent group sequential analyses." They therefore point out that "group sequential analysis should never be deliberately applied to post-market safety surveillance when the data is available in a continuous or near continuous fashion." However, this highly frequent analysis of safety data takes into account only statistical advantages (more power and earlier signaling) and may not be feasible in many practical circumstances as discussed in Zhao et al. (2012) who propose a new approach to monitoring rare adverse events based on group sequential testing methods, which are tailored for post-marketing safety surveillance to account for confounding. The proposed group sequential approach is more flexible and can even be more efficient than continuous sequential testing methods after adjusting for the special features of the observational data. In discussing the challenges in the design and analysis of sequential safety monitoring using electronic observational data, Nelson et al. (2012) point out that the design choices for observational safety surveillance should consider "the hypotheses, population, prevalence, and severity of the outcomes, implications of signaling, and costs of false positive and negative findings."

There are also many analytic challenges including confounding, missing data, misclassifications, and unpredictable changes in dynamically accrued data (such as product uptake, vaccine dosage distributions). Nelson et al. (2012) further note that these factors impact not only the variability of adverse events, but also the type I error probability that will be lower than planned if critical values for continuous sequential analysis are used but testing is not strictly continuous. Therefore, they propose that thresholds for type I error control in sequential testing should be adjusted over time to take into account these factors.

8.2.2 Frequency of analyses in sequential surveillance

The frequency of sequential analyses for safety surveillance usually depends on the nature of the adverse events (severity and rarity) under surveillance, the product of interest (e.g., drugs treating serious conditions or vaccines for healthy infants), public health importance, frequency of data accrued, and the monitored population. In general, a high-frequency or even near-continuous (say, weekly or biweekly) sequential analysis should be considered for severe adverse events (e.g., life-threatening events), or events with high prevalence or of public health importance, and/or healthy population, in which a safety signal can be detected earlier with a high statistical power, as illustrated in Nelson et al. (2012) who also discuss statistical tradeoffs among different frequencies of sequential analyses. In contrast, a lower-frequency or group sequential analysis can be applied to adverse events with less severity and of less public health importance and drugs treating serious health problems for which there are no alternative options. In addition to these factors, Nelson et al. (2012) note that the frequency of sequential analysis can also be planned using either calender scale or accrued sample size, with the latter being attractive since it is tied with type I error spending at each test. The frequency of sequential analyses for prospective surveillance in observational studies has also been discussed by Kulldorff (2012) who says:

> The frequency of analyses in a sequential setting is primarily determined by how frequently data can be obtained from the health plans or other data providers. It is important to note though that different data providers do not need to be synchronized. One health plan may provide data every Monday morning for the events that happened during the prior week while another health plan may only be able to provide data once a month with a 10-week delay. With a sequential statistical design, the data can be analyzed as it arrives to the data coordinating center independently of when the events happened and from where it arrived. With a continuous sequential method, the data can be analyzed as often as one likes, without having to worry about multiple testing. If the data are analyzed at discrete time points but still frequently,

such as once a week, a continuous sequential method will be only slightly conservative so that the true alpha level is slightly higher than the nominal one. If analyses are done less frequently, such as once or twice a year, the true and nominal alpha levels may differ greatly, and it is then better to use a group sequential method... The frequency at which new data arrive is often a design consideration that can be controlled by the investigators. Sooner and more frequent is always better than later and less frequent from an analytical and performance perspective, but the former may be more costly in terms of both money and effort. It is then a trade-off between cost of setting up the surveillance system and its timeliness to detect a safety problem.

8.2.3 Selection of comparison group and other design considerations

As in any comparative studies, a critical component in sequential safety surveillance using observational data is the selection of comparison groups that can be used in sequential testing for safety signaling. An inappropriate choice of a comparison group can lead to selection bias and consequently invalidate the results of the sequential analysis. Kulldorff (2012) discusses the strategies for selection of comparison groups with special consideration given to the sequential nature of the analysis, in which concurrent data are usually unavailable at the beginning of surveillance. Depending on the medical product and the adverse event under surveillance, the comparison group can be concurrent or historical population controls, matched unexposed individuals, or self-controls and can be drawn from the same database, other databases with similar population characteristics, or published information. He also discusses other statistical design considerations. He points out that, unlike clinical trials in which each observation is costly, it is relatively easy and cheap in post-marketing safety surveillance to "continue surveillance for a little longer" to increase the overall statistical power, but "it is costly to reduce the time until a signal occurs, which is of great importance," as "it is often costly to increase the rate–at which the sample size accrues, as one would have added additional data such as another health plan." Another design consideration is the choice of stopping boundaries, which he argues to be primarily a tradeoff between "timeliness-to-signal for modest versus high excess risks." Silva (2017, 2018) has carried out comparative studies of different types of error spending functions in terms of expected number of events to signal.

Population controls. All unexposed individuals in the database can serve a population-based concurrent control group that is typically large and suitable for monitoring rare adverse events and for eliminating temporal trends if confounding adjustment is appropriately performed at each of the sequential analysis. Kulldorff (2012) discusses the example of the quadrivalent vaccine MMRV (measles, mumps, rubella, varicella) replacing separate injections of the MMR and V vaccines (see Section 7.9.2) for which the surveillance focuses on whether the risk of an adverse event among those who receive the new vaccine is the same as among those who receive the old vaccine. In this example, he points out that historical data can be used "to calculate the number of adverse events after the old vaccine in various demographical population groups based on age, gender, study site" and covariate-adjusted expected number of events can be calculated for those who receive the new vaccine. He further notes that due to underlying differences in surveillance population and the comparison population with respect to disease risk and some confounding factors, selection bias may be inevitable.

Matched controls. For concurrent matched controls, one or more unexposed individuals can be selected as controls for each exposed subject based on their age, gender, geographical location, and medical history. The controls can be chosen from children with hospital visit during the same week of the exposed child being vaccinated for children's vaccine surveillance, or individuals receiving a different product at the same time when an exposed person being treated by the product under surveillance. Matched controls can also be selected from a historical population for which the past experiences are collected for comparisons. However, this historical matched control may increase secular bias due to seasonality of the adverse events of interest.

Self-controls. In a self-control study, the unexposed time before taking a medical product is compared with the exposed time after taking the product for the same individual. Self-controls may be able to avoid selection bias, but are subject to bias due to seasonal trends and time-varying covariate effects.

Regardless of which method is used for selection of the comparison group, selection bias is always a concern in observational surveillance. The FDA encourages the use of multiple comparison groups in safety surveillance based on electronic healthcare data to increase the validity of safety studies and suggests that the primary comparison group be identified with rationales for each group (FDA, 2013a). In conducting safety surveillance of vaccine products, special attention should be given to the *healthy vaccinee effect*, which refers to the fact that people receiving a vaccine tend to be healthier than those who don't or who receive the vaccine later because of illness or lack of access to primary care. In this case, the self-control design can be used to address this issue.

8.3 Adjustments for observational data and applications to sequential safety surveillance

8.3.1 Stratification

Li (2009) develops the conditional sequential sampling procedure (CSSP) to control for confounding bias in drug safety surveillance. CSSP partitions the study subjects into S subgroups based on discrete (or discretized) confounders. Such stratification attempts to result in approximately homogeneous patient subgroups for whom adverse event rates can be compared between treatment and control groups. It uses a group sequential test, with alpha-spending to control the overall type I error and a prescribed maximum number K of interim tests. Under the assumption that the study population can be divided into S homogeneous strata based on baseline confounders such as age and sex, denote by $n^1_{s,k}$ (respectively, $n^0_{s,k}$) the number of new AE cases for the subjects in stratum s receiving the drug of interest (respectively, drug of comparison) in time period between the $(k-1)$st and the kth interim analysis, and by $\tau^1_{s,k}$ (respectively, $\tau^0_{s,k}$) the corresponding exposure time. The drug of interest corresponds to the new treatment and is abbreviated by DOI, whereas the drug of comparison corresponds to the control and is abbreviated by DOC. As in CMaxSPRT described in Section 8.1.1, CSSP also assumes that the number of AEs has a Poisson($\mu^j_{s,k}$) distribution, where

$$\mu^j_{s,k} = (1-j)\lambda_{s,k}\tau^0_{s,k} + j\theta\lambda_{s,k}\tau^1_{s,k}, \quad j = 0,1, \tag{8.10}$$

where θ is the relative risk of AE for DOI with respect to DOC, and $\lambda_{s,k}$ is the baseline AE rate for each unit of exposure time of a subject in stratum s during the time period between the $(k-1)$st and the kth interim analysis. Let $T_k = \sum_{i=1}^{k}\sum_{s=1}^{S} n^1_{s,i}$ and $N_{s,k} = n^1_{s,k} + n^0_{s,k}$. Noting that $(T_k, N_{s,k})$ is a sufficient statistic for $(\theta, \lambda_{s,k})$, Li (2009) derives the conditional distribution of T_k given $\{N_{s,i} : 1 \geq s \geq S, 1 \geq i \geq k\}$ to test the null hypothesis $\theta = 1$. Under the null hypothesis, because $n^1_{s,k}|N_{s,k} \sim \text{Binomial}(N_{s,k}, \tau^1_{s,k}/(\tau^1_{s,k} + \tau^0_{s,k}))$, the conditional distribution of T_k is known and does not depend on the nuisance parameter $\lambda_{s,k}$. However, the joint distribution of $(T_1, \ldots, T_K)$ under the null hypothesis is difficult to express analytically. CSSP specifies the group sequential test by an error spending function and uses an iterative simulation procedure to carry out the test. It simulates B samples $\tilde{n}^1_{s,i:b} \sim$ Binomial($N_{s,i}, \tau^1_{s,i}/(\tau^1_{s,i} + \tau^0_{s,i})$), $1 \geq s \geq S$, to form $\tilde{T}_{k,b} \sum_{i=1}^{k}\sum_{s=1}^{S} \tilde{n}_{s,i:b}$ for $b = 1, \ldots, B$. The iterations proceed as follows, using the error spending function $\alpha_1 < \alpha_2 < \ldots < \alpha_K = \alpha$ of the type I error of a group sequential test:

Step 1: Stop and reject the null hypothesis if T_1 exceeds Q_1, which is the $(1 - \alpha_1)$-quartile of $\{\tilde{T}_{1,b} : b = 1, \ldots, B\}$. Else continue and remove $\tilde{T}_{1,b} > Q_1$ from the B simulated trajectories, leaving behind a subset $\mathcal{B}$ of $\{1, \ldots, B\}$.

Step k: Stop and reject the null hypothesis if T_k exceeds Q_k, which is the $(1 - \alpha_k)$-quartile of $\{\tilde{T}_{k,b} : b \in \mathcal{B}_{k-1}\}$. Else continue and remove $\tilde{T}_{k,b} > Q_k$ from $\mathcal{B}_{k-1}$, leaving behind a subset $\mathcal{B}_k$ of $\mathcal{B}_{k-1}$.

The procedure terminates with at most K steps. Cook et al. (2012) comment that the "CSSP approach is especially good when evaluating rare events" but that "it has limitations when there are too many strata and/or short intervals between analyses."

8.3.2 Matching and applications to VSD and Sentinel data

In their review of group sequential monitoring of postmarket safety surveillance, Cook et al. (2012) describe besides CSSP the following matching approach to adjust for confounding. This approach creates for each exposed subject M unexposed subjects who have the same categorical confounders. Let p denote the proportion of adverse events for the exposed group, which is $1/(M = 1)$ under the null hypothesis. The log GLR (generalized likelihood ratio) statistic at the kth interim analysis is

$$\ell_k = \log\left(\left(\frac{\hat{p}}{1/(M+1)}\right)^{m(k)} \left(\frac{1-\hat{p}}{M/(M+1)}\right)^{n(k)-m(k)}\right)$$
$$= m(k)\log\left((M+1)\hat{p}\right) + (n(k) - m(k))\log\left((M+1)(1-\hat{p})/M\right), \quad (8.11)$$

where $n(k)$ is the total number of adverse events up to the kth interim analysis, $m(k)$ is the corresponding number for the exposed group, and $\hat{p} = m(k)/n(k)$ is the maximum likelihood estimate of p. They propose to use the Pocock or O'Brien-Fleming boundary, or an error spending function, to apply the group sequential approach; see Supplement 1 in Section 8.4 for the background of these group sequential boundaries and error spending functions. Matching has been used earlier for the MaxSPRT by Kulldorff et al. (2011, Section 5) to adjust for confounding in comparing an exposed time period after vaccination with an exposed time period before vaccination from the same subject in a self-control design, for which they point out that this basically reduces the test to that for binomial data:

> We continue surveillance until either there is a signal rejecting the null hypothesis or when we have observed a total of N adverse events in the exposed and unexposed time periods combined. In essence, we have a number of coin tosses (adverse events), which may either turn up as head or tail (exposed or unexposed). Under the null hypothesis, the probability of a head is known to be p, where $p = 0.5$ for a 1:1 matching ratio when the exposed and

unexposed time periods are of the same length, $p = 0.25$ for a 1:3 matching ratio, etc.

They note that this idea also applies to matched control designs that "compare individuals exposed to the drug/vaccine with matched unexposed individuals", which is what Cook et al. (2012) review as a method to adjust for confounding, as described earlier in this paragraph.

Nelson et al. (2012, 2013) describe applications of these adaptations of group sequential methods to observational postmarketing safety surveillance, using electronic databases from the Vaccine Safety Datalink (VSD) described in Section 7.1.4. VSD "has created a population-based framework with which to conduct near real-time surveillance by weekly updating of vaccine and adverse event data on over 9 million members of 8 medical care organizations (MCOs) and has used this framework to monitor the safety of many new-vaccines since 2005," and in particular a pentavalent combination DTaP-IPV-Hib vaccine for which Nelson et al. (2013) conducted prospective group sequential Poisson-based likelihood ratio tests to compare the incidence of 7 adverse events in children aged 6 weeks to 4 years who received the vaccine with that in historical recipients of DTaP-containing vaccines. "To control for confounding, historical event rates were computed by MCO site, gender, and age group and used to compute stratum-specific expected counts," thereby using stratification to control for confounding, Nelson et al. (2012) note that VSD and the Sentinel System of the FDA (Behrman et al., 2011) "can provide a complementary middle group between traditional passive reporting databases, which are often used to generate hypotheses by searching for associations among a large number of product-event pairs," as we have described in Sections 7.3 and 7.4, "and phase IV observational studies and randomized trials, which provide more in-depth investigations of a single hypothesis using more accurate information and thus are designed to yield more definitive results." They point out that this middle group has "successfully detected an increased risk of seizure after receipt of the MMRV vaccine compared with separate injections of MMR and V vaccines." Kulldorff (2012, p. 850), however, gives a somewhat different account of how sequential analysis using VSD data detected this increased risk of seizure, saying after their review of using Poisson-based MaxSPRT, CMaxSPRT, and the binomial MaxSPRT in the VSD project:

> For the MMRV vaccine, weekly sequential analyses detected an increased risk of seizures among infants compared to users of the MMR vaccine. This statistical signal was investigated using temporal scan statistics and logistic regression and confirmed to be real. As a result, ACIP modified their vaccine recommendations in February 2008, no longer recommending MMRV over separate vaccinations of MMR and varicella, and the FDA and the manufacturer revised the product label.

They cite Klein et al. (2010), which we have noted in Section 7.9.2 to be the developments, after the ACIP meeting in 2008, of sequential monitoring of prespecified adverse events following vaccination using VSD surveillance systems for different vaccines. Thus, Klein et al. (2010), Nelson et al. (2012), and Kulldorff (2012) represent subsequent "successes" of sequential analysis methods for "early detection" of this increased risk of seizure, after the ACIP recommendation that was based on other post-licensure observational safety studies.

Supplements 2 and 3 in Section 8.4 provides further details on the sequential detection methods in the preceding quotation from Kulldorff (2012) and about logistic regression from Cook et al. (2015) who also introduce a group sequential approach that uses generalized estimating equations to adjust for confounding via regression. Indeed, the supplements and Section 8.3.3 provide details on a number of sequential testing and detection procedures, with adjustment for confounding and using the VSD and Sentinel System of the FDA as test beds, which were developed by Kulldorff and his collaborators (Brown et al., 2009; Yih et al., 2009; Greene et al., 2009; Belongia et al., 2010; Klein et al., 2010; Greene et al., 2011; Lee et al., 2011; Yih et al., 2011) and by Zhao et al. (2012), Cook et al. (2012), Nelson et al. (2012, 2013) and Leite et al. (2016).

8.3.3 Propensity scores and inverse probability weighting

PS-enhanced CSSP

Li et al. (2011) introduce a new sequential monitoring approach to using observational electronic healthcare databases for drug safety surveillance comparing two approved medical products. This new approach improves the confounding adjustment performance of the conditional sequential sampling procedure (CSSP) proposed earlier by Li (2009), which is described in Section 8.3.1. However, the CSSP method has limitations in controlling confounding bias, especially when the number of confounders is large and some confounders are continuous. Li et al. (2011) enhance the stratification of CSSP by using selected percentiles of the estimated propensity score (PS) that is defined as the conditional probability of receiving the treatment of interest given measured baseline confounding factors. The basic idea is to remove the confounding bias under the assumption of no unmeasured confounders. Specifically, let Z and $\mathbf{X}$ denote the treatment indicator and the vector of covariates, respectively, and assume that they are conditionally independent given the propensity score. Then, under the null hypothesis of no excess risk for the treatment group, the incidence rate of the adverse event does not depend on Z given the propensity score, which results in a binomial distribution for the number of adverse events in the treatment group given the total number of adverse events in both the treatment and control groups. As Li et al.

(2011) point out, the PS-enhanced CSSP (a) accommodates patient follow-up or exposure time, (b) allows highly frequent testing, and (c) adjusts for multiple quantitative and qualitative confounders.

Inverse probability weighting via the estimated PS

As pointed out by Røysland (2012), "it is common to re-weight the observational data in order to mimic observations coming from the counterfactual scenarios (involving a hypothetical randomized controlled trial, which is) referred to as inverse probability weighting (that) has occasionally been reported to be too unstable" by Cole and Hernán (2008) and others. Combining regression with weighting by the estimated PS has been widely used to address this problem, as pointed out in the last paragraph of Section 6.3.4 on "doubly robust" or "augmented inverse probability weighted (AIPW) estimators." Nelson et al. (2016, Section V) describe sequential analysis using the "Regression and IPTW" models (i.e., AIPW since IPTW stands for "inverse probability of treatment weighting" to emphasize the role of the propensity score in reweighting the observation) in the FDA's Mini-Sentinel projects on ACE (angiotensin-converting enzyme) inhibitors and ARBs (angiotensin receptor blockers) to treat hypertension; both drugs block the effect of the chemical angiotensin II that narrows blood vessels but work by different mechanisms. ARBs are usually prescribed to patients who cannot tolerate ACE inhibitors. By widening the blood vessels, they allow blood to flow more easily and thereby lower blood pressure. Another class of drugs that reduce blood pressure is called beta blockers, which block norepinephrine and epinephrine from binding to beta receptors. Both ACEs/ARBs and beta-blockers have side effects, and the aforementioned Mini-Sentinel projects is on sequential surveillance of the risk of angioedema (swelling of tissues) with ACEs and ARBs relative to beta-blockers. "The cohort included subjects who were 18 years and older at some point January 2003 (when ARBs came to the market) through December 2012" and who "were members from one of four health plans (Aetna, UnitedHealthcare, Group Health, Kaiser Permanente in North California)" satisfying certain inclusion-exclusion criteria mentioned in Section V B.1 of Nelson et al. (2016), whose Section V B.2 begins by saying : "This evaluation examines two medication classes of ACE inhibitors and ARBs" and "a comparator group of beta-blockers" so that "the cohort included new users of any of these three medication therapeutic classes", and ends with "We began surveillance on June 29, 2008, when all Data Partners (the four healthcare companies) had data available for analysis", carrying out the group sequential design (with four groups/lookc) described in their Section VI E, for which the analysis for ACE inhibitors "signaled at the first look" so that the secondary results for ARB were also analyzed but "no signal was detected at any of the four planned looks."

8.3.4 Signal diagnosis

Kulldorff (2012) points out that the preceding methods for sequential detection of safety signals only generates "alerts about potential vaccine or drug safety problems" and represents "only the first step," to be followed by "further investigations and analyses before making definite conclusions," and gives the following reasons for such caution:

(a) There are many potential sources of bias in observational data.

(b) Surveillance systems usually involve many drug-event pairs and adjust only for their common covariates/possible confounders such as age, gender, and seasonality in the sequential analysis, leaving drug-event specific covariates/confounders and sensitivity analysis to the signal investigation phase.

He also provides a number of methods for signal diagnosis, including the following:

- Adjust for a different and larger set of potential confounders using standard non-sequential pharmacoepidemiologic methods on the same data set. This may include age adjustments, adjustments for concomitant vaccines or medications, adjustments for seasonal trends and secular trends, for day-of-the-week effects, and for chronic disease conditions, etc.

- Compare the signal generated by a drug-event pair with results for subdiagnostic groups and with results from similar drugs and diagnostic events. For example, if there is a signal indicating an increased risk of febrile seizures, check if there is also an increased risk of fever, even if that by itself would not be of interest.

- Compare the results with other existing data sets, such as: Phase III clinical trials, Phase IV postmarketing trials, spontaneous adverse event reporting systems such as AERS and VAERS, and electronic health records from a different health plan.

- Use descriptive histograms for different time windows from initial exposure to the adverse event, to visualize if the distributions have changed. "Formal statistical inference can be done using the temporal scan statistic (see Supplement 3 of Section 7.10), which adjusts for the multiple testing inherent in the many windows" scanned.

Lai et al. (2018b), however, have recently shown how temporal scan statistics and inverse probability weighting in the framework of Røysland (2012) and Aalen et al. (2012) can be applied sequentially over time for safety signal detection and diagnosis.

8.3.5 Sequential likelihood ratio trend-in-trend design in the presence of unmeasured confounding

The trend-in-trend (TT) design has been introduced in Section 6.4.2 to address unmeasured confounding in observational studies as an alternative to instrumental variables for causal inference. Ertefaie et al. (2018) point out that "all existing sequential testing methods rely heavily on the assumption of no unmeasured confounding, which is untestable in non-randomized cohort studies" and then say: "Violations of this assumption can lead to erroneous causal inferences. The trend-in-trend (TT) design is a new non-experimental research design that can be used to study causal effects of treatments for which there are strong or moderate time trends, as in the case for newly approved drugs with a strong market uptake." They develop a sequential version of the TT design by coupling it to sequential GLR tests, and call it a sequential likelihood ratio trend-in-trend (SLR-TT) design. The data from n subjects in the observational study can be represented by n i.i.d trajectories of length T. The ith trajectory is the sequence $(\mathbf{X}_i, D_{i1}, Y_{i1}, \ldots, D_{iT}, Y_{iT})$, where $\mathbf{X}_i$ is a vector of measured baseline characteristics that follows a distribution F, D_{it} is the treatment status (equal to 1 for the new treatment, and 0 for the control) at time t, and Y_{it} is the indicator of whether an adverse event occurred between time $t - 1$ and t. Let $g(= 1, 2, \ldots, G)$ denote the stratum index after stratification based on the cumulative probability of exposure. Assuming the link function (6.15) for the Bernoulli outcome variable of the ith subject given the stratum index g and the treatment status D_{it} at time t, Ertefaie et al. (2018) derive the likelihood function $L_s(\beta_0, \beta_1, \beta_2)$ up to time s. Note that β_1 is the parameter of interest and null hypothesis can be written as $H_0 : \beta_1 = 0$. Following Shih et al. (2010), the stopping rule for the sequential GLR test is

$$\tau = \inf\left\{ 1 \leq s \leq T : \log \frac{L_s(\hat{\beta}_0, \hat{\beta}_1, \hat{\beta}_2)}{L_s(\hat{\beta}_0^{H_0}, 0, \hat{\beta}_2^{H_0})} > b \right\}, \qquad (8.12)$$

where $(\hat{\beta}_0, \hat{\beta}_1, \hat{\beta}_2)$ is the MLE of the parameter vector $(\beta_0, \beta_1, \beta_2)$ and $(\hat{\beta}_0^{H_0}, 0, \hat{\beta}_2^{H_0})$ is the MLE of the corresponding parameter vector under the null hypothesis $H_0 : \beta_1 = 0$, based on all the data up to time s. Ertefaie et al. (2018) provide an algorithm to determine b that satisfies a prescribed type I error for the sequential test.

8.4 Supplements and problems

1. *Repeated significance tests, likelihood ratio identities and sequential GLR tests for composite hypothesis, group sequential designs and error*

spending approach. Armitage, McPherson, and Rowe (1969) proposed a new alternative to the SPRT and its variants, called the *repeated significance test* (RST). The underlying motivation for the RST is that, since the strength of evidence in favor of a treatment from a clinical trial is conveniently indicated by the results of a conventional significance test, it is appealing to apply the significance test, with nominal significance level α, repeatedly during the trial. Noting that the overall significance level α^*, which is the probability that the nominal significance level is attained at some stage, is larger than α, they developed a recursive numerical algorithm to compute α^* in the case of testing a normal mean θ with known variance σ^2, for which the RST of $H_0 : \theta = 0$ is of the form

$$T = \inf\{n \le M : |S_n| \ge c\sigma\sqrt{n}\}, \tag{8.13}$$

rejecting H_0 if $T < M$ or if $T = M$ and $|S_M| \ge a\sigma\sqrt{M}$, where $S_n = X_1 + \cdots + X_n$. Haybittle (1971) proposed to modify the stopping rule of the RST to $T < M$ or $|S_M| \ge a\sigma\sqrt{M}$ to increase its power. The value $a(\le c)$ is so chosen that the overall significance level is equal to some prescribed number. In particular, $a = \infty$ gives the fixed sample size test while $a = c$ gives the RST. In double-blind multicenter clinical trials, it is not feasible to arrange for continuous examination of the data as they accumulate to perform the RST. This led Pocock (1977) to introduce a "group sequential" version of RST, in which the X_n represents an approximately normally distributed statistic of the data in the nth group (instead of the nth observation) and M represents the maximum number of groups. Instead of the square-root boundary $a\sigma\sqrt{n}$, O"Brien and Fleming (1979) proposed to use a constant stopping boundary in

$$T = \inf\{n \le M : |S_n| \ge b\}, \tag{8.14}$$

which corresponds to the group sequential version of an SPRT.

The Neyman-Pearson lemma says that among all tests whose type I error probabilities do not exceed α, the *likelihood ratio test* is most powerful in the sense that it maximizes the probability of rejecting the null hypothesis under the alternative hypothesis. For fixed sample size tests, a first step to extend the Neyman-Pearson theory from simple to composite hypotheses is to consider one-sided composite hypotheses of the form $H_0 : \theta \le \theta_0$ versus $H_1 : \theta > \theta_0$ in the case of parametric families with monotone likelihood ratio in a real parameter θ. In this case, the level-α Neyman-Pearson test of $H : \theta = \theta_0$ versus $K : \theta = \theta_1(> \theta_0)$ does not depend on θ_1 and therefore can be used to test H_0 versus H_1. In the sequential setting, however, we cannot reduce the optimality considerations for one-sided composite hypotheses to those for simple hypotheses even in the presence of the monotone likelihood ratio. This led Kiefer and Weiss (1957) to consider the problem of minimizing the expected sample size at a given parameter θ^* subject to error probability constraints at θ_0 and θ_1. Using dynamic programming arguments, Lorden (1976) showed that a nearly optimal solution to the KieferWeiss problem is a 2-SPRT with stopping rule of the form

$$T^* = \inf \left\{ n : \prod_{i=1}^{n} (f_{\theta^*}(X_i)/f_{\theta_0}(X_i)) \geq A_0 \text{ or } \prod_{i=1}^{n} (f_{\theta^*}(X_i)/f_{\theta_1}(X_i)) \geq A_1 \right\},$$

rejecting $H : \theta = \theta_0$ if $\prod_{i=1}^{T^*} (f_{\theta^*}(X_i)/f_{\theta_0}(Xi)) \geq A_0$ and rejecting $K : \theta = \theta_1$ if the other boundary is crossed upon stopping. Ideally, θ^* should be chosen to be the true parameter value θ, which is unknown. Replacing θ by its maximum likelihood ratio estimate $\hat{\theta}_n$ at stage n leads to the sequential GLR test of $H_0 : \theta \leq \theta_0$ versus $H_1 : \theta \geq \theta_1$ that stops sampling at stage

$$\tau = \inf \left\{ n : \hat{\theta}_n > \theta_0 \text{ and } \prod_{i=1}^{n} (f_{\hat{\theta}_n}(X_i)/f_{\theta_0}(X_i)) \geq A_0^{(n)} \text{ or } \right.$$

$$\left. \hat{\theta}_n < \theta_1 \text{ and } \prod_{i=1}^{n} (f_{\hat{\theta}_n}(X_i)/f_{\theta_1}(X_i)) \geq A_1^{(n)} \right\}, \qquad (8.15)$$

and rejects H_i if the GLR statistic for testing θ_i exceeds $A_i^{(n)}$ $(i = 0, 1)$.

This sequential GLR, with $A_0^{(\tau)} = A_1^{(n)} = 1/c$, was derived earlier by Schwarz (1962) as an asymptotic solution to the Bayes problem of testing H_0 versus H_1 with 0-1 loss and cost c per observation, as $c \to 0$ while θ_0 and θ_1 are fixed. For the case of a normal mean θ, Chernoff (1961, 1965) derived a different and considerably more complicated approximation to the Bayes test of $H_0' : \theta < \theta_0$ versus $H_1' : \theta > \theta_0$. In fact, setting $\theta_1 = \theta_0$ in Schwarz's test does not yield Chernoff's test. This disturbing discrepancy between the asymptotic approximations of Schwarz (assuming an indifference zone) and Chernoff (without an indifference zone separating the one-sided hypotheses) was resolved by Lai (1988), who gave a unified solution (to both problems) that uses a stopping rule of the form

$$N(g, c) = \inf \left\{ n : \max \left[\sum_{i=1}^{n} \log \frac{f_{\hat{\theta}_n}(X_i)}{f_{\theta_0}(X_i)}, \sum_{i=1}^{n} \log \frac{f_{\hat{\theta}_n}(X_i)}{f_{\theta_1}(X_i)} \right] \geq g(cn) \right\}.$$

The function g satisfies $g(t) \sim \log(1/t)$ as $t \to 0$ and is the boundary of an associated optimal stopping problem for the Brownian motion. By solving the latter problem numerically, Lai (1988) also gave a closed-form approximation to the function g. In practice, one often imposes an upper bound M and also a lower bound m on the total number of observations. With $M/m \to b > 1$ and $\log \alpha \sim \log \beta$, one can replace the time-varying boundary $g(cn)$ by a constant threshold c. The test of $H : \theta = \theta_0$ with stopping rule

$$\tilde{N} = \inf \left\{ n \geq m : \left[\prod_{i=1}^{n} f_{\hat{\theta}_n}(X_i) \right] \bigg/ \left[\prod_{i=1}^{n} f_{\theta_0}(X_i) \right] \geq e^c \right\} \wedge M \quad (8.16)$$

which corresponds to Lai's stopping rule with $\theta_1 = \theta_0$, $g(cn)$ replaced by c, and n restricted between m and M, is called a *repeated GLR test*. The test rejects H if the GLR statistic exceeds e^c upon stopping. It is straightforward to extend the repeated GLR test to multivariate θ and composite null hypothesis $H_0 : \theta \in \Theta_0$, by simply replacing $\prod_{i=1}^{n} f_{\theta_0}(X_i)$ by $\sup_{\theta \in \Theta_0} \prod_{i=1}^{n} f_{\theta_0}(X_i)$.

Details of the sequential GLR tests (8.15) and (8.16) and their connections to the Bayes tests of Schwarz and Chernoff are given in Chapter 3 of Bartroff et al. (2013), where likelihood ratio identities underlying (8.2) and the lower bounds on the expected sample size of a test with prescribed type I and type II error constraints are also given. Specifically, let F be an event that depends on the observations $X_1, \ldots, X_T$ up to a stopping time T; a positive integer-valued random variable is called a stopping time if for every $n \geq 1$, the event $\{T = n\}$ depends on $X_1, \ldots, X_n$. Let P (respectively, Q) be a probability measure such that X_i has conditional density function $p_i(\cdot | X_1, \ldots, X_{i-1})$ (respectively, $q_i(\cdot | X_1, \ldots, X_{i-1})$) with respect to some measure ν_i; for the case $i = 1$ the conditional density notation means the marginal density of X_1. Assuming $p_i(\cdot | X_1, \ldots, X_{i-1}) > 0$ whenever $q_i(\cdot | X_1, \ldots, X_{i-1}) > 0$ and vice versa, define the likelihood ratio of Q with respect to P based on $X_1, \ldots, X_n$ by

$$L_n = \prod_{i=1}^{n} \frac{q_i(X_i | X_1, \ldots, X_{i-1})}{p_i(X_i | X_1, \ldots, X_{i-1})}. \quad (8.17)$$

The likelihood ratio identities, introduced by Wald (1945), are

$$Q(F \cap \{T < \infty\}) = E_P(L_T I_{F \cap \{T < \infty\}})$$
$$P(F \cap \{T < \infty\}) = E_Q(L_T^{-1} I_{F \cap \{T < \infty\}}). \quad (8.18)$$

For the case of i.i.d. $X_1, X_2, \ldots$ with common density function F, Wald combined (8.18) with

$$E\left(\sum_{i=1}^{T} X_i \right) = \mu E(T), \text{ where } \mu = E(X_i), \quad (8.19)$$

to derive the lower bounds for the expected sample size under H_0 and H_1 of any test (sequential or otherwise) of $H_0 : f = p_0$ versus $H_1 : f = f_1$ that has error probabilities α and β. Hoeffding

(1960) extended this arguments to derive the expected sample size under a density function f with Kullback-Leibler information number $I(f, f_i) = E_f \left[\log \left(f(X_1) / f_i(X_1) \right) \right]$:

$$E_f(T) \geq \left\{ \left[-\zeta \log(\alpha + \beta) + (\sigma/4)^2 \right]^{1/2} - \sigma/4 \right\}^2 / \zeta^2, \qquad (8.20)$$

where $\zeta = \max \left\{ I(f, f_0), I(f, f_1) \right\}$ and

$$\sigma^2 = E_f \left(\left\{ \log \left(\frac{f_1(X_1)}{f_0(X_1)} \right) - I(f, f_0) + I(f, f_1) \right\}^2 \right).$$

Lorden (1976) showed that the 2-SPRT (described in the second paragraph above) asymptotically attains Hoeffding's lower bound.

Chapter 4 of Bartroff et al. (2013) modifies the relatively complete theory of fully sequential tests of composite hypotheses for group sequential tests, thereby deriving in their Section 4.2 flexible and efficient group sequential GLR tests which use modified Haybittle-Peto boundaries to self-tune to unknown parameters. Besides the Pocock and O'Brien-Fleming boundaries (8.13) and (8.14) for testing a normal mean θ under the assumption of equal group sizes, their Section 4.1 also describes the error spending approach introduced by Lan and DeMets (1983) to remove the assumption of equal group sizes. In practice, clinical trial protocols usually specify the calendar times of interim monitoring, for which the number of n_i of subjects for the ith interim analysis is unknown in advance and the group sizes $n_i - n_{i-1}$ may be quite uneven. Noting that $\left\{ S_n / \left(\sigma \sqrt{M} \right), 1 \leq n \leq M \right\}$ has the same distribution as $\{ B(n/M) : 1 \leq n \leq M \}$ under the null hypothesis, the Lan-DeMets method (a) regards $\pi(t) = P_0(\tau \leq t)$ for $t < 1$ as the type I error spent, up to time t, in early stopping to reject the null hypothesis for testing the null hypothesis of zero drift for the Brownian motion $B(\cdot)$, and (b) transforms the *error spending function* $\pi(t)$ to stopping boundaries a_i for S_{n_i} ($1 \leq i \leq k$, assuming $k - 1$ interim analyses) via

$$P_0 \left\{ |S_{n_i}| \geq a_i, |S_{n_j}| < a_j \text{ for } 1 \leq j < i \right\} = \pi(n_i/M) - \pi(n_{i-1}/M) \qquad (8.21)$$

for $1 \leq i \leq k$, with $\pi(1) = \alpha$, i.e., spending whatever is left in the kth analysis (with $n_k = M$, the maximum sample size) so that the overall type I error is α.

2. *Sequential testing and safety signal detection procedures in VSD and Mini-Sentinel projects.* Kulldorff (2012, pp. 859–860) reviews the work that he and his collaborators (whom we have cited in the references in the last paragraph of Section 8.3.2) have carried out for VSD project, saying:

Starting in 2004, the CDC-sponsored VSD project began pioneering the use of sequential statistical methods for near real-time safety surveillance of new vaccines, using weekly data from eight managed-care organizations. Using the MaxSPRT, seasonal influenza vaccine was monitored during the 2004/05 season. Subsequent vaccines for which surveillance has been performed in near real-time include Menactra, two tetanus-diphtheria-acellular pertussis vaccines Adacel and Boostrix, MMRV, RotaTeq (a pentavalent bovine-derived rotavirus vaccine for infants), Gardasil (a human papillomavirus vaccine for young women), and seasonal and H1N1 influenza vaccines. For each vaccine, a different set of five to ten plausible adverse events are monitored... The choice is based on biological plausibility, known safety problems with related vaccines, safety concerns from precensure clinical trials or other data sources, and a review of the existing literature.

He also says that "sequential analysis has also been considered for near real-time postmarketing (drug) surveillance", which is "more complex than vaccine safety surveillance for three main reasons":

- longer exposure time period for drugs, as opposed to a vaccination occurring on a known day,
- it is known "almost surely that a person actually got the vaccine as it is administered by a health-care worker, while drug exposure is usually estimated from dispensing or prescribing data without certain knowledge about if and how often the drug was actually taken",
- "most vaccines are given to a high proportion of a mostly healthy population" while "a drug is given to a selected patient population who may have pre-existing health conditions that could be related to the adverse event under surveillance."

Leite et al. (2016) give a more recent review of statistical methods for real-time vaccine safety surveillance.

Near real-time postmarketing drug (and other FDA-regulated medical product) surveillance is part of the Sentinel Initiative, "a multifaceted effort" by the FDA to develop "an active national surveillance system that leverages existing electronic health care data to proactively and rapidly assess medical product safety" and to "complement existing surveillance tools", as pointed out by Nelson et al. (2016). Mini-Sentinel is a pilot project sponsored by the FDA to improve and facilitate development of the Sentinel System, and the 2016 report by Nelson et al. (2016) describes their work on "signal refinement activities", which typically do not involve detailed protocols "with full adjustment for potential confounders tailored to each outcome" and which "have been a major focus of the Mini-Sentinel pilot." The report describes its purpose and scope as follows:

> Once the FDA has selected a particular productoutcome pair of interest and determined that Sentinel is an appropriate environment to conduct a safety assessment, it is important to understand what steps are needed to develop a detailed surveillance plan using the available tools. The purpose of this report is to provide suggestions about how to plan a safety assessment using the two tools (described and illustrated in the report) which can be applied as a one-time (Level 2) analysis or conducted repeatedly at multiple prespecified points in time, using a sequential monitoring framework (Level 3). A plan involving one-time analysis may make sense to assess safety for an existing medical product that has been on the market for many years...and so is already well powered to address the question of interest...A plan involving multiple assessments of the data over time could be employed for a newly marketed product or an existing product approved for new indications, with analyses conducted routinely as adequate amounts of new product uptake occurs so that safety signals of concern could be detected earlier. The scope of the planning recommendations assumes the following:
>
> - FDA has already determined that the productoutcome pair is suited for examination using Sentinel data,
> - The study design taxonomy has been consulted to suggest an appropriate epidemiological study design or designs (i.e., selfcontrolled or a cohort design), and
> - Either the Regression or IPTW regression tool has been preliminarily deemed appropriate.

The "IPTW regression" above refers to inverse probability weighted regression (with propensity score weighting), whereas "regression" refers to logistic or Poisson regression adjustment for confounders in the estimation of risk difference or relative risk. We have cited the work of Nelson and her collaborators related to the Sentinel Initiative that preceded this report in the references in the last paragraph of Section 8.3.2. The report provides an overview of fully sequential and group sequential methods in observational safety surveillance, including MaxSPRT and sequential GLR tests, and gives the following suggestions on planning sequential safety surveillance:

- Pre-specification of surveillance design and plans, including outcomes of interest, exposure and cohort eligibility, choices of comparator, subgroup analysis, duration of surveillance (in calendar time).

- Use of existing data to inform surveillance planning, e.g., related to sample size estimation, number and timing of sequential analyses, expected rates of update from Data Partners.

- Clear communication with FDA on the sequential design's operating characteristics so that the meaning of a safety signal is well understood if it should occur.

- Selection of confounders that need to be adjusted in the analyses.

3. *Generalized estimating equations in group sequential safety monitoring.* Cook et al. (2015) present a group sequential (GS) method based on generalized estimating equations (GEE) for safety monitoring using observational data and illustrate the method with VSD data. Their goal is to "test the overall hypothesis that there is a higher risk of an adverse event for those who receive...a new vaccine, compared with a comparable unexposed group after accounting for confounding" and the test is performed "repeatedly over time by conducting on-going surveillance for an elevated risk as more data accrue." A safety signal of an elevated rate for the target adverse event among vaccine recipients is declared if the test statistic at the tth analysis exceeds a predefined threshold value $c(t)$ that is determined by the null distribution of the test statistic and an error spending function $c(t) = au(t)$, where $u(t)$ is a specified function such as $u(t) = 1$ or $u(t) = \sqrt{n_t}$) and a is defined by type I error control at α. Let $X_i = 1$ (respectively, 0) denote that subject i receives the new vaccine (respectively, comparator vaccine) and $Y_i = 1$ (respectively, 0) denote that the same subject experiences (respectively, does not experience) the adverse event under surveillance. Furthermore, let $\mathbf{Z}_i = (Z_{i1}, \ldots, Z_{ip})$ denote a vector of baseline variables such as age, gender, health conditions, and possibly also interactions between the baseline variables. Cook et al. (2015) fit the logistic regression model

$$\text{logit}\,[P(Y_i|X_i, \mathbf{Z}_i)] = \beta_0 + \beta_X(t)X_i + \boldsymbol{\beta}_Z(t)\mathbf{Z}_i \qquad (8.22)$$

at $t = 1, \ldots, T$ to estimate the vaccine effect $\hat{\beta}_X(t)$ on the adverse event after adjusting for the covariate effects, and use the Wald statistic $W(t) = \hat{\beta}_X(t)/\sqrt{\text{Var}(\hat{\beta}_X(t))}$ to test the null hypothesis H_0 of no elevated risk of the event in vaccine recipients relative to those who receive the comparator vaccine. They point out that using the normal approximation to the Wald statistic under H_0 may not be reliable in the case of rare adverse events, and therefore consider a permutation approach instead. Specifically, under the null hypothesis $H_0 : \beta_X(t) = 0$ for all t, $Y_i|\mathbf{Z}_i$ is independent of X_i, which leads to their permutation approach:

Step 1. At each analysis time $t = 1, \ldots, T$, create a single complete permuted exposure vector $\mathbf{X}^{(j)}$ by permuting observed exposures $(X_{n_{t-1}+1}, \ldots, X_{n_t})$ to form $(X^{(j)}_{n_{t-1}+1}, \ldots, X^{(j)}_{n_t})$.

Step 2. For $t = 1, \ldots, T$,

(a) calculate the score statistic $S(t)$ based on the permuted exposure data $\mathbf{X}^{(j)}$ and observed outcome and confounder data $(\mathbf{Y}, \mathbf{Z})$ to form $S^{(j)}(t)$;

(b) if $S^{(j)}(t) \geq au(t)$ then let $C_j = 1$ and stop; otherwise let $C_j = 0$ and continue to $t + 1$ if $t < T$;

(c) if $t = T$ and $C_j = 0$, stop with no signal detected from permuted data $\mathbf{X}^{(j)}$.

The procedure repeats N times and α can be estimated by $\hat{\alpha} = \sum_{j=1}^{N} C_j / N$. Hence one can solve iteratively for a until $\hat{\alpha} \doteq \alpha$; see Cook et al. (2015) for details of their GSGEE approach, its application to VSD data, and a simulation study comparing GSGEE with other group sequential methods in terms of average time of signaling and power.

4. *Exercise.* Li et al. (2014) apply the MaxSPRT approach for sequential continuous surveillance of vaccine safety, in which they consider four different error spending functions that correspond to four sets of time-varying boundary values (also called critical value functions). Specifically, they consider the following critical value functions:

$$V_1(t) = c_1 e^{-t}, \ V_2(t) = c_2 \log(e + t), \ V_3(t) = c2^t, \ V_4 = \tilde{c}(0.2)^t \quad (8.23)$$

where $t = \mu_t / t^*$, t^* denotes the upper limit of the expected number of adverse events by the end of surveillance, and $c_1, c_2, c, \tilde{c}$ are constants.

(a) Use the numerical method described in Kulldorff et al. (2011, pp. 65-67) to compute the critical boundaries when the type I error is $\alpha = 0.05$ for the log-likelihood ratio test statistic LLR_n (p. 71 of their paper).

(b) Carry out simulation studies to compare the performance characteristics of the four critical value functions in terms of expected sample size and power.

Bibliography

Aalen, O. O., K. Røysland, J. M. Gran, and B. Ledergerber (2012). Causality, mediation and time: a dynamic viewpoint. *Journal of the Royal Statistical Society: Series A 175*(4), 831–861.

Abe, S. (2010). *Support Vector Machines for Pattern Classification.* Springer.

Acquavella, J., B. Bradbury, C. Critchlow, J. M. Sprafka, J. Sullivan, and J. B. Litten (2014). Pharmacoepidemiology as part of pharmacovigilance for biologic therapies. In E. Andres and N. Moore (Eds.), *Mann's Pharmacovigilance*, pp. 685–702. John Wiley & Sons, Ltd.

Acri, T. and R. Gross (2014). Studies of medication bias. In B. Strom, S. Kimmel, and S. Hennessy (Eds.), *Pharmacoepidemiology, 5th Edition*, pp. 795–806. Chichester, UK: John Wiley & Sons, Ltd.

Agresti, A. (2013). *Categorical Data Analysis.* John Wiley & Sons, Ltd.

Ahmed, I., B. Béguad, and P. Tubert-Bitter (2015). Evaluation of post-marketing safety using spontaneous reporting databases. In A. Gould (Ed.), *Statistical Methods for Evaluating Safety in Medical Product Development*, pp. 332–44. New York: Wiley.

Almenoff, J., J. Tonning, A. Gould, A. Szarfman, M. Hauben, R. Ouellet-Hellstrom, R. Ball, K. Hornbuckle, L. Walsh, and C. Yee (2005). Perspectives on the use of data mining in pharmacovigilance. *Drug Safety 28*(11), 981–1007.

Altman, D. G. (1998). Confidence intervals for the number needed to treat. *British Medical Journal 317*(7168), 1309.

Altman, N. S. (1992). An introduction to kernel and nearest-neighbor nonparametric regression. *The American Statistician 46*(3), 175–185.

Amit, Y. and D. Geman (1997). Shape quantization and recognition with randomized trees. *Neural Computation 9*(7), 1545–1588.

Amorim, L. D. and J. Cai (2015). Modelling recurrent events: a tutorial for analysis in epidemiology. *International Journal of Epidemiology 44*(1), 324–333.

Amur, S., L. LaVange, I. Zineh, S. Buckman-Garner, and J. Woodcock (2015). Biomarker qualification: toward a multiple stakeholder framework for biomarker development, regulatory acceptance, and utilization. *Clinical Pharmacology & Therapeutics 98*(1), 34–46.

Anadón, A., M. A. Martínez, V. Castellano, and M. R. Martínez-Larrañaga (2014). The role of in vitro methods as alternatives to animals in toxicity testing. *Expert Opinion on Drug Metabolism & Toxicology 10*(1), 67–79.

Andersen, G., T. Thybo, H. Cederberg, M. Orešič, M. Esteller, A. Zorzano, B. Carr, M. Walker, J. Cobb, and C. Clissmann (2014). The DEXLIFE study methods: identifying novel candidate biomarkers that predict progression to type 2 diabetes in high risk individuals. *Diabetes Research and Clinical Practice 106*(2), 383–389.

Andersson, S. A., D. Madigan, and M. D. Perlman (1997). A characterization of Markov equivalence classes for acyclic digraphs. *The Annals of Statistics 25*(2), 505–541.

Andersson, S. A., D. Madigan, and M. D. Perlman (2001). Alternative Markov properties for chain graphs. *Scandinavian Journal of Statistics 28*(1), 33–85.

Andridge, R. R. and R. J. Little (2011). Proxy pattern-mixture analysis for survey nonresponse. *Journal of Official Statistics 27*(2), 153–180.

Angrist, J. D. and J.-S. Pischke (2014). *Mastering Metrics: The Path from Cause to Effect*. Princeton University Press.

Ankley, G. T., R. S. Bennett, R. J. Erickson, D. J. Hoff, M. W. Hornung, R. D. Johnson, D. R. Mount, J. W. Nichols, C. L. Russom, and P. K. Schmieder (2010). Adverse outcome pathways: a conceptual framework to support ecotoxicology research and risk assessment. *Environmental Toxicology and Chemistry 29*(3), 730–741.

Annaert, P. P. and K. L. Brouwer (2005). Assessment of drug interactions in hepatobiliary transport using rhodamine 123 in sandwich-cultured rat hepatocytes. *Drug Metabolism and Disposition 33*(3), 388–394.

Aoyama, T., Y. Suzuki, and H. Ichikawa (1990). Neural networks applied to pharmaceutical problems. III. Neural networks applied to quantitative structure-activity relationship (QSAR) analysis. *Journal of Medicinal Chemistry 33*(9), 2583–2590.

Armitage, P. (1954). Sequential tests in prophylactic and therapeutic trials. *Quarterly Journal of Medicine 23*(91), 255–74.

Armitage, P. (1955). Tests for linear trends in proportions and frequencies. *Biometrics 11*(3), 375–386.

Armitage, P., C. McPherson, and B. Rowe (1969). Repeated significance tests on accumulating data. *Journal of the Royal Statistical Society. Series A (General) 132*(2), 235–244.

Arvidson, K. B. (2008). FDA toxicity databases and real-time data entry. *Toxicology and Applied Pharmacology 233*(1), 17–19.

Attene-Ramos, M. S., R. Huang, M. Sam, K. L. Witt, A. Richard, R. R. Tice, A. Simeonov, C. P. Austin, and M. Xia (2015). Profiling of the Tox21 chemical collection for mitochondrial function to identify compounds that acutely decrease mitochondrial membrane potential. *Environmental Health Perspectives (Online) 123*(1), 49–56.

Babb, J., A. Rogatko, and S. Zacks (1998). Cancer phase I clinical trials: efficient dose escalation with overdose control. *Statistics in Medicine 17*(10), 1103–1120.

Baetschmann, G. and R. Winkelmann (2013). Modeling zero-inflated count data when exposure varies: With an application to tumor counts. *Biometrical Journal 55*(5), 679–686.

Bailer, A. J. and C. J. Portier (1988). Effects of treatment-induced mortality and tumor-induced mortality on tests for carcinogenicity in small samples. *Biometrics 44*(2), 417–431.

Bailey, S., A. Singh, R. Azadian, P. Huber, and M. Blum (2010). Prospective data mining of six products in the US FDA Adverse Event Reporting System. *Drug Safety 33*(2), 139–146.

Baiocchi, M., J. Cheng, and D. S. Small (2014). Instrumental variable methods for causal inference. *Statistics in Medicine 33*(13), 2297–2340.

Baker, S. G. and B. S. Kramer (2002). The transitive fallacy for randomized trials: if A bests B and B bests C in separate trials, is A better than C? *BMC Medical Research Methodology 2*(1), 13.

Bal-Price, A. and P. Jennings (2014). *In Vitro Toxicology Systems.* Springer.

Bale, S. S., L. Vernetti, N. Senutovitch, R. Jindal, M. Hegde, A. Gough, W. J. McCarty, A. Bakan, A. Bhushan, and T. Y. Shun (2014). *In vitro* platforms for evaluating liver toxicity. *Experimental Biology and Medicine 239*(9), 1180–1191.

Ball, R., M. Robb, S. Anderson, and G. Dal Pan (2016). The FDA's sentinel initiativeA comprehensive approach to medical product surveillance. *Clinical Pharmacology & Therapeutics 99*(3), 265–268.

Ballman, K. V. (2015). Biomarker: predictive or prognostic? *Journal of Clinical Oncology 33*(33), 3968–3971.

Barlow, W. E., R. L. Davis, J. W. Glasser, P. H. Rhodes, R. S. Thompson, J. P. Mullooly, S. B. Black, H. R. Shinefield, J. I. Ward, and S. M. Marcy (2001). The risk of seizures after receipt of whole-cell pertussis or measles, mumps, and rubella vaccine. *New England Journal of Medicine 345*(9), 656–661.

Bartholomay, A. (1957). The sequential probability ratio test applied to the design of clinical experiments. *New England Journal of Medicine 256*(11), 498–505.

Bartroff, J., T. Lai, and M. Shih (2013). *Sequential Experimentation in Clinical Trials*. Springer.

Bartroff, J. and T. L. Lai (2010). Approximate dynamic programming and its applications to the design of phase I cancer trials. *Statistical Science 25*(2), 245–257.

Bartroff, J. and T. L. Lai (2011). Incorporating individual and collective ethics into phase I cancer trial designs. *Biometrics 67*(2), 596–603.

Bartroff, J., T. L. Lai, and B. Narasimhan (2014). A new approach to designing phase I-II cancer trials for cytotoxic chemotherapies. *Statistics in Medicine 33*(16), 2718–2735.

Basant, N., S. Gupta, and K. P. Singh (2016). QSAR modeling for predicting reproductive toxicity of chemicals in rats for regulatory purposes. *Toxicology Research 5*(4), 1029–1038.

Baskin, I. I., V. A. Palyulin, and N. S. Zefirov (2009). Neural networks in building QSAR models. In D. J. Livingstone (Ed.), *Artificial Neural Networks: Methods and Applications*, pp. 133–154. Springer.

Bate, A., M. Lindquist, I. Edwards, S. Olsson, R. Orre, A. Lansner, and R. De Freitas (1998). A Bayesian neural network method for adverse drug reaction signal generation. *European Journal of Clinical Pharmacology 54*(4), 315–321.

Bate, A., A. Pariente, M. Hauben, and B. Bégaud (2014). Quantitative signal detection and analysis in pharmacovigilance. In E. Andres and N. Moore (Eds.), *Mann's Pharmacovigilance*, Chapter 20, pp. 331–354. John Wiley & Sons, Ltd.

Behrman, R. E., J. S. Benner, J. S. Brown, M. McClellan, J. Woodcock, and R. Platt (2011). Developing the sentinel systema national resource for evidence development. *New England Journal of Medicine 364*(6), 498–499.

Belongia, E. A., S. A. Irving, I. M. Shui, M. Kulldorff, E. Lewis, R. Yin,

T. A. Lieu, E. Weintraub, W. K. Yih, and R. Li (2010). Real-time surveillance to assess risk of intussusception and other adverse events after pentavalent, bovine-derived rotavirus vaccine. *The Pediatric Infectious Disease Journal 29*(1), 1–5.

Benfenati, E. (2016). *In Silico Methods for Predicting Drug Toxicity.* Springer.

Benigni, R. (2016). Predictive toxicology today: the transition from biological knowledge to practicable models. *Expert Opinion on Drug Metabolism & Toxicology 12*(9), 989–992.

Benigni, R., A. Giuliani, R. Franke, and A. Gruska (2000). Quantitative structure-activity relationships of mutagenic and carcinogenic aromatic amines. *Chemical Reviews 100*(10), 3697–3714.

Benjamini, Y. and Y. Hochberg (1995). Controlling the false discovery rate: A practical and powerful approach to multiple testing. *Journal of the Royal Statistical Society: Series B 57*(1), 289–300.

Benjamini, Y. and D. Yekutieli (2001). The control of the false discovery rate in multiple testing under dependence. *The Annals of Statistics 29*, 1165–1188.

Benz, R. D. (2007). Toxicological and clinical computational analysis and the US FDA/CDER. *Expert Opinion on Drug Metabolism & Toxicology 3*(1), 109–124.

Bergstralh, E. J., J. L. Kosanke, and S. J. Jacobsen (1996). Software for optimal matching in observational studies. *Epidemiology 7*(3), 331–332.

Berlin, J. A., S. Cepeda, and C. J. Kim (2012). The use of meta-analysis in pharmacoepidemiology. In B. L. Strom, S. E. Kimmel, and S. Hennessy (Eds.), *Pharmacoepidemiology, Fifth Edition*, pp. 7239–756. John Wiley & Sons.

Berlin, J. A., B. Crowe, and H. A. Xia (2014). The evaluation of adverse events in clinical trials (with a particular focus on the use of meta-analysis). In E. B. Andrews and N. Moore (Eds.), *Mann's Pharmacovigilance*, pp. 109–119. John Wiley & Sons.

Berry, S. (2000). Meta-analysis versus large trials: Resolving the controversy. In D. Stangl and D. Berry (Eds.), *Meta-Analysis in Medicine and Health Policy*, pp. 65–82. CRC Press.

Berry, S. and D. Berry (2004). Accounting for multiplicities in assessing drug safety: A three-level hierarchical mixture model. *Biometrics 60*(2), 418–426.

Bhaumik, D. K., A. Amatya, S.-L. T. Normand, J. Greenhouse, E. Kaizar, B. Neelon, and R. D. Gibbons (2012). Meta-analysis of rare binary adverse event data. *Journal of the American Statistical Association 107*(498), 555–567.

Bie, S., P. M. Coloma, C. Ferrajolo, K. Verhamme, G. Trifirò, M. J. Schuemie, S. M. Straus, R. Gini, R. Herings, and G. Mazzaglia (2015). The role of electronic healthcare record databases in paediatric drug safety surveillance: a retrospective cohort study. *British Journal of Clinical Pharmacology 80*(2), 304–314.

Bisgin, H., Z. Liu, H. Fang, X. Xu, and W. Tong (2011). Mining FDA drug labels using an unsupervised learning technique-topic modeling. *BMC Bioinformatics 12*(10), S11.

Blom, T. and J. M. Mooij (2018). Generalized strucutral causal models. *arXiv*. preprint arXiv:1805.06539.

Blyth, C. R. (1972). On simpson's paradox and the sure-thing principle. *Journal of the American Statistical Association 67*(338), 364–366.

Bonate, P. L. (2011). *Pharmacokinetic-Pharmacodynamic Modeling and Simulation*. Springer.

Bongers, S., J. Peters, B. Schölkopf, and J. M. Mooij (2016). Structural causal models: Cycles, marginalizations, exogenous reparametrizations and reductions. *arXiv*. (preprint arXiv:1611.06221).

Borenstein, M., L. V. Hedges, J. Higgins, and H. R. Rothstein (2009). *Introduction to Meta-analysis*. John Wiley & Sons, Ltd.

Boverhof, D. R. and B. B. Gollapudi (2011). *Applications of Toxicogenomics in Safety Evaluation and Risk Assessment*. John Wiley & Sons.

Braña, I., E. Zamora, and J. Tabernero (2013). Cardiotoxicity. In M. A. Dicato (Ed.), *Side Effects of Medical Cancer Therapy*, pp. 483–530. Springer.

Braun, T. M. (2002). The bivariate continual reassessment method: extending the crm to phase I trials of two competing outcomes. *Controlled Clinical Trials 23*(3), 240–256.

Braun, T. M. and S. Wang (2010). A hierarchical Bayesian design for phase I trials of novel combinations of cancer therapeutic agents. *Biometrics 66*(3), 805–812.

Breiman, L. (1996). Bagging predictors. *Machine Learning 24*(2), 123–140.

Breiman, L. (1998). Arcing classifier (with discussion and a rejoinder by the author). *The Annals of Statistics 26*(3), 801–849.

Breiman, L. (2001). Random forests. *Machine Learning 45*(1), 5–32.

Briggs, K., C. Barber, M. Cases, P. Marc, and T. Steger-Hartmann (2015). Value of shared preclinical safety studies–The eTOX database. *Toxicology Reports 2*, 210–221.

Briggs, K., M. Cases, D. J. Heard, M. Pastor, F. Pognan, F. Sanz, C. H. Schwab, T. Steger-Hartmann, A. Sutter, and D. K. Watson (2012). Inroads to predict in vivo toxicologyłan introduction to the eTOX project. *International Journal of Molecular Sciences 13*(3), 3820–3846.

Brock, W. J., K. L. Hastings, and K. M. McGown (2013). *Nonclinical Safety Assessment: A Guide to International Pharmaceutical Regulations*. John Wiley & Sons.

Brockhaus, A. C., R. Bender, and G. Skipka (2014). The peto odds ratio viewed as a new effect measure. *Statistics in Medicine 33*(28), 4861–4874.

Brookhart, M. A., T. Stürmer, R. J. Glynn, J. Rassen, and S. Schneeweiss (2010). Confounding control in healthcare database research: challenges and potential approaches. *Medical Care 48*(6 0), S114.

Brown, E. (2004a). Dictionaries and coding in pharmacovigilance. In J. Talbot and P. Waller (Eds.), *Stephens' Detection of New Adverse Drug Reactions* (5th ed.)., pp. 533–57. Chichester, UK: John Wiley & Sons Ltd.

Brown, E. G. (2004b). Using MedDRA. *Drug Safety 27*(8), 591–602.

Brown, E. G., L. Wood, and S. Wood (1999). The medical dictionary for regulatory activities (MedDRA). *Drug Safety 20*(2), 109–117.

Brown, J. S., M. Kulldorff, K. R. Petronis, R. Reynolds, K. A. Chan, R. L. Davis, D. Graham, S. E. Andrade, M. A. Raebel, and L. Herrinton (2009). Early adverse drug event signal detection within population-based health networks using sequential methods: key methodologic considerations. *Pharmacoepidemiology and Drug Safety 18*(3), 226–234.

Brown, J. S., K. R. Petronis, A. Bate, F. Zhang, I. Dashevsky, M. Kulldorff, T. R. Avery, R. L. Davis, K. A. Chan, and S. E. Andrade (2013). Drug adverse event detection in health plan data using the gamma poisson shrinker and comparison to the tree-based scan statistic. *Pharmaceutics 5*(1), 179–200.

Brumback, B. A., R. J. Cook, and L. M. Ryan (2000). A meta-analysis of case-control and cohort studies with interval-censored exposure data: application to chorionic villus sampling. *Biostatistics 1*(2), 203–217.

Bucher, H. C., G. H. Guyatt, L. E. Griffith, and S. D. Walter (1997). The results of direct and indirect treatment comparisons in meta-analysis of randomized controlled trials. *Journal of clinical epidemiology 50*(6), 683–691.

Bühlmann, P. (2012). Bagging, boosting and ensemble methods. In J. E. Gentle, W. K. Hrdle, and Y. Mori (Eds.), *Handbook of Computational Statistics*, pp. 985–1022. Springer.

Bühlmann, P. and T. Hothorn (2007). Boosting algorithms: Regularization, prediction and model fitting. *Statistical Science 22*(4), 477–505.

Bühlmann, P. and B. Yu (2003). Boosting with the l 2 loss: regression and classification. *Journal of the American Statistical Association 98*(462), 324–339.

Burden, F. R. (2001). Quantitative structure- activity relationship studies using Gaussian processes. *Journal of Chemical Information and Computer Sciences 41*(3), 830–835.

Burke, D. L., J. Ensor, and R. D. Riley (2017). Meta-analysis using individual participant data: one-stage and two-stage approaches, and why they may differ. *Statistics in Medicine 36*(5), 855–875.

Burke, S. P., K. Stratton, and A. Baciu (2007). *The Future of Drug Safety: Promoting and Protecting the Health of the Public*. National Academies Press.

Cai, T., L. Parast, and L. Ryan (2010). Meta-analysis for rare events. *Statistics in Medicine 29*(20), 2078–2089.

Cai, T., L. Tian, P. H. Wong, and L. Wei (2011). Analysis of randomized comparative clinical trial data for personalized treatment selections. *Biostatistics 12*(2), 270–282.

Calabrese, R., B. Casl, and S. A. Osmetti (2011). Generalized extreme value regression: an application to credit defaults. In *Bulletin of the ISI 58th World Statistics Congress of the International Statistical Institute*. ISI 2011 National Organising Committee.

Cameron, A. C. and P. K. Trivedi (2013). *Regression Analysis of Count Data*, Volume 53. Cambridge University Press.

Campion, S., J. Aubrecht, K. Boekelheide, D. W. Brewster, V. S. Vaidya, L. Anderson, D. Burt, E. Dere, K. Hwang, and S. Pacheco (2013). The current status of biomarkers for predicting toxicity. *Expert Opinion on Drug Metabolism & Toxicology 9*(11), 1391–1408.

Canida, T. and J. Ihrie (2017). openEBGM: An R Implementation of the Gamma-Poisson Shrinker Data Mining Model. *The R Journal 9*(2), 499–519.

Carlin, B. P. and T. A. Louis (2000). *Bayes and Empirical Bayes Methods for Data Analysis*. Chapman & Hall/CRC Boca Raton, FL.

Caruso, D., A. B. Claiborne, R. A. English, A. B. Claiborne, R. A. English, and D. Caruso (2014). *Characterizing and Communicating Uncertainty in the Assessment of Benefits and Risks of Pharmaceutical Products: Workshop Summary*. National Academies Press (https://doi.org/10.17226/18870).

Cases, M., K. Briggs, T. Steger-Hartmann, F. Pognan, P. Marc, T. Kleinöder, C. H. Schwab, M. Pastor, J. Wichard, and F. Sanz (2014). The eTOX data-sharing project to advance *In silico* drug-induced toxicity prediction. *International Journal of Molecular Sciences 15*(11), 21136–21154.

Casey, W. (2013). Tox21 Overview and Update. *In Vitro Cellular & Developmental Biology–Animal 49*, S7–S8.

Cash, G. G. (2001). Prediction of the genotoxicity of aromatic and heteroaromatic amines using electrotopological state indices. *Mutation Research / Genetic Toxicology and Environmental Mutagenesis 491*(1), 31–37.

Catalano, P. J. and L. M. Ryan (1994). Statistical methods in developmental toxicology. In G. P. Patil and C. R. Rao (Eds.), *Handbook of Statistics, Volume 12 - Environmental Statistics*, pp. 507–533. Elsevier.

CDC (2008). Update: recommendations from the advisory committee on immunization practices (acip) regarding administration of combination mmrv vaccine. *MMWR. Morbidity and Mortality Weekly Report 57*(10), 258.

CDC (2012). *Vaccine Adverse Event Reporting System (VAERS)*. Centers for Disease Control and Prevention.

Chakra, C. N. A., A. Pariente, M. Pinet, L. Nkeng, N. Moore, and Y. Moride (2010). Case series in drug safety. *Drug Safety 33*(12), 1081–1088.

Chakraborty, B. and E. Moodie (2013). *Statistical Methods for Dynamic Treatment Regimes*. Springer.

Chakravarty, A. G. (2010). Sentinel Initiative - Monitoring Medical Product Safety . Presentation at the 2010 FDA/Industry Statistics Workshop, Washington DC, 2010.

Chakravarty, A. G., R. Izem, S. Keeton, C. Y. Kim, M. S. Levenson, and M. Soukup (2016). The role of quantitative safety evaluation in regulatory decision making of drugs. *Journal of Biopharmaceutical Statistics 26*(1), 17–29.

Chavan, S., A. Abdelaziz, J. G. Wiklander, and I. A. Nicholls (2016). A *k*-nearest neighbor classification of hERG K+ channel blockers. *Journal of Computer-Aided Molecular Design 30*(3), 229–236.

Chen, C., T. Garrido, D. Chock, G. Okawa, and L. Liang (2009). The Kaiser Permanente Electronic Health Record: transforming and streamlining modalities of care. *Health Affairs 28*(2), 323–333.

Chen, C.-h., W. K. Härdle, and A. Unwin (2007). *Handbook of Data Visualization*. Springer.

Chen, J. J. (2005). Statistical analysis for developmental and reproductive toxicologists. In R. D. Hood (Ed.), *Developmental and Reproductive Toxicology: A Practical Approach, Second Edition*, pp. 697–711. Taylor & Francis.

Chen, J. J., R. L. Kodell, R. B. Howe, and D. W. Gaylor (1991). Analysis of trinomial responses from reproductive and developmental toxicity experiments. *Biometrics 47*(3), 1049–1058.

Chen, M., H. Hong, H. Fang, R. Kelly, G. Zhou, J. Borlak, and W. Tong (2013). Quantitative structure-activity relationship models for predicting drug-induced liver injury based on FDA-approved drug labeling annotation and using a large collection of drugs. *Toxicological Sciences 136*(1), 242–249.

Chen, M.-H. (1994). Importance-weighted marginal Bayesian posterior density estimation. *Journal of the American Statistical Association 89*, 818–824.

Chen, P.-Y. and A. A. Tsiatis (2001). Causal inference on the difference of the restricted mean lifetime between two groups. *Biometrics 57*(4), 1030–1038.

Chen, R. T., J. W. Glasser, P. H. Rhodes, R. L. Davis, W. E. Barlow, R. S. Thompson, J. P. Mullooly, S. B. Black, H. R. Shinefield, and C. M. Vadheim (1997). Vaccine Safety Datalink project: a new tool for improving vaccine safety monitoring in the United States. *Pediatrics 99*(6), 765–773.

Chen, R. T., S. C. Rastogi, J. R. Mullen, S. W. Hayes, S. L. Cochi, J. A. Donlon, and S. G. Wassilak (1994). The vaccine adverse event reporting system (VAERS). *Vaccine 12*(6), 542–550.

Chen, X., T. Christensen, and E. T. Tamer (2018). MCMC confidence sets for identified sets. *Econometrica*. (forthcoming).

Chernoff, H. (1961). Sequential tests for the mean of a normal distribution. In *Proc. Fourth Berkeley Symp. Math. Statist. Probab*, Volume 1, pp. 79–91.

Chernoff, H. (1965). Sequential tests for the mean of a normal distribution iv (discrete case). *The Annals of Mathematical Statistics*, 55–68.

Cheung, Y. K. (2011). *Dose Finding by the Continual Reassessment Method*. CRC Press.

Cheung, Y. K. and R. Chappell (2000). Sequential designs for phase I clinical trials with late-onset toxicities. *Biometrics 56*(4), 1177–1182.

Chuang-Stein, C. (1994). A new proposal for benefit-less-risk analysis in clinical trials. *Controlled Clinical Trials 15*(1), 30–43.

Chuang-Stein, C. (1998). Laboratory data in clinical trials: a statistician's perspective. *Controlled Clinical Trials 19*(2), 167–177.

Chuang-Stein, C., N. R. Mohberg, and M. S. Sinkula (1991). Three measures for simultaneously evaluating benefits and risks using categorical data from clinical trials. *Statistics in Medicine 10*(9), 1349–1359.

Chuang-Stein, C. and H. A. Xia (2013). The practice of pre-marketing safety assessment in drug development. *Journal of Biopharmaceutical Statistics 23*(1), 3–25.

CIOMS (1999). *Reporting of Adverse Drug Reactions: Definitions of Terms and Criteria for Their Use*. Council for International Organizations of Medical Sciences (CIOMS), Geneva. (https://cioms.ch/wp-content/uploads/2017/01/reporting_adverse_drug.pdf).

CIOMS (2016). *Evidence Synthesis and Meta-Analysis for Drug Safety*. Council for International Organizations of Medical Sciences (CIOMS), Geneva.

Cipriani, A., J. P. Higgins, J. R. Geddes, and G. Salanti (2013). Conceptual and technical challenges in network meta-analysis. *Annals of Internal Medicine 159*(2), 130–137.

Claggett, B., L. Tian, D. Castagno, and L.-J. Wei (2014). Treatment selections using risk–benefit profiles based on data from comparative randomized clinical trials with multiple endpoints. *Biostatistics 16*(1), 60–72.

Cleophas, T. J., A. H. Zwinderman, and H. I. Cleophas-Allers (2013). *Machine Learning in Medicine*. Springer.

Cochran, W. G. (1954). Some methods for strengthening the common χ^2 tests. *Biometrics 10*(4), 417–451.

Cocos, A., A. G. Fiks, and A. J. Masino (2017). Deep learning for pharmacovigilance: recurrent neural network architectures for labeling adverse drug reactions in twitter posts. *Journal of the American Medical Informatics Association 24*(4), 813–821.

Cohen, J. (1960). A coefficient of agreement for nominal scales. *Educational and Psychological Measurement 20*(1), 37–46.

Colatsky, T., B. Fermini, G. Gintant, J. B. Pierson, P. Sager, Y. Sekino, D. G. Strauss, and N. Stockbridge (2016). The comprehensive in vitro proarrhythmia assay (CiPA) initiative–update on progress. *Journal of Pharmacological and Toxicological Methods 81*, 15–20.

Cole, S. R. and M. A. Hernán (2008). Constructing inverse probability weights for marginal structural models. *American Journal of Epidemiology 168*(6), 656–664.

Collins, J. M., C. K. Grieshaber, and B. A. Chabner (1990). Pharmacologically guided phase I clinical trials based upon preclinical drug development. *Journal of the National Cancer Institute 82*(16), 1321–1326.

Cook, A. J., R. C. Tiwari, R. D. Wellman, S. R. Heckbert, L. Li, P. Heagerty, T. Marsh, and J. C. Nelson (2012). Statistical approaches to group sequential monitoring of postmarket safety surveillance data: current state of the art for use in the mini-sentinel pilot. *Pharmacoepidemiology and Drug Safety 21*(S1), 72–81.

Cook, A. J., R. D. Wellman, J. C. Nelson, L. A. Jackson, and R. C. Tiwari (2015). Group sequential method for observational data by using generalized estimating equations: application to vaccine safety datalink. *Journal of the Royal Statistical Society: Series C (Applied Statistics) 64*(2), 319–338.

Cook, N., A. R. Hansen, L. L. Siu, and A. R. Abdul Razak (2015). Early phase clinical trials to identify optimal dosing and safety. *Molecular Oncology 9*(5), 997–1007.

Cook, R. J. and J. Lawless (2007). *The Statistical Analysis of Recurrent Events*. Springer.

Cook, R. J. and D. L. Sackett (1995). The number needed to treat: a clinically useful measure of treatment effect. *British Medical Journal 310*(6977), 452.

Cordeiro, G. M. and P. McCullagh (1991). Bias correction in generalized linear models. *Journal of the Royal Statistical Society: Series B 53*(3), 629–643.

Cortes, C. and V. Vapnik (1995). Support-vector networks. *Machine Learning 20*(3), 273–297.

Cox, D. (1972). Regression models and life-tables. *Journal of the Royal Statistical Society: Series B 34*(2), 187–220.

Cox, D. R. and D. Oakes (1984). *Analysis of survival data. 1984.* Chapman&Hall, London.

Crowe, B., A. Brueckner, C. Beasley, and P. Kulkarni (2013). Current practices, challenges, and statistical issues with product safety labeling. *Statistics in Biopharmaceutical Research 5*(3), 180–193.

Crowe, B., H. Xia, J. Berlin, D. Watson, H. Shi, S. Lin, J. Kuebler, R. Schriver, N. Santanello, G. Rochester, J. Porter, M. Oster, D. Mehrotra, L. Zhengqing, E. King, E. Harpur, and D. Hall (2009). Recommendations for the safety planning, data collection, evaluation and reporting during drug, biologic and vaccine development: a report of the safety planning, evaluation and reporting team. *Clinical Trials 6*, 430–40.

Dancey, J., B. Freidlin, and L. Rubinstein (2006). Accelerated titration designs. In S. Chevret (Ed.), *Statistical Methods for Dose-Finding Experiments*, pp. 91–114. Wiley.

Darpo, B., C. Benson, C. Dota, G. Ferber, C. Garnett, C. Green, V. Jarugula, L. Johannesen, J. Keirns, and K. Krudys (2015). Results from the IQ-CSRC prospective study support replacement of the thorough QT study by QT assessment in the early clinical phase. *Clinical Pharmacology & Therapeutics 97*(4), 326–335.

Darpo, B., C. Garnett, C. T. Benson, J. Keirns, D. Leishman, M. Malik, N. Mehrotra, K. Prasad, S. Riley, and I. Rodriguez (2014). Cardiac Safety Research Consortium: can the thorough QT/QTc study be replaced by early QT assessment in routine clinical pharmacology studies? Scientific update and a research proposal for a path forward. *American Heart Journal 168*(3), 262–272.

Darroch, J. N., S. L. Lauritzen, and T. P. Speed (1980). Markov fields and log-linear interaction models for contingency tables. *The Annals of Statistics 8*(3), 522–539.

Davidian, M. (2009). Nonlinear mixed effects models. In G. Fitzmaurice, M. Davidian, G. Verbeke, and G. Molenberghs (Eds.), *Longitudinal Data Analysis*, pp. 107–142. Chapman & Hall.

Davis, B. and H. Southworth (2016). Statistical analysis of cumulative serious adverse event data from development safety update reports. *Therapeutic Innovation & Regulatory Science 50*(2), 188–194.

Davis, R., M. Kolczak, E. Lewis, J. Nordin, M. Goodman, D. Shay, R. Platt, S. Black, H. Shinefield, and R. Chen (2005). Active Surveillance of Vaccine Safety: A System to Detect Early Signs of Adverse Events. *Epidemiology 16*(3), 336–341.

Dawid, A., M. Musio, and S. Fienberg (2016). From statistical evidence to evidence of causality. *Bayesian Analysis 11*(3), 725–752.

Dawid, A. P. (1979). Conditional independence in statistical theory. *Journal of the Royal Statistical Society: Series B*, 1–31.

de Kleijn, D. P., F. L. Moll, W. E. Hellings, G. Ozsarlak-Sozer, P. de Bruin, P. A. Doevendans, A. Vink, L. M. Catanzariti, A. H. Schoneveld, and A. Algra (2010). Local atherosclerotic plaques are a source of prognostic biomarkers for adverse cardiovascular events. *Arteriosclerosis, Thrombosis, and Vascular Biology 30*(3), 612–619.

Deeks, J. J., D. G. Altman, and M. J. Bradburn (2008). Statistical methods for examining heterogeneity and combining results from several studies in meta-analysis. In M. Egger, G. D. Smith, and D. G. Altman (Eds.), *Systematic Reviews in Health Care: Meta-Analysis in Context, Second Edition*, pp. 285–312. BMJ Publishing Group.

Deeks, J. J. and J. P. Higgins (2010). Statistical algorithms in review manager 5. *Statistical Methods Group of The Cochrane Collaboration*, 1–11.

Dehejia, R. and S. Wahba (1999). Causal effects in nonexperimental studies: Reevaluating the evaluation of training programs. *Journal of the American Statistical Association 94*(448), 1053–62.

Dehejia, R. and S. Wahba (2004). Causal inference with general treatment regimes. *Journal of the American Statistical Association 99*, 854–66.

Delage, G. (2000). Rotavirus vaccine withdrawal in the United States: The role of postmarketing surveillance. *The Canadian Journal of Infectious Diseases 11*(1), 10–12.

Dellicour, S., F. O. Ter Kuile, and A. Stergachis (2008). Pregnancy exposure registries for assessing antimalarial drug safety in pregnancy in malaria-endemic countries. *PLoS Medicine 5*(9), e187.

Demetri, G. D., M. von Mehren, R. L. Jones, M. L. Hensley, S. M. Schuetze, A. Staddon, M. Milhem, A. Elias, K. Ganjoo, and H. Tawbi (2015). Efficacy and safety of trabectedin or dacarbazine for metastatic liposarcoma or leiomyosarcoma after failure of conventional chemotherapy: results of a phase III randomized multicenter clinical trial. *Journal of Clinical Oncology 34*(8), 786–793.

DerSimonian, R. and N. Laird (1986). Meta-analysis in clinical trials. *Controlled Clinical Trials* 7(3), 177–188.

DerSimonian, R. and N. Laird (2015). Meta-analysis in clinical trials revisited. *Contemporary Clinical Trials* 45, 139–145.

DeStefano, F. (2001). The Vaccine Safety Datalink project. *Pharmacoepidemiology and Drug Safety* 10(5), 403–406.

Di Veroli, G. Y., M. R. Davies, H. Zhang, N. Abi-Gerges, and M. R. Boyett (2014). hERG inhibitors with similar potency but different binding kinetics do not pose the same proarrhythmic risk: implications for drug safety assessment. *Journal of Cardiovascular Electrophysiology* 25(2), 197–207.

Dias, S., A. Ades, N. J. Welton, J. P. Jansen, and A. J. Sutton (2018). *Network Meta-Analysis for Decision-Making*. John Wiley & Sons.

Dietterich, T. G. (1998). Approximate statistical tests for comparing supervised classification learning algorithms. *Neural Computation* 10(7), 1895–1923.

Dore, D. D., J. D. Seeger, and K. Arnold Chan (2009). Use of a claims-based active drug safety surveillance system to assess the risk of acute pancreatitis with exenatide or sitagliptin compared to metformin or glyburide. *Current Medical Research and Opinion* 25(4), 1019–1027.

Dragalin, V., V. Fedorov, and Y. Wu (2008). Adaptive designs for selecting drug combinations based on efficacy–toxicity response. *Journal of Statistical Planning and Inference* 138(2), 352–373.

Du, J., J. Xu, H.-Y. Song, and C. Tao (2017). Leveraging machine learning-based approaches to assess human papillomavirus vaccination sentiment trends with twitter data. *BMC Medical Informatics and Decision Making* 17(2), 69.

DuMouchel, W. (1999). Bayesian data mining in large frequency tables, with an application to the FDA spontaneous reporting system, with discussions by O'Neill and Szarbman, Louis and Shen, Madigan and author's rejoinder. *The American Statistician 53*, 177–202.

DuMouchel, W. (2007). Statistical issues in the analysis of spontaneous report databases. Speaker presentation at the Institute of Medicine Workshop on Emerging Safety Science.

DuMouchel, W. and R. Harpaz (2012). Regression-adjusted GPS algorithm (RGPS). *ORACLE Health Sciences*.

DuMouchel, W. and D. Pregibon (2001). Empirical Bayes screening for multi-item associations. In *Proceedings of the Seventh ACM SIGKDD International Conference on Knowledge Discovery and Data Mining*, pp. 67–76. ACM.

DuMouchel, W., P. B. Ryan, M. J. Schuemie, and D. Madigan (2013). Evaluation of disproportionality safety signaling applied to healthcare databases. *Drug Safety 36*(1), 123–132.

Edwards, I. R. and J. K. Aronson (2000). Adverse drug reactions: definitions, diagnosis, and management. *The Lancet 356*(9237), 1255–1259.

Efron, B. (2003). Robbins, empirical Bayes and microarrays. *The Annals of Statistics 31*(2), 366–378.

Efron, B. (2004). Large-scale simultaneous hypothesis testing. *Journal of American Statistics Association 99*.

Efron, B. (2007). Size, power and false discovery rate. *The Annals of Statistics 35*(4), 1351–77.

EMA (2009). *Reflection Paper on Benefit-Risk Assessment Methods in the Context of the Evaluation of Marketing Authorisation Applications of Medicinal Products for Human Use*. EMEA/CHMP. London, 19 March 2008.

Embrechts, P., C. Klüppelberg, and T. Mikosch (1997). *Modelling Extremal Events for Finance and Insurance*. Springer-Verlag, New-York.

Ernster, V. L. (1994). Nested case-control studies. *Preventive Medicine 23*(5), 587–590.

Ertefaie, A., X. Ji, L. C. E, S. Hennessy, and D. Small (2018). Sequential drug safety surveillance in the presence of unmeasured confounding using the trend-in-trend design. Technical report, Center for Clinical Epidemiology and Biostatistics, Perelman School of Medicine, University of Pennsylvania. (doi: 10.1111/j.1541-0420.2005.000).

Evans, S. R. and D. Follmann (2016). Using outcomes to analyze patients rather than patients to analyze outcomes: a step toward pragmatism in benefit: risk evaluation. *Statistics in Biopharmaceutical Research 8*(4), 386–393.

Fan, S. K., Y. Lu, and Y.-G. Wang (2012). A simple Bayesian decision-theoretic design for dose-finding trials. *Statistics in Medicine 31*(28), 3719–3730.

Farrington, C. (1995). Relative incidence estimation from case series for vaccine safety evaluation. *Biometrics 51*(1), 228–235.

Farrington, C., J. Nash, and E. Miller (1996). Case series analysis of adverse reactions to vaccines: a comparative evaluation. *American Journal of Epidemiology 143*(11), 1165–1173.

Farrington, P., M. Rush, E. Miller, S. Pugh, A. Colville, A. Flower, J. Nash, and P. Morgan-Capner (1995). A new method for active surveillance of adverse events from diphtheria/tetanus/pertussis and measles/mumps/rubella vaccines. *The Lancet 345*(8949), 567–569.

FDA (1988). *Guideline for the Format and Content of the Clinical and Statistical Sections of an Application*. Rockville, MD: US Food and Drug Administration.

FDA (1995). *Coding Symbols for Thesaurus of Adverse Reaction Terms*. Rockville, MD: United States Food and Drug Administration.

FDA (2001). *Guidance for Industry: Statistical Aspects of the Design, Analysis, and Interpretation of Chronic Rodent Carcinogenicity Studies of Pharmaceuticals*. US Food and Drug Administration.

FDA (2008a). *Genotoxic and Carcinogenic Impurities in Drug Substances and Products*. US Food and Drug Administration.

FDA (2008b). *The Sentinel Initiative: National Strategy for Monitoring Medical Product Safety*. US Food and Drug Administration.

FDA (2010a). *Guidance for Industry and Investigators: Safety Reporting Requirements for INDs and BA / BE Studies*. US Food and Drug Administration.

FDA (2010b). *The Sentinel Initiative: An update on FDA's progress in building a national electronic system for monitoring the postmarket safety of FDA-approved drugs and other medical products*. US Food and Drug Administration.

FDA (2011a). *Advancing Regulatory Science at FDA: A Strategic Plan*. US Food and Drug Administration.

FDA (2011b). *Guidance for Industry: E2F Development Safety Update Report*. US Food and Drug Administration.

FDA (2011c). *Guidance for Industry: Reproductive and Developmental Toxicities–Integrating Study Results to Assess Concerns*. US Food and Drug Administration.

FDA (2012). *Guidance for Industry: Postmarketing Studies and Clinical Trials–Implementation of Section 505 (o)(3) of the Federal Food, Drug, and Cosmetic Act*. US Food and Drug Administration.

FDA (2013a). *Best Practices for Conducting and Reporting Pharmacoepidemiologic Safety Studies Using Electronic Healthcare Data.* US Food and Drug Administration, Washington DC.

FDA (2013b). *Structured Approach to Benefit-Risk Assessment in Drug Regulatory Decision-Making.* US Food and Drug Administration.

FDA (2014a). *FDA Adverse Event Reporting System (FAERS) (formerly AERS). US Food and Drug Administration.* US Food and Drug Administration.

FDA (2014b). *Medical Device Reporting (MDR).* US Food and Drug Administration.

FDA (2014c). *Qualification Process for Drug Development Tools.* US Food and Drug Administration.

FDA (2015a). *Adverse Reactions Section of Labeling for Human Prescription Drug and Biological Products - Content and Format.* US Food and Drug Administration.

FDA (2015b). *Guidance for Industry: Developing Products for Weight Management.* US Food and Drug Administration.

FDA (2016). *Safety Testing of Drug Metabolites Guidance for Industry.* US Food and Drug Administration.

FDA (2017a). *Factors to Consider When Making Benefit-Risk Determinations for Medical Device Investigational Device Exemptions.* US Food and Drug Administration.

FDA (2017b). *FDA Briefing Document: Pharmaceutical Science and Clinical Pharmacology Advisory Committee Meeting–Strategies, Approaches, and Challenges in Model-Informed Drug Development (MIDD).* US Food and Drug Administration.

FDAAA (2007). *Food and Drug Administration Amendments Act.* US Department of Health and Human Services, Washington DC.

Feinberg, E. A. and A. Shwartz (2002). *Handbook of Markov Decision Processes: Methods and Applications.* Springer Science & Business Media.

Feng, J., L. Lurati, H. Ouyang, T. Robinson, Y. Wang, S. Yuan, and S. S. Young (2003). Predictive toxicology: benchmarking molecular descriptors and statistical methods. *Journal of Chemical Information and Computer Sciences 43*(5), 1463–1470.

Ferrari, T., G. Gini, and E. Benfenati (2009). Support vector machines in the prediction of mutagenicity of chemical compounds. In *Fuzzy Information Processing Society, Annual Meeting of the North American*, pp. 1–6. IEEE.

Ferri, N., P. Siegl, A. Corsini, J. Herrmann, A. Lerman, and R. Benghozi (2013). Drug attrition during pre-clinical and clinical development: understanding and managing drug-induced cardiotoxicity. *Pharmacology & Therapeutics 138*(3), 470–484.

Festing, M. F. (2014). The extended statistical analysis of toxicity tests using standardised effect sizes (SESs): A comparison of nine published papers. *PloS One 9*(11), 1–15.

Fielden, M. R. and T. R. Zacharewski (2001). Challenges and limitations of gene expression profiling in mechanistic and predictive toxicology. *Toxicological Sciences 60*(1), 6–10.

Florian, J., C. Garnett, S. Nallani, B. Rappaport, and D. Throckmorton (2012). A modeling and simulation approach to characterize methadone QT prolongation using pooled data from five clinical trials in MMT patients. *Clinical Pharmacology & Therapeutics 91*(4), 666–672.

Freedman, D. (2005). *Statistical Models: Theory and Practice*. Cambridge University Press, Cambridge, U.K.

Freidlin, B. and R. Simon (2005). Adaptive signature design: an adaptive clinical trial design for generating and prospectively testing a gene expression signature for sensitive patients. *Clinical Cancer Research 11*(21), 7872–7878.

Freund, Y. and R. E. Schapire (1995). A decision-theoretic generalization of on-line learning and an application to boosting. In P. Vitányi (Ed.), *European Conference on Computational Learning Theory*, pp. 23–37. Second European Conference, EuroCOLT '95 Barcelona, Spain, March 1315, 1995 Proceedings. Springer.

Friedman, J. H. (2001). Greedy function approximation: a gradient boosting machine. *The Annals of Statistics 29*(5), 1189–1232.

Friendly, M. (1994a). A fourfold display for 2 by 2 by k tables. Technical report, Technical Report 217, Psychology Department, York University.

Friendly, M. (1994b). Mosaic displays for multi-way contingency tables. *Journal of the American Statistical Association 89*(425), 190–200.

Friendly, M. (2000). *Visualizing Categorical Data*. SAS Institute. Cary, NC.

Frisch, R. (1934). *Statistical confluence analysis by means of complete regression systems*, Volume 5. Universitetets Økonomiske Instituut.

Frome, E. L. (1983). The analysis of rates using poisson regression models. *Biometrics*, 665–674.

Frome, E. L. and H. Checkoway (1985). Use of poisson regression models in estimating incidence rates and ratios. *American Journal of Epidemiology 121*(2), 309–323.

Frydenberg, M. (1990). Marginalization and collapsibility in graphical interaction models. *The Annals of Statistics 18*(2), 790–805.

Funk, M. J., D. Westreich, C. Wiesen, T. Stürmer, M. A. Brookhart, and M. Davidian (2011). Doubly robust estimation of causal effects. *American Journal of Epidemiology 173*(7), 761–767.

Furey, T. S., N. Cristianini, N. Duffy, D. W. Bednarski, M. Schummer, and D. Haussler (2000). Support vector machine classification and validation of cancer tissue samples using microarray expression data. *Bioinformatics 16*(10), 906–914.

Gadaleta, D., F. Pizzo, A. Lombardo, A. Carotti, S. E. Escher, O. Nicolotti, and E. Benfenati (2014). A *k*-NN algorithm for predicting oral subchronic toxicity in the rat. *Altex 31*(4), 423–432.

Gail, M. H., J. P. Costantino, J. Bryant, R. Croyle, L. Freedman, K. Helzlsouer, and V. Vogel (1999). Weighing the risks and benefits of tamoxifen treatment for preventing breast cancer. *Journal of the National Cancer Institute 91*(21), 1829–1846.

Gao, M., H. Igata, A. Takeuchi, K. Sato, and Y. Ikegaya (2017). Machine learning-based prediction of adverse drug effects: An example of seizure-inducing compounds. *Journal of pharmacological sciences 133*(2), 70–78.

Garnett, C., K. Needleman, J. Liu, R. Brundage, and Y. Wang (2016). Operational Characteristics of Linear Concentration-QT Models for Assessing QTc Interval in the Thorough QT and Phase I Clinical Studies. *Clinical Pharmacology & Therapeutics 100*(2), 170–178.

Garrison, L. P. J., A. Towse, and B. W. Bresnahan (2007). Assessing a structured, quantitative health outcomes approach to drug risk-benefit analysis. *Health Affairs 26*(5), 684–695.

Geladi, P. and B. R. Kowalski (1986). Partial least-squares regression: a tutorial. *Analytica Chimica Acta 185*, 1–17.

Gelber, R. D., B. F. Cole, S. Gelber, and A. Goldhirsch (1995). Comparing treatments using quality-adjusted survival: the Q-TWiST method. *The American Statistician 49*(2), 161–169.

Gelber, R. D., A. Goldhirsch, B. F. Cole, H. S. Wieand, G. Schroeder, and

J. E. Krook (1996). A quality-adjusted time without symptoms or toxicity (Q-TWiST) analysis of adjuvant radiation therapy and chemotherapy for resectable rectal cancer. *Journal of the National Cancer Institute 88*(15), 1039–1045.

Genovese, C. R. and L. Wasserman (2004). A stochastic process approach to false discovery control. *The Annals of Statistics 32*(3), 1035–1061.

Genovese, C. R. and L. Wasserman (2006). Exceedance control of the false discovery proportion. *Journal of the American Statistical Association 101*(476), 1408–1417.

Ghorbanzadeh, M., J. Zhang, and P. L. Andersson (2016). Binary classification model to predict developmental toxicity of industrial chemicals in zebrafish. *Journal of Chemometrics 30*(6), 298–307.

Ghosh, A. K. (2006). On optimum choice of k in nearest neighbor classification. *Computational Statistics & Data Analysis 50*(11), 3113–3123.

Ghosh, D. and D. Lin (2000). Nonparametric analysis of recurrent events and death. *Biometrics 56*(2), 554–562.

Gibofsky, A., W. R. Palmer, E. C. Keystone, M. H. Schiff, J. Feng, P. McCroskery, S. W. Baumgartner, and J. A. Markenson (2011). Rheumatoid arthritis disease-modifying antirheumatic drug intervention and utilization study: safety and etanercept utilization analyses from the radius 1 and radius 2 registries. *The Journal of Rheumatology 38*(1), 1–8.

Gilbert, P. B. (2005). A modified false discovery rate multiple-comparisons procedure for discrete data, applied to human immunodeficiency virus genetics. *Journal of the Royal Statistical Society: Series C 54*(1), 143–158.

Gilks, W. R., S. Richardson, and D. Spiegelhalter (1995). *Markov Chain Monte Carlo in Practice*. CRC Press.

Gintant, G., P. T. Sager, and N. Stockbridge (2016). Evolution of strategies to improve preclinical cardiac safety testing. *Nature Reviews Drug Discovery*.

Giusti, C. and R. J. Little (2011). An analysis of nonignorable nonresponse to income in a survey with a rotating panel design. *Journal of Official Statistics 27*(2), 211–229.

Glaz, J., J. I. Naus, and S. Wallenstein (2001). *Scan statistics*. Springer: New York.

Goodman, S. N., M. L. Zahurak, and S. Piantadosi (1995). Some practical improvements in the continual reassessment method for phase I studies. *Statistics in Medicine 14*(11), 1149–1161.

Gooley, T. A., P. J. Martin, L. D. Fisher, and M. Pettinger (1994). Simulation as a design tool for phase I/II clinical trials: an example from bone marrow transplantation. *Controlled Clinical Trials 15*(6), 450–462.

Gorodkin, J. (2004). Comparing two k-category assignments by a k-category correlation coefficient. *Computational Biology and Chemistry 28*(5), 367–374.

Gould, A. (2002). Drug safety evaluation in and after clinical trials. In *Deming Conference, Atlantic City*, Volume 3.

Gould, A. (2007). Accounting for multiplicity in the evaluation of signals obtained by data mining from spontaneous report adverse event databases. *Biometrical Journal 49*, 151–65.

Gould, A. (2008). Detecting potential safety issues in clinical trials by Bayesian screening. *Biometrical Journal 50*(5), 837–51.

Gould, A. L. (2013). Detecting potential safety issues in large clinical or observational trials by Bayesian screening when event counts arise from Poisson distributions. *Journal of Biopharmaceutical Statistics 23*(4), 829–847.

Gould, A. L. (2015a). Pharmacovigilance using observational/longitudinal databases and web-based information. In A. L. Gould (Ed.), *Statistical Methods for Evaluating Safety in Medical Product Development*, pp. 345–360. John Wiley & Sons, Ltd.

Gould, A. L. (2015b). *Statistical Methods for Evaluating Safety in Medical Product Development*. John Wiley & Sons.

Gould, A. L. (2018). Unified screening for potential elevated adverse event risk and other associations. *Statistics in Medicine.* https://doi.org/10.1002/sim.7686.

Gramatica, P. (2007). Principles of QSAR models validation: Internal and external. *Molecular Informatics 26*(5), 694–701.

Gramatica, P. and A. Sangion (2016). A historical excursus on the statistical validation parameters for QSAR models: A clarification concerning metrics and terminology. *Journal of Chemical Information and Modeling 56*(6), 1127–1131.

Greco, T., A. Zangrillo, G. Biondi-Zoccai, and G. Landoni (2013). Meta-analysis: pitfalls and hints. *Heart Lung Vessel 5*(4), 219–25.

Greene, S. K., M. Kulldorff, E. M. Lewis, R. Li, R. Yin, E. S. Weintraub, B. H. Fireman, T. A. Lieu, J. D. Nordin, and J. M. Glanz (2009). Near real-time surveillance for influenza vaccine safety: proof-of-concept in the vaccine safety datalink project. *American Journal of Epidemiology 171*(2), 177–188.

Greene, S. K., M. Kulldorff, R. Yin, W. K. Yih, T. A. Lieu, E. S. Weintraub, and G. M. Lee (2011). Near real-time vaccine safety surveillance with partially accrued data. *Pharmacoepidemiology and drug safety 20*(6), 583–590.

Griffin, M. R., W. A. Ray, E. A. Mortimer, G. M. Fenichel, and W. Schaffner (1991). Risk of seizures after measles-mumps-rubella immunization. *Pediatrics 88*(5), 881–885.

Guo, J. J., S. Pandey, J. Doyle, B. Bian, Y. Lis, and D. W. Raisch (2010). A review of quantitative risk–benefit methodologies for assessing drug safety and efficacy–report of the ISPOR risk–benefit management working group. *Value in Health 13*(5), 657–666.

Guo, X., T. Lai, H. Shek, and S. Way (2017). *Quantitative Trading: Algorithms, Analytics, Data, Models, Optimizations*. Chapman & Hall (CRC Press), Boca Raton, FL.

Gupta, R. C. (2014). *Biomarkers in Toxicology*. Academic Press.

Gurtcheff, S. E. (2008). Introduction to the MAUDE database. *Clinical Obstetrics and Gynecology 51*(1), 120–123.

Haidich, A.-B. (2010). Meta-analysis in medical research. *Hippokratia (Suppl.) 14*(1), 29.

Haines, L. M., I. Perevozskaya, and W. F. Rosenberger (2003). Bayesian optimal designs for phase I clinical trials. *Biometrics 59*(3), 591–600.

Hallas, J. (1996). Evidence of depression provoked by cardiovascular medication: a prescription sequence symmetry analysis. *Epidemiology 7*(5), 478–484.

Hammad, T. A. and C. A. Pinto (2016). Key changes in benefit–risk assessment guidelines and implications for data analysis in drug development. *Statistics in Biopharmaceutical Research 8*(4), 366–372.

Hannan, J. F. and H. Robbins (1955). Asymptotic solutions of the compound decision problem for two completely specified distributions. *The Annals of Mathematical Statistics 26*(1), 37–51.

Hansen, S. N., M. Overgaard, P. K. Andersen, and E. T. Parner (2017). Estimating a population cumulative incidence under calendar time trends. *BMC Medical Research Methodology 17*(1), 7. (DOI 10.1186/s12874-016-0280-6).

Harrington, J. A., G. M. Wheeler, M. J. Sweeting, A. P. Mander, and D. I. Jodrell (2013). Adaptive designs for dual-agent phase I dose-escalation studies. *Nature Reviews Clinical Oncology 10*(5), 277–288.

Hartigan-Go, K. Y. and J. Q. Wong (2000). Inclusion of therapeutic failures as adverse drug reactions. *Side Effects of Drugs Essay 23*, xxvii–xxxiii.

Hartzema, A. G., J. A. Racoosin, T. E. MaCurdy, J. M. Gibbs, and J. A. Kelman (2011). Utilizing Medicare claims data for real-time drug safety evaluations: is it feasible? *Pharmacoepidemiology and Drug Safety 20*(7), 684–688.

Hastie, T. and R. Tibshirani (1990). *Generalized Additive Models*. John Wiley & Son, Ltd.

Hastie, T. and R. Tibshirani (1996). Discriminant adaptive nearest neighbor classification. *IEEE Transactions on Pattern Analysis and Machine Intelligence 18*(6), 607–616.

Hastie, T., R. Tibshirani, and J. Friedman (2009). *The Elements of Statistical Learning* (2nd ed.). New York: Springer. (Original edition, 2001).

Haybittle, J. (1971). Repeated assessment of results in clinical trials of cancer treatment. *The British Journal of Radiology 44*(526), 793–797.

He, Y.-Y., W. Yan, C.-L. Liu, X. Li, R.-J. Li, Y. Mu, Q. Jia, F.-F. Wu, L.-L. Wang, and K.-L. He (2015). Usefulness of S100A12 as a prognostic biomarker for adverse events in patients with heart failure. *Clinical Biochemistry 48*(4), 329–333.

Heckerman, D. (1997). Bayesian networks for data mining. *Data Mining and Knowledge Discovery 1*(1), 79–119.

Heitjan, D. F. and S. Basu (1996). Distinguishing "missing at random" and "missing completely at random". *The American Statistician 50*(3), 207–213.

Helma, C. (2005a). A brief introduction to predictive toxicology. In C. Helma (Ed.), *Predictive Toxicology*, pp. 1–9. CRC Press.

Helma, C. (2005b). *Predictive Toxicology*. CRC Press.

Helma, C., R. D. King, S. Kramer, and A. Srinivasan (2001). The predictive toxicology challenge 2000–2001. *Bioinformatics 17*(1), 107–108.

Henegar, C., C. Bousquet, A. Lillo-Le Louët, P. Degoulet, and M. Jaulent (2004). A knowledge based approach for automated signal generation in pharmacovigilance. In *MedInfo*, pp. 626–630. Amsterdam: IOS Press.

Hengelbrock, J., J. Gillhaus, S. Kloss, and F. Leverkus (2016). Safety data from randomized controlled trials: applying models for recurrent events. *Pharmaceutical Statistics 15*(4), 315–323.

Hennessy, S. and B. L. Strom (2007). PDUFA reauthorization–drug safety's golden moment of opportunity? *New England Journal of Medicine 356*(17), 1703–1704.

Heyd, J. M. and B. P. Carlin (1999). Adaptive design improvements in the continual reassessment method for phase I studies. *Statistics in Medicine 18*(11), 1307–1321.

Heyse, J., B. Kuter, M. Dallas, and P. Heaton (2008). Evaluating the safety of a rotavirus vaccine: the REST of the story. *Clinical Trials 5*(2), 131–139.

Heyse, J. F. (2011). A false discovery rate procedure for categorical data. In M. Bhattacharjee, S. K. Dhar, and S. Subramanian (Eds.), *Recent Advances in Biostatistics: False Discovery Rates, Survival Analysis, and Related Topics*, pp. 43–58. World Scientific.

Higgin, J., S. Thompson, J. Deeks, and D. Altman (2003). Measuring inconsistency in meta-analysis. *British Medical Journal 327*, 557–560.

Higgins, J. and S. G. Thompson (2002). Quantifying heterogeneity in a meta-analysis. *Statistics in medicine 21*(11), 1539–1558.

Higgins, J. P. and S. Green (2011). *Cochrane Handbook for Systematic Reviews of Interventions*, Volume 4. John Wiley & Sons.

Hilbe, J. M. (2011). *Negative Binomial Regression*. Cambridge University Press.

Hill, A. (1965). The environment and disease: Association or causation? *Proceedings of the Royal Society of Medicine 58*(5), 295–300.

Ho, T. K. (1995). Random decision forests. In *Proceedings of the third international conference on document analysis and recognition, 1995.*, Volume 1, pp. 278–282. IEEE.

Ho, T. K. (1998). The random subspace method for constructing decision forests. *IEEE Transactions on Pattern Analysis and Machine Intelligence 20*(8), 832–844.

Hoeffding, W. (1960). Lower bounds for the expected sample size and the average risk of a sequential procedure. *The Annals of Mathematical Statistics 31*(2), 352–368.

Holford, N. (2006). Dose response: Pharmacokinetic–pharmacodynamic approach. In N. Ting (Ed.), *Dose Finding in Drug Development*, pp. 73–88. Springer.

Holland, B. S. and M. D. Copenhaver (1987). An improved sequentially rejective bonferroni test procedure. *Biometrics 43*(2), 417–423.

Holland, P. (1986). Statistics and causal inference (with comments by D.B. Rubin, D.R. Cox, C. Glymor, C.Granyor, and author's rejoinder). *Journal of the American Statistical Association 81*(396), 945–970.

Holm, S. (1979). A simple sequentially rejective multiple test procedure. *Scandinavian Journal of Statistics 6*, 65–70.

Hong, H., M. Chen, H. W. Ng, and W. Tong (2016). QSAR Models at the US FDA/NCTR. In E. Benfenati (Ed.), *In silico Methods for Predicting Drug Toxicity*, pp. 431–459. Springer.

Hothorn, L. A. (2014). Statistical evaluation of toxicological bioassays–a review. *Toxicology Research 3*(6), 418–432.

Houede, N., P. F. Thall, H. Nguyen, X. Paoletti, and A. Kramar (2010). Utility-based optimization of combination therapy using ordinal toxicity and efficacy in phase I/II trials. *Biometrics 66*(2), 532–540.

Howard, R. and J. Matheson (1984). Influence diagrams. In R. Howard and J. Matheson (Eds.), *Readings on the Principles and Applications of Decision Analysis*. Menlo Park, CA: Strategic Decisions Group.

Huang, L., J. Zalkikar, and R. C. Tiwari (2011). A likelihood ratio test based method for signal detection with application to FDA's drug safety data. *Journal of the American Statistical Association 106*(496), 1230–1241.

Huang, M., Q. Liang, P. Li, J. Xia, Y. Wang, P. Hu, Z. Jiang, Y. He, L. Pang, and L. Han (2013). Biomarkers for early diagnosis of type 2 diabetic nephropathy: a study based on an integrated biomarker system. *Molecular BioSystems 9*(8), 2134–2141.

Huang, R., M. Xia, S. Sakamuru, J. Zhao, S. A. Shahane, M. Attene-Ramos, T. Zhao, C. P. Austin, and A. Simeonov (2016). Modelling the Tox21 10 K chemical profiles for in vivo toxicity prediction and mechanism characterization. *Nature Communications 7*, 1–10.

Hug, C., M. Sievers, R. Ottermanns, H. Hollert, W. Brack, and M. Krauss (2015). Linking mutagenic activity to micropollutant concentrations in wastewater samples by partial least square regression and subsequent identification of variables. *Chemosphere 138*, 176–182.

Hughes, D., E. Waddingham, S. Mt-Isa, A. Goginsky, E. Chan, G. Downey, C. E. Hallgreen, K. S. Hockley, J. Juhaeri, and A. Lieftucht (2014). *IMI-PROTECT Benefit-Risk Group Recommendations Report: Recommendations for the methodology and visualisation techniques to be used in the assessment of benefit and risk of medicines.* PROTECT Consortium, London.

Hughes, S., A. Hughes, C. Brothers, W. Spreen, and D. Thorborn (2008). PREDICT-1 (CNA106030): the first powered, prospective trial of pharmacogenetic screening to reduce drug adverse events. *Pharmaceutical Statistics 7*(2), 121–129.

Hunt, D. L. and C.-S. Li (2006). A regression spline model for developmental toxicity data. *Toxicological Sciences 92*(1), 329–334.

Huynh, T., Y. He, A. Willis, and S. Rüger (2016). Adverse drug reaction classification with deep neural networks. In *Proceedings of COLING 2016, the 26th International Conference on Computational Linguistics: Technical Papers*, pp. 877–887.

ICH (1998). *Statistical Principles for Clinical Trials.* International Conference on Harmonisation. London, UK.

ICH (2001). *Maintenance of the ICH Guideline on Clinical Safety Data Management: Data Elements for Transmission of Individual Case Safety Reports E2B(R2).* ICH Harmonised Tripartite.

ICH (2003). *Post-Approval Safety Data Management: Definitions and Standards for Expedited Reporting.* ICH Harmonised Tripartite.

ICH (2005a). *The Clinical Evaluation of QT/QTc Interval Prolongation and Proarrhythmic Potential for Non-antiarrhythmic Drugs - E14.* ICH Harmonised Tripartite.

ICH (2005b). *The Non-Clinical Evaluation of the Potential for Delayed Ventricular Repolarization (QT Interval Prolongation) by Human Pharmaceuticals.* ICH Harmonised Tripartite.

ICH (2008). *Nonclinical Safety Studies for the Conduct of Human Clinical Trials and Marketing Authorization for Pharmaceuticals. M3 (R2).* ICH Harmonised Tripartite.

ICH (2015). *ICH E14 Guideline: The Clinical Evaluation of QT/QTc Interval Prolongation and Proarrhythmic Potential for Non-Antiarrhythmic Drugs. Questions & Answers (R3).* ICH Harmonised Tripartite.

Ing, C.-K. and T. L. Lai (2011). A stepwise regression method and consistent model selection for high-dimensional sparse linear models. *Statistica Sinica 21*(4), 1473–1513.

Institute of Medicine (2012). *Ethical and Scientific Issues in Studying the Safety of Approved Drugs.* The National Academics Press, Washington, D.C.

Ioannidis, J. (2016). The mass production of redundant, misleading, and conflicted systematic reviews and meta-analyses. *The Milbank Quarterly 94*(3), 485–514.

Iskander, J. K., E. R. Miller, and R. T. Chen (2004). Vaccine adverse event reporting system (VAERS). *Pediatr Ann 33*, 599.

Ivanova, A. (2003). A new dose-finding design for bivariate outcomes. *Biometrics 59*(4), 1001–1007.

Jacobsen, S. J., B. K. Ackerson, L. S. Sy, T. N. Tran, T. L. Jones, J. F. Yao, F. Xie, T. C. Cheetham, and P. Saddier (2009). Observational safety study of febrile convulsion following first dose mmrv vaccination in a managed care setting. *Vaccine 27*(34), 4656–4661.

Ji, X., D. S. Small, C. E. Leonard, and S. Hennessy (2017). The trend-in-trend research design for causal inference. *Epidemiology 28*(4), 529–536.

Ji, Y., Y. Li, and B. N. Bekele (2007). Dose-finding in phase I clinical trials based on toxicity probability intervals. *Clinical Trials 4*(3), 235–244.

Jiang, Q. and W. He (2016). *Benefit-Risk Assessment Methods in Medical Product Development: Bridging Qualitative and Quantitative Assessments*. CRC Press.

Jin, X., M. Jin, and L. Sheng (2014). Three dimensional quantitative structure–toxicity relationship modeling and prediction of acute toxicity for organic contaminants to algae. *Computers in Biology and Medicine 51*, 205–213.

Johannesen, L., J. Vicente, M. Hosseini, and D. G. Strauss (2016). Automated Algorithm for J-Tpeak and Tpeak-Tend Assessment of Drug-Induced Proarrhythmia Risk. *PloS One 11*(12), 1–18.

Johannesen, L., J. Vicente, J. Mason, C. Sanabria, K. Waite-Labott, M. Hong, P. Guo, J. Lin, J. S. Sørensen, and L. Galeotti (2014). Differentiating drug-induced multichannel block on the electrocardiogram: randomized study of dofetilide, quinidine, ranolazine, and verapamil. *Clinical Pharmacology & Therapeutics 96*(5), 549–558.

Jones, B., J. Roger, P. W. Lane, A. Lawton, C. Fletcher, J. C. Cappelleri, H. Tate, P. Moneuse, and PSI Health Technology Special Interest Group, Evidence Synthesis sub-team (2011). Statistical approaches for conducting network meta-analysis in drug development. *Pharmaceutical Statistics 10*(6), 523–531.

Jones, J. K. (2012). Assessing causality of case reports of suspected adverse events. In B. L. Strom, S. E. Kimmel, and S. Hennessy (Eds.),

Pharmacoepidemiology, Fifth Edition, pp. 581–600. John Wiley & Sons, Ltd.

Jones, J. K. and E. Kingery (2014). How we assess causality. In E. Andres and N. Moore (Eds.), *Mann's Pharmacovigilance*, pp. 319–330. John Wiley & Sons, Ltd.

Julious, S. A., D. Machin, and S.-B. Tan (2010). *An Introduction to Statistics in Early Phase Trials*. John Wiley & Sons, Ltd.

Kachuck, N. (2011). Registries, research, and regrets: is the FDA's postmarketing REMS process not adequately protecting patients? *Therapeutic Advances in Neurological Disorders 4*(6), 339–347.

Kalbfleisch, J. and R. Prentice (1980). *The Statistical Analysis of Failure Time Data*.

Kaplan, K., S. Rusche, H. Lakkis, G. Bottenfield, F. Guerra, J. Guerrero, H. Keyserling, E. Felicione, T. Hesley, and J. Boslego (2002). Postlicensure comparative study of unusual high-pitched crying following COMVAX and placebo versus PedvaxHIB and RECOMBIVAX in healthy infants. *Vaccine 21*, 181–87.

Karp, N. A., T. F. Meehan, H. Morgan, J. C. Mason, A. Blake, N. Kurbatova, D. Smedley, J. Jacobsen, R. F. Mott, and V. Iyer (2015). Applying the ARRIVE guidelines to an in vivo database. *PLoS Biol 13*(5), e1002151.

Kavlock, R. J., G. Ankley, J. Blancato, M. Breen, R. Conolly, D. Dix, K. Houck, E. Hubal, R. Judson, and J. Rabinowitz (2007). Computational toxicology–A state of the science mini review. *Toxicological Sciences 103*(1), 14–27.

Keeney, R. L. and H. Raiffa (1993). *Decisions with Multiple Objectives: Preferences and Value Trade-offs*. Cambridge University Press.

Keiding, N. and D. Clayton (2014). Standardization and control for confounding in observational studies: A historical perspective. *Statistical Science 29*(4), 529–58.

Kiefer, J. and L. Weiss (1957). Some properties of generalized sequential probability ratio tests. *The Annals of Mathematical Statistics 28*(1), 57–74.

Kilpatrick, S. (1962). Occupational mortality indices. *Population Studies 16*(2), 175–188.

King, E. N. and T. P. Ryan (2002). A preliminary investigation of maximum likelihood logistic regression versus exact logistic regression. *The American Statistician 56*(3), 163–170.

Bibliography

King, G. and L. Zeng (2001). Logistic regression in rare events data. *Political Analysis*, 137–163.

Kinsner-Ovaskainen, A., R. Rzepka, R. Rudowski, S. Coecke, T. Cole, and P. Prieto (2009). Acutoxbase, an innovative database for *in vitro* acute toxicity studies. *Toxicology in Vitro 23*(3), 476–485.

Klein, N. P., B. Fireman, W. K. Yih, E. Lewis, M. Kulldorff, P. Ray, R. Baxter, S. Hambidge, J. Nordin, and A. Naleway (2010). Measles-mumps-rubella-varicella combination vaccine and the risk of febrile seizures. *Pediatrics 126*(1), e1–e8.

Knudsen, T. B., D. A. Keller, M. Sander, E. W. Carney, N. G. Doerrer, D. L. Eaton, S. C. Fitzpatrick, K. L. Hastings, D. L. Mendrick, and R. R. Tice (2015). FutureTox II: in vitro data and *In silico* models for predictive toxicology. *Toxicological Sciences 143*(2), 256–267.

Koller, D. and N. Friedman (2009). *Probabilistic graphical models: principles and techniques*. MIT press.

Koopmans, T. C. and O. Reiersol (1950). The identification of structural characteristics. *The Annals of Mathematical Statistics 21*(2), 165–181.

Korn, E. L., S. G. Arbuck, J. M. Pluda, R. Simon, R. S. Kaplan, and M. C. Christian (2001). Clinical trial designs for cytostatic agents: are new approaches needed? *Journal of Clinical Oncology 19*(1), 265–272.

Koster, J. T. (1996). Markov properties of nonrecursive causal models. *The Annals of Statistics 24*(5), 2148–2177.

Koster, J. T. (2002). Marginalizing and conditioning in graphical models. *Bernoulli 8*(6), 817–840.

Kotz, S. and S. Nadarajah (2000). *Extreme Value Distributions: Theory and Applications*. World Scientific.

Koutsoukas, A., J. St Amand, M. Mishra, and J. Huan (2016). Predictive toxicology: Modeling chemical induced toxicological response combining circular fingerprints with random forest and support vector machine. *Frontiers in Environmental Science 4*, 11.

Krause, A. and M. O'Connell (2012). *A Picture Is Worth a Thousand Tables: Graphics in Life Sciences*. Springer.

Kubota, K., T. Hida, S. Ishikura, J. Mizusawa, M. Nishio, M. Kawahara, A. Yokoyama, F. Imamura, K. Takeda, and S. Negoro (2014). Etoposide and cisplatin versus irinotecan and cisplatin in patients with limited-stage small-cell lung cancer treated with etoposide and cisplatin plus concurrent accelerated hyperfractionated thoracic radiotherapy (JCOG0202): a randomised phase 3 study. *The Lancet Oncology 15*(1), 106–113.

Kuderer, N. M. and A. C. Wolff (2014). Enhancing therapeutic decision making when options abound: Toxicities matter. *Journal of Clinical Oncology 32*(19), 1990–1993.

Kulldorff, M. (1997). A spatial scan statistic. *Communications in Statistics-Theory and methods 26*(6), 1481–1496.

Kulldorff, M. (2011). Sequential statistical methods for prospective post-marketing safety surveillance. *Pharmacoepidemiology, Fifth Edition*, 852–867.

Kulldorff, M. (2012). Sequential statistical methods for prospective post-marketing safety surveillance. In B. L. Strom, S. E. Kimmel, and S. Hennessy (Eds.), *Pharmacoepidemiology, Fifth Edition*, pp. 852–867. Wiley Online Library.

Kulldorff, M., W. F. Athas, E. J. Feurer, B. A. Miller, and C. R. Key (1998). Evaluating cluster alarms: a space-time scan statistic and brain cancer in Los Alamos, New Mexico. *American Journal of Public Health 88*(9), 1377–1380.

Kulldorff, M., I. Dashevsky, T. R. Avery, A. K. Chan, R. L. Davis, D. Graham, R. Platt, S. E. Andrade, D. Boudreau, and M. J. Gunter (2013). Drug safety data mining with a tree-based scan statistic. *Pharmacoepidemiology and Drug Safety 22*(5), 517–523.

Kulldorff, M., R. Davis, M. Kolczak, E. Lewis, T. Lieu, and R. Platt (2011). A maximized sequential probability ratio test for drug and vaccine safety surveillance. *Sequential Analysis 30*(1), 58–78.

Kulldorff, M., Z. Fang, and S. J. Walsh (2003). A tree-based scan statistic for database disease surveillance. *Biometrics 59*(2), 323–331.

Kuramoto, L., B. G. Sobolev, and M. G. Donaldson (2008). On reporting results from randomized controlled trials with recurrent events. *BMC Medical Research Methodology 8*(1), 35.

Kuter, B. J., M. L. Hoffman Brown, J. Hartzel, W. R. Williams, K. A. Eves, S. Black, H. Shinefield, K. S. Reisinger, C. D. Marchant, and B. J. Sullivan (2006). Safety and immunogenicity of a combination: Measles, mumps, rubella and varicella vaccine (proquad®). *Human Vaccines 2*(5), 205–214.

Lahdelma, R. and P. Salminen (2010). Stochastic multicriteria acceptability analysis (SMAA). In M. Ehrgott, J. R. Figueira, and S. Greco (Eds.), *Trends in Multiple Criteria Decision Analysis*, pp. 285–315. Springer.

Lai, E. C.-C., N. Pratt, C.-Y. Hsieh, S.-J. Lin, A. Pottegård, E. E. Roughead, Y.-H. K. Yang, and J. Hallas (2017). Sequence symmetry analysis in pharmacovigilance and pharmacoepidemiologic studies. *European Journal of Epidemiology 32*(7), 567–582.

Lai, T. (1988). Nearly optimal sequential tests of composite hypotheses. *Ann. Statist 16*(2), 856–886.

Lai, T. L. and O. Y.-W. Liao (2012). Efficient adaptive randomization and stopping rules in multi-arm clinical trials for testing a new treatment. *Sequential Analysis 31*(4), 441–457.

Lai, T. L., O. Y.-W. Liao, and D. W. Kim (2013). Group sequential designs for developing and testing biomarker-guided personalized therapies in comparative effectiveness research. *Contemporary Clinical Trials 36*(2), 651–663.

Lai, T. L. and J. Miao (2017). Compound decisions and an empirical Bayesian approach to false discovery rates. Technical report, Center for Innovative Study Design, Stanford University.

Lai, T. L., J. Miao, and K. W. Tsang (2018a). Control of false rejections in multiple testing following hierarchical selection: Theory and applications. Technical report, Center for Innovative Study Design, Stanford University.

Lai, T. L., J. Miao, and K. W. Tsang (2018b). Sequential detection and diagnosis in the presence of confounding and/or censoring. Technical report, Center for Innovative Study Design, Stanford University.

Lai, T. L., T. Xia, and H. Yuan (2017). Modified gradient boosting in high-dimensional nonlinear regression. Technical report, Center for Innovative Study Design, Stanford University.

Lai, T. L., H. Xing, and Z. Chen (2011). Mean-variance portfolio optimization when means and covariances are unknown. *The Annals of Applied Statistics 5*(2A), 798–823.

Lai, T. L. and Z. Ying (1991). Rank regression methods for left-truncated and right-censored data. *The Annals of Statistics 19*(2), 531–556.

Lampa, E., L. Lind, P. M. Lind, and A. Bornefalk-Hermansson (2014). The identification of complex interactions in epidemiology and toxicology: a simulation study of boosted regression trees. *Environmental Health 13*(1), 57.

Lan, G. K. and D. L. DeMets (1983). Discrete sequential boundaries for clinical trials. *Biometrika 70*(3), 659–663.

Lanes, S. F. and C. de Luise (2006). Bias due to false-positive diagnoses in an automated health insurance claims database. *Drug Safety 29*(11), 1069–1075.

Lao, K. S., C. S. Chui, K. K. Man, W. C. Lau, E. W. Chan, and I. C. Wong (2016). Medication safety research by observational study design. *International Journal of Clinical Pharmacy 38*(3), 676–684.

Laupacis, A., D. L. Sackett, and R. S. Roberts (1988). An assessment of clinically useful measures of the consequences of treatment. *New England Journal of Medicine 318*(26), 1728–1733.

Lauritzen, S. L. and N. Wermuth (1989). Graphical models for associations between variables, some of which are qualitative and some quantitative. *The annals of Statistics 17*(1), 31–57.

Le Tourneau, C., J. J. Lee, and L. L. Siu (2009). Dose escalation methods in phase I cancer clinical trials. *Journal of the National Cancer Institute 101*(10), 708–720.

Lee, B., J. Lessler, and E. Stuart (2010). Improving propensity score weighting using machine learning. *Statistics in Medicine 29*(3), 337–46.

Lee, B. L., S. K. Fan, and Y. Lu (2017). A curve-free Bayesian decision-theoretic design for two-agent phase I trials. *Journal of Biopharmaceutical Statistics 27*(1), 34–43.

Lee, G. M., S. K. Greene, E. S. Weintraub, J. Baggs, M. Kulldorff, B. H. Fireman, R. Baxter, S. J. Jacobsen, S. Irving, and M. F. Daley (2011). H1n1 and seasonal influenza vaccine safety in the vaccine safety datalink project. *American Journal of Preventive Medicine 41*(2), 121–128.

Lehman, H., J. Chen, A. Gould, R. Kassekert, P. Beninger, R. Carney, M. Goldberg, M. Goss, K. Kidos, and R. Sharrar (2007). An evaluation of computer-aided disproportionality analysis for post-marketing signal detection. *Clinical Pharmacology & Therapeutics 82*(2), 173–180.

Lehmann, E. L. and J. P. Romano (2006). *Testing Statistical Hypotheses* (3rd ed.). New York: Springer.

Leite, A., N. J. Andrews, and S. L. Thomas (2016). Near real-time vaccine safety surveillance using electronic health records: a systematic review of the application of statistical methods. *Pharmacoepidemiology and Drug Safety 25*(3), 225–237.

Leitgöb, H. (2013). The problem of modeling rare events in ML-based logistic regression. Paper presented at the European Survey Research Association. Ljubljana, Slovenia.

Levinson, D. (2006). Adverse event reporting for medical devices. Technical report, Inspector General, Department of Health and Human Services.

Lewis, D. (1973). *Counterfactuals.* Harvard University Press, Cambridge, MA.

Li, A. P. (2005). Preclinical in vitro screening assays for drug-like properties. *Drug Discovery Today: Technologies 2*(2), 179–185.

Li, L. (2009). A conditional sequential sampling procedure for drug safety surveillance. *Statistics in Medicine 28*(25), 3124–3138.

Li, L. and M. Kulldorff (2010). A conditional maximized sequential probability ratio test for pharmacovigilance. *Statistics in Medicine 29*(2), 284–295.

Li, L., M. Kulldorff, J. C. Nelson, and A. J. Cook (2011). A propensity score-enhanced sequential analytic method for comparative drug safety surveillance. *Statistics in Biosciences 3*(1), 45–62.

Li, R., B. Stewart, E. Weintraub, and M. M. McNeil (2014). Continuous sequential boundaries for vaccine safety surveillance. *Statistics in Medicine 33*(19), 3387–3397.

Li, R., E. Weintraub, M. M. McNeil, M. Kulldorff, E. M. Lewis, J. Nelson, S. Xu, L. Qian, N. P. Klein, and F. Destefano (2018). Meningococcal conjugate vaccine safety surveillance in the vaccine safety datalink using a tree-temporal scan data mining method. *Pharmacoepidemiology and drug safety 27*(4), 391–397.

Li, Z., S. Dutta, J. Sheng, P. N. Tran, W. Wu, K. Chang, T. Mdluli, D. G. Strauss, and T. Colatsky (2017). Improving the *In silico* assessment of proarrhythmia risk by combining hERG (Human Ether-à-go-go-Related Gene) channel–Drug binding kinetics and multichannel pharmacology. *Circulation: Arrhythmia and Electrophysiology 10*(2), e004628.

Li, Z., S. Dutta, J. Sheng, P. N. Tran, W. Wu, and T. Colatsky (2016). A temperature–dependent *In silico* model of the human ether-à-go-go-related (hERG) gene channel. *Journal of Pharmacological and Toxicological Methods 81*, 233–239.

Liaw, A. and V. Svetnik (2015). QSAR modeling: Prediction of biological activity from chemical structure. In A. L. Gould (Ed.), *Statistical Methods for Evaluating Safety in Medical Product Development*, pp. 66–83. John Wiley & Sons.

Lieberman, J. M., W. R. Williams, J. M. Miller, S. Black, H. Shinefield, F. Henderson, C. D. Marchant, A. Werzberger, S. Halperin, and J. Hartzel (2006). The safety and immunogenicity of a quadrivalent measles, mumps, rubella and varicella vaccine in healthy children: a study of manufacturing consistency and persistence of antibody. *The Pediatric Infectious Disease Journal 25*(7), 615–622.

Lifschitz, V. (1997). On the logic of causal explanation. *Artificial Intelligence 96*(2), 451–465.

Lindquist, M. (2008). Vigibase, the WHO global icsr database system: basic facts. *Drug Information Journal 42*(5), 409–419.

Little, R. and H. An (2004). Robust likelihood-based analysis of multivariate data with missing values. *Statistica Sinica 14*(3), 949–968.

Little, R. and D. Rubin (2000). Causal effects in clinical and epidemiological studies via potential outcomes: Concepts and analytical approaches. *Annual Review of Public Health 21*, 121–45.

Little, R. J. (2002). *Statistical analysis with missing data*. John Wiley & Sons.

Little, R. J. and D. B. Rubin (2014). *Statistical analysis with missing data*, Volume 333. John Wiley & Sons.

Liu, G. F. (2013). On analysis of low incidence adverse events in clinical trials. In M. Hu, Y. Liu, and J. Lin (Eds.), *Topics in Applied Statistics*, pp. 273–282. Springer.

Liu, G. F., J. Wang, K. Liu, and D. B. Snavely (2006). Confidence intervals for an exposure adjusted incidence rate difference with applications to clinical trials. *Statistics in Medicine 25*(8), 1275–1286.

Liu, R., G. Tawa, and A. Wallqvist (2012). Locally weighted learning methods for predicting dose-dependent toxicity with application to the human maximum recommended daily dose. *Chemical Research in Toxicology 25*(10), 2216–2226.

Liu, S. and Y. Yuan (2015). Bayesian optimal interval designs for phase I clinical trials. *Journal of the Royal Statistical Society: Series C 64*(3), 507–523.

López-Fernández, T. and P. Thavendiranathan (2017). Emerging cardiac imaging modalities for the early detection of cardiotoxicity due to anticancer therapies. *Revista Española de Cardiología (English Edition) 70*(6), 487–495.

Lorden, G. (1976). 2-SPRT's and the modified Kiefer-Weiss problem of minimizing an expected sample size. *The Annals of Statistics 4*(2), 281–291.

Lynd, L. D., M. Najafzadeh, L. Colley, M. F. Byrne, A. R. Willan, M. J. Sculpher, F. R. Johnson, and A. B. Hauber (2010). Using the incremental net benefit framework for quantitative benefit–risk analysis in regulatory decision–making: A case study of alosetron in rrritable bowel syndrome. *Value in Health 13*(4), 411–417.

Ma, H., Q. Jiang, C. Chuang-Stein, S. R. Evans, W. He, G. Quartey, J. Scott, S. Wen, and R. Arani (2016). Considerations on endpoint selection, weighting determination, and uncertainty evaluation in the benefit-risk assessment of medical product. *Statistics in Biopharmaceutical Research 8*(4), 417–425.

Madigan, D., P. E. Stang, J. A. Berlin, M. Schuemie, J. M. Overhage, M. A. Suchard, B. Dumouchel, A. G. Hartzema, and P. B. Ryan (2014). A systematic statistical approach to evaluating evidence from observational studies. *Annual Review of Statistics and Its Application 1*, 11–39.

Mandrekar, S. J., Y. Cui, and D. J. Sargent (2007). An adaptive phase I design for identifying a biologically optimal dose for dual agent drug combinations. *Statistics in Medicine 26*(11), 2317–2330.

Mannhold, R., H. Kubinyi, G. Folkers, F. Pfannkuch, and L. Suter-Dick (2014). *Predictive Toxicology: From Vision to Reality*, Volume 64. John Wiley & Sons.

Manski, C. (2003). *Partial Identification of Probability Distributions*. Springer, New York.

Mantel, N. (1966). Evaluation of survival data and two new rank order statistics arising in its consideration. *Cancer Chemotherapy Reports 50*(3), 163–170.

Mantel, N. and W. Haenszel (1959). Statistical aspects of the analysis of data from retrospective studies of disease. *J Nat C Inst 22*, 719–748.

Markowitz, H. (1952). Portfolio selection. *The Journal of Finance 7*(1), 77–91.

Marschak, J. and W. H. Andrews (1944). Random simultaneous equations and the theory of production. *Econometrica, Journal of the Econometric Society*, 143–205.

Martin, R., D. Rose, K. Yu, and S. Barros (2006). Toxicogenomics strategies for predicting drug toxicity. *Pharmacogenomics 7*(7), 1003–1016.

Mauri, A., V. Consonni, and R. Todeschini (2016). Molecular descriptors. In *Handbook of Computational Chemistry*, pp. 1–29. Springer.

McCain, N. and H. Turner (1997). On relating causal theories to other formalisms. *Proceedings of the Association for Advancement of Artificual Intelligence*, 460–465.

McCullagh, P. (1987). *Tensor Methods in Statistics*. Chapman & Hall, London.

McNaughton, R., G. Huet, and S. Shakir (2014). An investigation into drug products withdrawn from the EU market between 2002 and 2011 for safety reasons and the evidence used to support the decision-making. *British Medical Journal 4*(1), e004221.

MedDRA-MSSO (2015). *Introductory Guide: MedDRA Version 18.0.* MedDRA Maintenance and Support Services Organization.

Mehrotra, D. and J. Heyse (2004a). Use of the false discovery rate for evaluating clinical safety data. *Statistical Methods in Medical Research 13*(3), 227–38.

Mehrotra, D. V. and A. J. Adewale (2012). Flagging clinical adverse experiences: reducing false discoveries without materially compromising power for detecting true signals. *Statistics in Medicine 31*(18), 1918–1930.

Mehrotra, D. V. and J. F. Heyse (2004b). Use of false discovery rate for evaluating clinical safety data. *Statistical Methods in Medical Research 13*, 227–238.

Mehta, C. R. and N. R. Patel (1995). Exact logistic regression: theory and examples. *Statistics in Medicine 14*(19), 2143–2160.

Mehta, S., A. Shelling, A. Muthukaruppan, A. Lasham, C. Blenkiron, G. Laking, and C. Print (2010). Predictive and prognostic molecular markers for cancer medicine. *Therapeutic Advances in Medical Oncology 2*(2), 125–148.

Miettinen, O. and M. Nurminen (1985). Comparative analysis of two rates. *Statistics in Medicine 4*(2), 213–226.

Millar, A. W. and K. P. Lynch (2003). Opinion: Rethinking clinical trials for cytostatic drugs. *Nature Reviews. Cancer 3*(7), 540–545.

Millard, D. C., M. Clements, and J. D. Ross (2017). The CiPA Microelectrode Array Assay with hSC-Derived Cardiomyocytes: Current Protocol, Future Potential. *Stem Cell-Derived Models in Toxicology*, 83–107.

Miller, D. R., S. A. Oliveria, D. R. Berlowitz, B. G. Fincke, P. Stang, and D. E. Lillienfeld (2008). Angioedema incidence in US veterans initiating angiotensin-converting enzyme inhibitors. *Hypertension 51*(6), 1624–1630.

Miller, L. E. (2013). Lorcaserin for weight loss: insights into US Food and Drug Administration approval. *J Acad Nutr Diet 113*(1), 25–30.

Miotto, R., F. Wang, S. Wang, X. Jiang, and J. T. Dudley (2017). Deep learning for healthcare: review, opportunities and challenges. *Briefings in Bioinformatics*, 1–1–1. (doi:10.1093/bib/bbx044).

Modi, M. (2006). Dose-finding studies in phase I and estimation of maximally tolerated dose. In N. Ting (Ed.), *Dose Finding in Drug Development*, pp. 30–48. Springer.

Møller, S. (1995). An extension of the continual reassessment methods using a preliminary up-and-down design in a dose finding study in cancer patients, in order to investigate a greater range of doses. *Statistics in Medicine 14*(9), 911–922.

Moon, H., H. Ahn, R. L. Kodell, and J. J. Lee (2003). Estimation of k for the poly-k test with application to animal carcinogenicity studies. *Statistics in Medicine 22*(16), 2619–2636.

Morrato, E. H. and D. B. Allison (2012). FDA approval of obesity drugs: a difference in risk-benefit perceptions. *JAMA 308*(11), 1097–1098.

Mosier, P. D. and P. C. Jurs (2002). QSAR/QSPR studies using probabilistic neural networks and generalized regression neural networks. *Journal of Chemical Information and Computer Sciences 42*(6), 1460–1470.

Mozzicato, P. (2007). Standardised MedDRA Queries: Their Role in Signal Detection. *Drug Safety 30*, 617–619.

Mt-Isa, S., C. E. Hallgreen, N. Wang, T. Callréus, G. Genov, I. Hirsch, S. F. Hobbiger, K. S. Hockley, D. Luciani, and L. D. Phillips (2014). Balancing benefit and risk of medicines: a systematic review and classification of available methodologies. *Pharmacoepidemiology and Drug Safety 23*(7), 667–678.

Munsaka, M. S. (2017). Leveraging machine learning in the analysis of safety data in drug research and healthcare infromatics. In *Proceedings of the Joint Statistical Meetings – Section for Statistical Programmers and Analysis*, pp. 326–334. Americal Statistical Association.

Murphy, T. (2001). Strong association between oral rotavirus vaccine and intussusception. *Reactions 841*, 3.

Murphy, T., P. Gargiullo, M. Massoudi, D. Nelson, A. Jumaan, C. Okoro, L. Zanardi, S. Setia, E. Fair, C. LeBaron, B. Schwartz, M. Wharton, and J. Livinggood (2001). Intussusception among infants given an oral rotavirus vaccine. *New England Journal of Medicine 344*(8), 564–72.

Murphy, T. V., P. J. Smith, P. M. Gargiullo, and B. Schwartz (2003). The first rotavirus vaccine and intussusception: epidemiological studies and policy decisions. *Journal of Infectious Diseases 187*(8), 1309–1313.

Murray, S. and A. A. Tsiatis (1999). Sequential methods for comparing years of life saved in the two-sample censored data problem. *Biometrics 55*(4), 1085–1092.

Mussen, F., S. Salek, and S. Walker (2007). A quantitative approach to benefit-risk assessment of medicines–Part 1: the development of a new model using multi-criteria decision analysis. *Pharmacoepidemiology and Drug Safety (Suppl.) 16*, 2–15.

Nahler, G. (2009). WHO-adverse reaction terminology (WHO-ART). *Dictionary of Pharmaceutical Medicine*, 192–193.

Najafzadeh, M., S. Schneeweiss, N. Choudhry, K. Bykov, K. H. Kahler, D. P. Martin, and J. J. Gagne (2015). A unified framework for classification of methods for benefit-risk assessment. *Value in Health 18*, 250–259.

Nandedkar, S. B. and Y. C. Waykole (2016). Toxicogenomics and its applications. *World Journal of Pharmacy and Pharmaceutical Sciences 5*, 699–707.

National Research Council (2007). *Applications of Toxicogenomic Technologies to Predictive Toxicology and Risk Assessment.* National Academies Press.

Naus, J. I. (1965a). the distribution of the size of the maximum cluster of points on a line. *Journal of the American Statistical Association 60*(310), 532–538.

Naus, J. I. (1965b). clustering of random points in two dimensions. *Biometrika 52*(1-2), 263–266.

NCI (2009). *Common Terminology Criteria for Adverse Events (CTCAE) version 4.0.* Number 09-5410. National Cancer Institute.

Nelson, C., L. Wang, L. Fang, W. Weng, F. Cheng, M. Hepner, J. Lin, C. Garnett, and S. Ramanathan (2015). A Quantitative Framework to Evaluate Proarrhythmic Risk in a First-in-Human Study to Support Waiver of a Thorough QT Study. *Clinical Pharmacology & Therapeutics 98*(6), 630–638.

Nelson, J., A. Cook, and O. Yu (2009). Evaluation of signal detection methods for use in prospective postlicensure medical product safety surveillance. Technical report, FDA Sentinel Initiative Safety Signal Identification contract (http://www.fda.gov/OHRMS/DOCKETS/98fr/FDA-2009-N-0192-rpt.pdf).

Nelson, J. C., D. Boudreau, R. Wellman, O. Yu, A. J. Cook, J. Maro, R. Ouellet-hellstrom, J. Flyod, S. R. Heckbert, S. Pinheiro, M. Reichman, and A. Shoaibi (2016). Improving sequential safety surveillance planning methods for routine assessment that use regression adjustment or weighting to control confounding. Technical report, The Sentinel System.

https://www.sentinelinitiative.org/sites/default/files/Methods/Mini-Sentinel_Methods_Improving-Sequential-Safety-Surveillance_Report.pdf.

Nelson, J. C., A. J. Cook, O. Yu, C. Dominguez, S. Zhao, S. K. Greene, B. H. Fireman, S. J. Jacobsen, E. S. Weintraub, and L. A. Jackson (2012). Challenges in the design and analysis of sequentially monitored postmarket safety surveillance evaluations using electronic observational health care data. *Pharmacoepidemiology and Drug Safety 21*(S1), 62–71.

Nelson, J. C., O. Yu, C. P. Dominguez-Islas, A. J. Cook, D. Peterson, S. K. Greene, W. K. Yih, M. F. Daley, S. J. Jacobsen, and N. P. Klein (2013). Adapting group sequential methods to observational postlicensure vaccine safety surveillance: results of a pentavalent combination dtap-ipv-hib vaccine safety study. *American Journal of Epidemiology 177*(2), 131–141.

Nelson, W. B. (2003). *Recurrent Events Data Analysis for Product Repairs, Disease Recurrences, and Other Applications*. SIAM.

Neyman, J. (1923). On the application of probability theory to agricultural experiments. Essay on principles. Section 9. *Roczniki Nauk Rolniczych Tom X* (5), 465–480. English Translation in Statistical Science.

Neyman, J. (1962). Two breakthroughs in the theory of statistical decision making. *Reviews of International Statistical Institute 30*(1), 11–27.

Niraula, S., B. Seruga, A. Ocana, T. Shao, R. Goldstein, I. F. Tannock, and E. Amir (2012). The price we pay for progress: a meta-analysis of harms of newly approved anticancer drugs. *Journal of Clinical Oncology 30*(24), 3012–3019.

Nissen, S. E. and K. Wolski (2007). Effect of rosiglitazone on the risk of myocardial infarction and death from cardiovascular causes. *New England Journal of Medicine 356*(24), 2457–2471.

Obrezanova, O., G. Csányi, J. M. Gola, and M. D. Segall (2007). Gaussian processes: a method for automatic QSAR modeling of ADME properties. *Journal of Chemical Information and Modeling 47*(5), 1847–1857.

O"Brien, P. C. and T. R. Fleming (1979). A multiple testing procedure for clinical trials. *Biometrics 35*(3), 549–556.

Odani, M., S. Fukimbara, and T. Sato (2017). A Bayesian meta-analytic approach for safety signal detection in randomized clinical trials. *Clinical Trials 14*(2), 192–200.

O'Hara, T., L. Virág, A. Varró, and Y. Rudy (2011). Simulation of the undiseased human cardiac ventricular action potential: model formulation and experimental validation. *PLoS Comput Biol 7*(5), e1002061.

Olkin, I. and H. Saner (2001). Approximations for trimmed Fisher procedures in research synthesis. *Statistical Methods in Medical Research 10*(4), 267–276.

Onakpoya, I. J., C. J. Heneghan, and J. K. Aronson (2016). Worldwide withdrawal of medicinal products because of adverse drug reactions: A systematic review and analysis. *Critical Reviews in Toxicology 46*(6), 477–489.

O'Neill, R. T. and A. Szarfman (1999). Discussion (on "Bayesian Data Mining in Large Frequency Tables, with an Application to the FDA Spontaneous Reporting System" by W. Dumouchel. *The American Statistician 53*(3), 190–196.

O'Quigley, J. and M. Conaway (2010). Continual reassessment and related dose-finding designs. *Statistical Science 25*(2), 202–216.

O'Quigley, J., M. Pepe, and L. Fisher (1990). Continual reassessment method: A practical design for phase I clinical trials in cancer. *Biometrics 46*(1), 33–48.

Oziolor, E. M., J. W. Bickham, and C. W. Matson (2017). Evolutionary toxicology in an omics world. *Evolutionary Applications 10*, 752–761.

Pacurariu, A. C., S. M. Straus, G. Trifiro, M. J. Schuemie, R. Gini, R. Herings, G. Mazzaglia, G. Picelli, L. Scotti, and L. Pedersen (2015). Useful interplay between spontaneous ADR reports and electronic healthcare records in signal detection. *Drug Safety 38*(12), 1201–1210.

Paliwal, S. K., M. Pal, and A. A. Siddiqui (2010). Quantitative structure activity relationship analysis of angiotensin II AT1 receptor antagonists. *Medicinal Chemistry Research 19*(5), 475–489.

Park, B. K., M. Pirmohamed, and N. R. Kitteringham (1998). Role of drug disposition in drug hypersensitivity: a chemical, molecular, and clinical perspective. *Chemical Research in Toxicology 11*(9), 969–988.

Parker, R. M. and R. Hood (2006). Testing for reproductive toxicity. In R. D. Hood (Ed.), *Developmental and Reproductive Toxicology. A Practical Approach*, pp. 425–487. Taylor & Francis Group, LLC.

Patadia, V. K., M. J. Schuemie, P. Coloma, R. Herings, J. van der Lei, S. Straus, M. Sturkenboom, and G. Trifirò (2015). Evaluating performance of electronic healthcare records and spontaneous reporting data in drug safety signal detection. *International Journal of Clinical Pharmacy 37*(1), 94–104.

Pearl, J. (1995). Causal diagrams for empirical research. *Biometrika* 82(4), 669–710.

Pearl, J. (2005). Influence diagrams: Historical and personal perspectives. *Decision Analysis* 2(4), 232–234.

Pearl, J. (2009a). Causal inference in statistics: An overview. *Statistics Surveys 3*, 96–146.

Pearl, J. (2009b). *Causality: Models, Reasoning, and Inference* (2nd ed.). Cambridge University Press, New York. (Original edition, 2000).

Pearl, J. and E. Bareinboim (2014). External validity: From do-calculus to transportability across populations. *Statistical Science* 29(4), 579–595.

Pearl, J., M. Glymour, and N. Jewell (2016). *Causal Inference in Statistics. A Primer*. John Wiley & Sons.

Pena, E. A., R. L. Strawderman, and M. Hollander (2001). Nonparametric estimation with recurrent event data. *Journal of the American Statistical Association* 96(456), 1299–1315.

Perkins, E., N. Garcia-Reyero, S. Edwards, C. Wittwehr, D. Villeneuve, D. Lyons, and G. Ankley (2015). The adverse outcome pathway: A conceptual framework to support toxicity testing in the twenty-first century. *Computational Systems Toxicology*, 1–26.

Perkins, R., H. Fang, W. Tong, and W. J. Welsh (2003). Quantitative structure-activity relationship methods: Perspectives on drug discovery and toxicology. *Environmental Toxicology and Chemistry* 22(8), 1666–1679.

Petitti, D. B. (2000). *Meta-Analysis, Decision Analysis, and Cost-Effectiveness Analysis: Methods for Quantitative Synthesis in Medicine*. OUP USA.

Peto, R. (1974). Editorial: Guidelines on the analysis of tumour rates and death rates in experimental animals. *British Journal of Cancer* 29(2), 101.

Peto, R., M. Pike, N. Day, R. Gray, P. Lee, S. Parish, J. Peto, S. Richards, and J. Wahrendorf (1979). Guidelines for simple, sensitive significance tests for carcinogenic effects in long-term animal experiments. *IARC Monographs on the Evaluation of the Carcinogenic Risk of Chemicals to Humans* (Suppl. 2), 311–426.

Petri, H., H. De Vet, J. Naus, and J. Urquhart (1988). Prescription sequence analysis: a new and fast method for assessing certain adverse reactions of prescription drugs in large populations. *Statistics in Medicine* 7(11), 1171–1175.

Phillips, L. D. (2011). *Benefit-Risk Methodology Project: Work Package 2 Report: Applicability of Current Tools and Processes for Regulatory Benefit–Risk Assessment*. European Medicines Agency.

Phillips, L. D., A. Sashegyi, J. Felli, and R. Noel (2013). Benefit-risk modeling of medicinal products: Methods and applications. In A. Sashegyi, J. Felli, and R. Noel (Eds.), *Benefit-Risk Assessment in Pharmaceutical Research and Development*, pp. 59–96. Chapman and Hall/CRC, Boca Raton, FL.

Pigott, T. D. (2001). A review of methods for missing data. *Educational research and evaluation* 7(4), 353–383.

Platt, R. and R. Carnahan (2012). The US Food and Drug Administration's Mini-Sentinel Program. *Pharmacoepidemiology and Drug Safety* 21(S1), 1–303.

Pocock, S. J. (1977). Group sequential methods in the design and analysis of clinical trials. *Biometrika* 64(2), 191–199.

Pocock, S. J., C. A. Ariti, T. J. Collier, and D. Wang (2011). The win ratio: a new approach to the analysis of composite endpoints in clinical trials based on clinical priorities. *European Heart Journal* 33(2), 176–182.

Polishchuk, P. G., E. N. Muratov, A. G. Artemenko, O. G. Kolumbin, N. N. Muratov, and V. E. Kuzmin (2009). Application of random forest approach to QSAR prediction of aquatic toxicity. *Journal of Chemical Information and Modeling* 49(11), 2481–2488.

Pratt, N., E. W. Chan, N.-K. Choi, M. Kimura, T. Kimura, K. Kubota, E. C.-C. Lai, K. K. Man, N. Ooba, and B.-J. Park (2015). Prescription sequence symmetry analysis: assessing risk, temporality, and consistency for adverse drug reactions across datasets in five countries. *Pharmacoepidemiology and Drug Safety* 24(8), 858–864.

Psaty, B. and S. Burke (2006). Protecting the health of the public–Institute of Medicine recommendations on drug safety. *The New England Journal of Medicine* 355(17), 1753–1755.

Pugsley, M. K., S. Authier, and M. Curtis (2008). Principles of safety pharmacology. *British Journal of Pharmacology* 154(7), 1382–1399.

Qin, C., K. Q. Tanis, A. A. Podtelezhnikov, W. E. Glaab, F. D. Sistare, and J. J. DeGeorge (2016). Toxicogenomics in drug development: a match made in heaven? *Expert Opinion on Drug Metabolism & Toxicology* 12(8), 847–849.

Qureshi, Z. P., E. Seoane-Vazquez, R. Rodriguez-Monguio, K. B. Stevenson, and S. L. Szeinbach (2011). Market withdrawal of new molecular entities approved in the United States from 1980 to 2009. *Pharmacoepidemiology and Drug Safety 20*(7), 772–777.

Racoosin, J. A., M. A. Robb, R. E. Sherman, and J. Woodcock (2012). FDA's Sentinel Initiative: Active Surveillance to Identify Safety Signals. In B. L. Strom, S. E. Kimmel, and S. Hennessy (Eds.), *Pharmacoepidemiology, Fifth Edition*, pp. 534–554. John Wiley & Sons, Ltd.

Raju, G., K. Gurumurthi, R. Domike, D. Kazandjian, G. Blumenthal, R. Pazdur, and J. Woodcock (2016). A benefit–risk analysis approach to capture regulatory decision-making: Non-small cell lung cancer. *Clinical Pharmacology & Therapeutics 100*(6), 672–684.

Ransohoff, R. M. (2007). Natalizumab for multiple sclerosis. *New England Journal of Medicine 356*(25), 2622–2629.

Rasmussen, C. and C. Williams (2006). *Gaussian Processes for Machine Learning*. The MIT Press, Cambridge.

Rawson, N. S. (2016). Drug safety: withdrawn medications are only part of the picture. *BMC Medicine 14*(1), 28.

Reisinger, K. S., M. L. H. Brown, J. Xu, B. J. Sullivan, G. S. Marshall, B. Nauert, D. O. Matson, P. E. Silas, F. Schödel, and J. O. Gress (2006). A combination measles, mumps, rubella, and varicella vaccine (proquad) given to 4-to 6-year-old healthy children vaccinated previously with mm-rii and varivax. *Pediatrics 117*(2), 265–272.

Renganathan, M., H. Wei, and Y. Zhao (2017). Cardiac Action Potential Measurement in Human Embryonic Stem Cell Cardiomyocytes for Cardiac Safety Studies Using Manual Patch-Clamp Electrophysiology. *Stem Cell-Derived Models in Toxicology*, 37–56.

Richardson, T. and P. Spirtes (2002). Ancestral graph Markov models. *Annals of Statistics 30*(4), 962–1030.

Riley, R. D., P. C. Lambert, and G. Abo-Zaid (2010). Meta-analysis of individual participant data: rationale, conduct, and reporting. *British Medical Journal 340*, c221. (doi: 10.1136/bmj.c221).

Ring, M. and B. M. Eskofier (2015). Data mining in the US National Toxicology Program (NTP) database reveals a potential bias regarding liver tumors in rodents irrespective of the test agent. *PloS One 10*(2), e0116488. (doi.org/10.1371/journal.pone.0116488).

Robb, M. A., J. A. Racoosin, C. Worrall, S. Chapman, T. Coster, and F. E. Cunningham (2012). Active surveillance of postmarket medical product safety in the federal partners' collaboration. *Medical Care 50*(11), 948–953.

Robbins, H. (1951). Asymptotically subminimax solutions of compound statistical decision problems. In J. Neyman (Ed.), *Proceedings of the Second Berkeley Symposium on Mathematical Statistics and Probability*. University of California Press, Mountain View, CA.

Robbins, H. (1964). The empirical Bayes approach to statistical decision problems. *The Annals of Mathematical Statistics 35*(1), 1–20.

Robins, J. (1986). A new approach to causal inference in mortality studies with a sustained exposure period — application to control of the healthy worker survivor effect. *Mathematical Modelling 7*(9-12), 1393–512.

Robins, J. (1987). A graphical approach to the identification and estimation of causal parameters in mortality studies with sustained exposure periods. *Journal of Chronic Diseases 40*, 139S–161S.

Robins, J. (1992). Estimation of the time-dependent accelerated failure time model in the presence of confounding factors. *Biometrika 79*(2), 321–334.

Robins, J., M. Sued, Q. Lei-Gomez, and A. Rotnitzky (2007). Comment: Performance of double-robust estimators when" inverse probability" weights are highly variable. *Statistical Science 22*(4), 544–559.

Robins, J. and A. Tsiatis (1992). Semiparametric estimation of an accelerated failure time model with time-dependent covariates. *Biometrics 48*, 479–95.

Robins, J. M., M. A. Hernan, and B. Brumback (2000). Marginal structural models and causal inference in epidemiology. *Epidemiology 11*(5), 550–560.

Robins, J. M. and A. Rotnitzky (1992). Recovery of information and adjustment for dependent censoring using surrogate markers. In N. P. Jewell, K. Dietz, and V. T. Farewell (Eds.), *AIDS Epidemiology: Methodological Issues*, pp. 297–331. Springer.

Robins, J. M., A. Rotnitzky, and L. P. Zhao (1994). Estimation of regression coefficients when some regressors are not always observed. *Journal of the American Statistical Association 89*(427), 846–866.

Robins, J. M., A. Rotnitzky, and L. P. Zhao (1995). Analysis of semiparametric regression models for repeated outcomes in the presence of missing data. *Journal of the American Statistical Association 90*(429), 106–121.

Rodriguez, E. M., J. A. Staffa, and D. J. Graham (2001). The role of databases in drug postmarketing surveillance. *Pharmacoepidemiology and Drug Safety 10*(5), 407–410.

Roggen, E. L. (2011). In vitro toxicity testing in the twenty-first century. *Frontiers in Pharmacology 2.* (doi: 10.3389/fphar.2011.00003).

Rondeau, V. (2010). Statistical models for recurrent events and death: Application to cancer events. *Mathematical and Computer Modelling 52*(7), 949–955.

Roquemore, L., M. A. Kauss, C. Hather, N. Thomas, and H. Uppal (2017). In Vitro Cardiotoxicity Investigation Using High Content Analysis and Human Stem Cell-Derived Models. In M. Clements and L. Roquemore (Eds.), *Stem Cell-Derived Models in Toxicology*, pp. 247–269. Springer.

Rose, C. E., S. W. Martin, K. A. Wannemuehler, and B. D. Plikaytis (2006). On the use of zero-inflated and hurdle models for modeling vaccine adverse event count data. *Journal of Biopharmaceutical Statistics 16*(4), 463–481.

Rosenbaum, P. and D. Rubin (1983). The central role of the propensity score in observational studies for causal effects. *Biometrika 70*(1), 41–55.

Rosenbaum, P. and D. Rubin (1984). Reducing bias in observational studies using subclassification on the propensity score. *Journal of the American Statistical Association 79*(387), 516–524.

Rosenbaum, P. R. and D. B. Rubin (1985). Constructing a control group using multivariate matched sampling methods that incorporate the propensity score. *The American Statistician 39*(1), 33–38.

Rosenblatt, M. (2017). The changing face of clinical trials: The large pharmaceutical company perspective. *New England Journal of Medicine 376*(1), 52–60.

Rosenkranz, G. K. (2009). Modeling laboratory data from clinical trials. *Computational Statistics & Data Analysis 53*(3), 812–819.

Rosner, G. L., W. Stadler, and M. J. Ratain (2002). Randomized discontinuation design: application to cytostatic antineoplastic agents. *Journal of Clinical Oncology 20*(22), 4478–4484.

Rothman, K. (1986). *Modern Epidemiology*. Little & Brown, Boston.

Roy, K., S. Kar, and R. N. Das (2015). *A Primer on QSAR / QSPR Modeling: Fundamental Concepts*. Springer.

Roy, K. and I. Mitra (2011). On various metrics used for validation of predictive QSAR models with applications in virtual screening and focused library design. *Combinatorial Chemistry & High Throughput Screening 14*(6), 450–474.

Roy, P. P. and K. Roy (2009). QSAR studies of CYP2D6 inhibitor aryloxypropanolamines using 2D and 3D descriptors. *Chemical Biology & Drug Design 73*(4), 442–455.

Røysland, K. (2012). Counterfactual analyses with graphical models based on local independence. *The Annals of Statistics 40*(4), 2162–2194.

Rubin, D. (1974). Estimating causal effects of treatments in randomized and nonrandomized studies. *Journal of Educational Psychology 66*(5), 688–701.

Rubin, D. (1978). Bayesian inference for causal effects: The role of randomization . *The Annals of Statistics* (1), 34–58.

Rubin, D. (2005). Causal inference using potential outcomes: design, modeling, decisions. *Journal of the American Statistical Association 100*(469), 322–331.

Rubin, D. B. (1976). Inference and missing data. *Biometrika 63*(3), 581–592.

Rubin, D. B. (1987). *Multiple imputation for nonresponse in surveys*. John Wiley & Sons.

Rubin, D. B. (2001). Using propensity scores to help design observational studies: application to the tobacco litigation. *Health Services and Outcomes Research Methodology 2*(3-4), 169–188.

Ryan, L. and G. Molenberghs (1999). Statistical methods for developmental toxicity: Analysis of clustered multivariate binary data. *Annals of the New York Academy of Sciences 895*(1), 196–211.

Ryan, P. B., D. Madigan, P. E. Stang, J. Marc Overhage, J. A. Racoosin, and A. G. Hartzema (2012). Empirical assessment of methods for risk identification in healthcare data: results from the experiments of the Observational Medical Outcomes Partnership. *Statistics in Medicine 31*(30), 4401–4415.

Sarkar, S. K. (1998). Some probability inequalities for ordered MTP2 random variables: a proof of the Simes conjecture. *Annals of Statistics 26*(2), 494–504.

Sarkar, S. K. and C.-K. Chang (1997). The simes method for multiple hypothesis testing with positively dependent test statistics. *Journal of the American Statistical Association 92*(440), 1601–1608.

Schafer, J. L. (1997). *Analysis of incomplete multivariate data*. Chapman and Hall/CRC.

Schafer, J. L. (1999). Multiple imputation: a primer. *Statistical methods in medical research 8*(1), 3–15.

Schneeweiss, S. and S. Suissa (2012). Advanced approaches to controlling confounding in pharmacoepidemiologic studies. In B. L. Strom, S. E. Kimmel, and S. Hennessy (Eds.), *Pharmacoepidemiology, Fifth Edition*, pp. 868–891. John Wiley & Sons, Ltd.

Schoenfeld, D. A. (1983). Sample-size formula for the proportional-hazards regression model. *Biometrics 39*(2), 499–503.

Schuemie, M. J., P. M. Coloma, H. Straatman, R. M. Herings, G. Trifirò, J. N. Matthews, D. Prieto-Merino, M. Molokhia, L. Pedersen, and R. Gini (2012). Using electronic health care records for drug safety signal detection: a comparative evaluation of statistical methods. *Medical Care 50*(10), 890–897.

Schüürmann, G., R.-U. Ebert, J. Chen, B. Wang, and R. Kühne (2008). External validation and prediction employing the predictive squared correlation coefficient–Test set activity mean vs training set activity mean. *Journal of Chemical Information and Modeling 48*(11), 2140–2145.

Schwaighofer, A., T. Schroeter, S. Mika, J. Laub, A. Ter Laak, D. Sülzle, U. Ganzer, N. Heinrich, and K.-R. Müller (2007). Accurate solubility prediction with error bars for electrolytes: A machine learning approach. *Journal of Chemical Information and Modeling 47*(2), 407–424.

Schwarz, G. (1962). Asymptotic shapes of bayes sequential testing regions. *The Annals of Mathematical Statistics*, 224–236.

Schwarzer, G., J. R. Carpenter, and G. Rücker (2015). *Meta-Analysis with R*. Springer.

Sébastien, B., D. Hoffman, C. Rigaux, F. Pellissier, and J. Msihid (2016). Model averaging in concentration–QT analyses. *Pharmaceutical Statistics 15*(6), 450–458.

Sedgwick, P. (2014). Retrospective cohort studies: advantages and disadvantages. *British Medical Journal 348*, g1072.

Seidling, H. and D. Bates (2014). The pharmacoepidemiology of medication error. In B. Strom, S. Kimmel, and S. Hennessy (Eds.), *Pharmacoepidemiology, 5th Edition*, pp. 840–51. Chichester, UK: John Wiley & Sons, Ltd.

Setoguchi, S., S. Schneeweiss, M. A. Brookhart, R. J. Glynn, and E. F. Cook (2008). Evaluating uses of data mining techniques in propensity score estimation: a simulation study. *Pharmacoepidemiology and drug safety 17*(6), 546–555.

Shaffer, J. P. (1986). Modified sequentially rejective multiple test procedures. *Journal of the American Statistical Association 81*(395), 826–831.

Shickel, B., P. J. Tighe, A. Bihorac, and P. Rashidi (2017). Deep EHR: A survey of recent advances in deep learning techniques for electronic health record (EHR) analysis. *IEEE Journal of Biomedical and Health Informatics*.

Shih, M., T. Lai, J. Heyse, and J. Chen (2010). Sequential generalized likelihood ratio tests for vaccine safety evaluation. *Statistics in Medicine 29*(26), 2698–2708.

Shinde, S. and S. Y. Crawford (2016). The science of safety–an emerging concept in medication use and research. *INNOVATIONS in Pharmacy 7*(3), 1–9.

Shinefield, H., S. Black, M. Thear, D. Coury, K. Reisinger, E. Rothstein, J. Xu, J. Hartzel, B. Evans, and L. Digilio (2006). Safety and immunogenicity of a measles, mumps, rubella and varicella vaccine given with combined haemophilus influenzae type b conjugate/hepatitis b vaccines and combined diphtheria-tetanus-acellular pertussis vaccines. *The Pediatric Infectious Disease Journal 25*(4), 287–292.

Sills, J. M. (1989). World Health Organization Adverse Reaction Terminology Dictionary. *Drug Information Journal 23*(2), 211–216.

Silva, I. R. (2017). Type i error probability spending for post-market drug and vaccine safety surveillance with poisson data. *Methodology and Computing in Applied Probability*, 1–12.

Silva, I. R. (2018). Type i error probability spending for post–market drug and vaccine safety surveillance with binomial data. *Statistics in Medicine 37*(1), 107–118.

Silva, I. R. and M. Kulldorff (2015). Continuous versus group sequential analysis for post-market drug and vaccine safety surveillance. *Biometrics 71*, 851–858.

Simmonds, M. C., J. P. Higginsa, L. A. Stewartb, J. F. Tierneyb, M. J. Clarke, and S. G. Thompson (2005). Meta-analysis of individual patient data from randomized trials: a review of methods used in practice. *Clinical Trials 2*(3), 209–217.

Simon, R., L. Rubinstein, S. G. Arbuck, M. C. Christian, B. Freidlin, and J. Collins (1997). Accelerated titration designs for phase I clinical trials in oncology. *Journal of the National Cancer Institute 89*(15), 1138–1147.

Simpson, E. H. (1951). The interpretation of interaction in contingency tables. *Journal of the Royal Statistical Society. Series B (Methodological) 13*(2), 238–241.

Simpson, S. E. (2013). A positive event dependence model for self-controlled case series with applications in postmarketing surveillance. *Biometrics 69*(1), 128–136.

Singh, S. and Y. K. Loke (2012). Drug safety assessment in clinical trials: methodological challenges and opportunities. *Trials 13*(1), 138.

Singleton, J. A., J. C. Lloyd, G. T. Mootrey, M. E. Salive, and R. T. Chen (1999). An overview of the vaccine adverse event reporting system (VAERS) as a surveillance system. *Vaccine 17*(22), 2908–2917.

Sioutos, N., S. de Coronado, M. W. Haber, F. W. Hartel, W.-L. Shaiu, and L. W. Wright (2007). NCI thesaurus: a semantic model integrating cancer-related clinical and molecular information. *Journal of Biomedical Informatics 40*(1), 30–43.

Slater, E. E. (2005). Today's FDA. *The New England Journal of Medicine 352*(3), 293.

Smith, S. W. (2007). Sidelining safety–The FDA's inadequate response to the IOM. *New England Journal of Medicine 357*(10), 960–963.

Soldatow, V. Y., E. L. LeCluyse, L. G. Griffith, and I. Rusyn (2013). In vitro models for liver toxicity testing. *Toxicology Research 2*(1), 23–39.

Sonesson, C. and D. Bock (2003). A review and discussion of prospective statistical surveillance in public health. *Journal of the Royal Statistical Society: Series A 166*(1), 5–21.

Soric, B. (1989). Statistical discoveries and effect size estimation. *Journal of the American Statistical Association 84*, 608–10.

Souayah, N., H. A. Yacoub, H. M. Khan, K. Farhad, L. S. Mehyar, L. Maybodi, D. L. Menkes, and A. I. Qureshi (2012). Guillain–Barré syndrome after influenza vaccination in the United States, a report from the CDC/FDA vaccine adverse event reporting system (1990–2009). *Journal of Clinical Neuromuscular Disease 14*(2), 66–71.

Southworth, H. and J. E. Heffernan (2012a). Extreme value modelling of laboratory safety data from clinical studies. *Pharmaceutical Statistics 11*(5), 361–366.

Southworth, H. and J. E. Heffernan (2012b). Multivariate extreme value modelling of laboratory safety data from clinical studies. *Pharmaceutical Statistics 11*(5), 367–372.

Spiegelhalter, D., O. Grigg, R. Kinsman, and T. Treasure (2003). Risk-adjusted sequential probability ratio tests: applications to bristol, shipman and adult cardiac surgery. *International Journal for Quality in Health Care 15*(1), 7–13.

Ståhle, L. and S. Wold (1987). Partial least squares analysis with cross-validation for the two-class problem: A Monte Carlo study. *Journal of Chemometrics 1*(3), 185–196.

Stang, P., P. Ryan, A. G. Hartzema, D. Madigan, J. Marc Overhage, E. Welebob, C. G. Reich, and T. Scarnecchia (2014). Development and evaluation of infrastructure and analytic methods for systematic drug safety surveillance: lessons and resources from the observational medical outcomes partnership. In E. Andres and N. Moore (Eds.), *Mann's Pharmacovigilance*, pp. 453–461. John Wiley & Sons, Ltd.

Steiner, S., R. Cook, V. Farewell, and T. Treasure (2000). Monitoring surgical performance using risk-adjusted cumulative sum charts. *Biostatistics 1*(4), 441–452.

Stinnett, A. A. and J. Mullahy (1998). Net health benefits: a new framework for the analysis of uncertainty in cost-effectiveness analysis. *Medical Decision Making (Suppl.) 18*(2), S68–S80.

Stockbridge, N., J. Morganroth, R. R. Shah, and C. Garnett (2013). Dealing with global safety issues. *Drug Safety 36*(3), 167–182.

Stone, A., C. Wheeler, and A. Barge (2007). Improving the design of phase II trials of cytostatic anticancer agents. *Contemporary Clinical Trials 28*(2), 138–145.

Storer, B. (1989). Design and analysis of phase I clinical trials. *Biometrics 45*(3), 925–37.

Storey, J. (2002). A direct approach to false discovery rates. *Journal of the Royal Statistical Society: Series B 64*, 479–498.

Storey, J. (2003). The positive false discovery rate: A Bayesian interpretation of the q-value. *The Annals of Statistics 31*, 2013–35.

Strom, B. L. (2006). *Pharmacoepidemiology*. John Wiley & Sons.

Stuart, E. (2010). Matching methods for causal inference: A review and a look forward. *Statistical Science 25*(1), 1–21.

Stuart, E. A., E. DuGoff, M. Abrams, D. Salkever, and D. Steinwachs (2013). Estimating causal effects in observational studies using electronic health data: challenges and (some) solutions. *Egems 1*(3).

Suchard, M. A., I. Zorych, S. E. Simpson, M. J. Schuemie, P. B. Ryan, and D. Madigan (2013). Empirical performance of the self-controlled case series design: lessons for developing a risk identification and analysis system. *Drug Safety 36*(1), 83–93.

Sun, W. (2016). Cardiotoxicity testing in drug development. *SM Journal of Cardiovascular Disorders 1*(1), 1–4.

Suter, L., L. E. Babiss, and E. B. Wheeldon (2004). Toxicogenomics in predictive toxicology in drug development. *Chemistry & Biology 11*(2), 161–171.

Svetnik, V., A. Liaw, C. Tong, J. C. Culberson, R. P. Sheridan, and B. P. Feuston (2003). Random forest: a classification and regression tool for compound classification and QSAR modeling. *Journal of Chemical Information and Computer Sciences 43*(6), 1947–1958.

Svetnik, V., T. Wang, C. Tong, A. Liaw, R. P. Sheridan, and Q. Song (2005). Boosting: An ensemble learning tool for compound classification and QSAR modeling. *Journal of Chemical Information and Modeling 45*(3), 786–799.

Sweeting, M. J., A. J. Sutton, and P. C. Lambert (2004). What to add to nothing? Use and avoidance of continuity corrections in meta-analysis of sparse data. *Statistics in Medicine 23*(9), 1351–1375.

Szarfman, A. and J. Levine (2006). Memorandum: NDA 21-144 KETEK (telithromycin) 400MG tablets®(Sanofi-Aventis): data mining analysis of adverse events and outcomes reported for telithromycin and 15 comparator drugs (AERS data). (https://www.fda.gov/ohrms/dockets/ac/06/briefing/2006-4266b1-02-06-FDA-appendic-f.pdf).

Szarfman, A., S. G. Machado, and R. T. ONeill (2002). Use of screening algorithms and computer systems to efficiently signal higher-than-expected combinations of drugs and events in the US FDA's spontaneous reports database. *Drug Safety 25*(6), 381–392.

Takeuchi, Y., T. Shinozaki, and Y. Matsuyama (2018). A comparison of estimators from self-controlled case series, case-crossover design, and sequence symmetry analysis for pharmacoepidemiological studies. *BMC Medical Research Methodology 18*(1), 4.

Tamer, E. (2010). Partial identification in econometrics. *Annual Review of Econometrics 2*(1), 167–195.

Tarlow, D., K. Swersky, L. Charlin, I. Sutskever, and R. Zemel (2013). Stochastic k-neighborhood selection for supervised and unsupervised learning. In *Proceedings of the 30th International Conference on Machine Learning*, pp. 199–207. Atlanta, Georgia, USA.

Tarone, R. (1990). A modified Bonferroni method for discrete data. *Biometrics 46*, 515–22.

Tatonetti, N. P., G. H. Fernald, and R. B. Altman (2011). A novel signal detection algorithm for identifying hidden drug-drug interactions in adverse event reports. *Journal of the American Medical Informatics Association 19*(1), 79–85.

Temlyakov, V. N. (2000). Weak greedy algorithms. *Advances in Computational Mathematics 12*(2), 213–227.

Temple, R. J. (1991). The regulatory evolution of the integrated safety summary. *Drug Information Journal 25*(4), 485–492.

Tervonen, T. and J. R. Figueira (2008). A survey on stochastic multicriteria acceptability analysis methods. *Journal of Multi-Criteria Decision Analysis 15*(1-2), 1–14.

Tervonen, T. and R. Lahdelma (2007). Implementing stochastic multicriteria acceptability analysis. *European Journal of Operational Research 178*(2), 500–513.

Tervonen, T., G. van Valkenhoef, E. Buskens, H. L. Hillege, and D. Postmus (2011). A stochastic multicriteria model for evidence-based decision making in drug benefit-risk analysis. *Statistics in Medicine 30*(12), 1419–1428.

Thall, P. F. and J. D. Cook (2006). Using both efficacy and toxicity for dose-finding. In S. Chevret (Ed.), *Statistical Methods for Dose-Finding Experiments*, pp. 275–285. Wiley Online Library.

Thall, P. F., H. Q. Nguyen, and E. H. Estey (2008). Patient-specific dose finding based on bivariate outcomes and covariates. *Biometrics 64*(4), 1126–1136.

Thall, P. F. and K. E. Russell (1998). A strategy for dose-finding and safety monitoring based on efficacy and adverse outcomes in phase I/II clinical trials. *Biometrics*, 251–264.

Thomas, R. S. and M. D. Waters (2016). *Toxicogenomics in Predictive Carcinogenicity*. Royal Society of Chemistry.

Tian, L., T. Cai, M. A. Pfeffer, N. Piankov, P.-Y. Cremieux, and L. Wei (2009). Exact and efficient inference procedure for meta-analysis and its application to the analysis of independent 2×2 tables with all available data but without artificial continuity correction. *Biostatistics 10*(2), 275–281.

Tibshirani, R. (1996). Regression shrinkage and selection via the lasso. *Journal of the Royal Statistical Society: Series B 58*(1), 267–288.

Tighiouart, M., Y. Liu, and A. Rogatko (2014). Escalation with overdose control using time to toxicity for cancer phase I clinical trials. *PloS One 9*(3), e93070.

Ting, N. (2006). *Dose Finding in Drug Development*. Springer.

Todeschini, R. and V. Consonni (2008). *Handbook of Molecular Descriptors*, Volume 11. John Wiley & Sons.

Todeschini, R. and V. Consonni (2009). *Molecular Descriptors for Chemoinformatics*, Volume 41. John Wiley & Sons.

Tong, W., Q. Xie, H. Hong, L. Shi, H. Fang, and R. Perkins (2004). Assessment of prediction confidence and domain extrapolation of two structure-activity relationship models for predicting estrogen receptor binding activity. *Environmental health perspectives*, 1249–1254.

Trontell, A. (2004). Expecting the unexpected–Drug safety, pharmacovigilance, and the prepared mind. *New England Journal of Medicine 351*(14), 1385–1387.

Tsiatis, A. A. (1990). Estimating regression parameters using linear rank tests for censored data. *The Annals of Statistics 18*(1), 354–372.

Tsiropoulos, I., M. Andersen, and J. Hallas (2009). Adverse events with use of antiepileptic drugs: a prescription and event symmetry analysis. *Pharmacoepidemiology and Drug Safety 18*(6), 483–491.

Tsong, Y., M. Shen, J. Zhong, and J. Zhang (2008). Statistical Issues of QT Prolongation Assessment Based on Linear Concentration Modeling. *Journal of Biopharmaceutical Statistics 18*(3), 564–584.

Turnbull, B. W., E. J. Iwano, W. S. Burnett, H. L. Howe, and L. C. Clark (1989). Monitoring for clusters of disease: application to leukemia incidence in upstate new york. *American Journal of Epidemiology 132*(Suppl. 1), 136–143.

Turner, J. R., D. R. Karnad, and S. Kothari (2017). *Cardiovascular Safety in Drug Development and Therapeutic Use*. Springer.

Tyl, R. W. and M. C. Marr (2006). Developmental toxicity testing–methodology. In R. D. Hood (Ed.), *Developmental and Reproductive Toxicology-A Practical Approach*, pp. 201–254. Taylor & Francis Group, LLC.

Uehara, T., C. Kondo, Y. Morikawa, H. Hanafusa, S. Ueda, Y. Minowa, N. Nakatsu, A. Ono, T. Maruyama, and I. Kato (2013). Toxicogenomic biomarkers for renal papillary injury in rats. *Toxicology 303*, 1–8.

Uehara, T., Y. Wang, and W. Tong (2015). Toxicogenomic and pharma-cogenomic biomarkers for drug discovery and personalized medicine. In V. Preedy and V. Patel (Eds.), *General Methods in Biomarker Research and Their Applications*, pp. 75–109. Springer.

Valerio, L. G. (2011). *In silico* toxicology models and databases as FDA Critical Path Initiative toolkits. *Human Genomics 5*(3), 200.

Valerio, L. G. and K. P. Cross (2012). Characterization and validation of an in silico toxicology model to predict the mutagenic potential of drug impurities. *Toxicology and Applied Pharmacology 260*(3), 209–221.

Van Houwelingen, H. C., L. R. Arends, and T. Stijnen (2002). Advanced methods in meta-analysis: multivariate approach and meta-regression. *Statistics in Medicine 21*(4), 589–624.

Vandenberk, B., E. Vandael, T. Robyns, J. Vandenberghe, C. Garweg, V. Foulon, J. Ector, and R. Willems (2016). Which qt correction for-mulae to use for qt monitoring? *Journal of the American Heart Associ-ation 5*(6), e003264.

Vareki, S. M., C. Garrigós, and I. Duran (2017). Biomarkers of Response to PD-1/PD-L1 Inhibition. *Critical Reviews in Oncology/Hematology 116*, 116–124.

Veerasamy, R., H. Rajak, A. Jain, S. Sivadasan, C. P. Varghese, and R. K. Agrawal (2011). Validation of QSAR models–Strategies and impor-tance. *International Journal of Drug Design & Discovery 3*, 511–519.

Velonas, V. M., H. H. Woo, C. G. d. Remedios, and S. J. Assinder (2013). Current status of biomarkers for prostate cancer. *International Journal of Molecular Sciences 14*(6), 11034–11060.

Vesikari, T., D. O. Matson, P. Dennehy, P. Van Damme, M. Santosham, Z. Rodriguez, M. J. Dallas, J. F. Heyse, M. G. Goveia, and S. B. Black (2006). Safety and efficacy of a pentavalent human–bovine (wc3) re-assortant rotavirus vaccine. *New England Journal of Medicine 354*(1), 23–33.

Vestergaard, M., A. Hviid, K. M. Madsen, J. Wohlfahrt, P. Thorsen, D. Schendel, M. Melbye, and J. Olsen (2004). Mmr vaccination and febrile seizures: evaluation of susceptible subgroups and long-term prognosis. *Jama 292*(3), 351–357.

Vesterinen, H., E. Sena, K. Egan, T. Hirst, L. Churolov, G. Currie, A. An-tonic, D. Howells, and M. Macleod (2014). Meta-analysis of data from animal studies: a practical guide. *Journal of Neuroscience Methods 221*, 92–102.

Vicente, J., L. Johannesen, M. Hosseini, J. W. Mason, P. T. Sager, E. Pueyo, and D. G. Strauss (2016). Electrocardiographic Biomarkers for Detection of Drug-Induced Late Sodium Current Block. *PloS One 11*(12), e0163619.

Vicente, J., N. Stockbridge, and D. G. Strauss (2016). Evolving regulatory paradigm for proarrhythmic risk assessment for new drugs. *Journal of Electrocardiology 49*(6), 837–842.

Villeneuve, D. L., D. Crump, N. Garcia-Reyero, M. Hecker, T. H. Hutchinson, C. A. LaLone, B. Landesmann, T. Lettieri, S. Munn, and M. Nepelska (2014a). Adverse outcome pathway (aop) development I: strategies and principles. *Toxicological Sciences 142*(2), 312–320.

Villeneuve, D. L., D. Crump, N. Garcia-Reyero, M. Hecker, T. H. Hutchinson, C. A. LaLone, B. Landesmann, T. Lettieri, S. Munn, and M. Nepelska (2014b). Adverse outcome pathway development II: best practices. *Toxicological Sciences 142*(2), 321–330.

Vinken, M. (2013). The adverse outcome pathway concept: a pragmatic tool in toxicology. *Toxicology 312*, 158–165.

Vinzi, V. E., W. W. Chin, J. Henseler, and H. Wang (2010). *Handbook of Partial Least Squares: Concepts, Methods and Applications.* Springer.

Waddingham, E., S. Mt-Isa, R. Nixon, and D. Ashby (2016). A Bayesian approach to probabilistic sensitivity analysis in structured benefit-risk assessment. *Biometrical Journal 58*(1), 28–42.

Wages, N. A., M. R. Conaway, and J. O'Quigley (2011). Continual reassessment method for partial ordering. *Biometrics 67*(4), 1555–1563.

Wahab, I. A., N. L. Pratt, M. D. Wiese, L. M. Kalisch, and E. E. Roughead (2013). The validity of sequence symmetry analysis (SSA) for adverse drug reaction signal detection. *Pharmacoepidemiology and Drug Safety 22*(5), 496–502.

Wald, A. (1945). Sequential tests of statistical hypotheses. *The Annals of Mathematical Statistics 16*(2), 117–186.

Wald, A. (1947). *Sequential Analysis.* Wiley New York.

Walker, T., K. Harris, E. Maifoshie, and K. Chaudhary (2017). Human stem cell-derived cardiomyocyte in vitro models for cardiotoxicity screening. *Stem Cells in Toxicology and Medicine*, 85–121.

Wallace, M. P., E. E. Moodie, and D. A. Stephens (2016). Smart thinking: a review of recent developments in sequential multiple assignment randomized trials. *Current Epidemiology Reports 3*(3), 225–232.

Wallenstein, S., J. Naus, and J. Glaz (1994). Power of the scan statistic in detecting a changed segment in a bernoulli sequence. *Biometrika 81*(3), 595–601.

Wang, J., P. Neskovic, and L. N. Cooper (2006). Neighborhood size selection in the k-nearest-neighbor rule using statistical confidence. *Pattern Recognition 39*(3), 417–423.

Wang, X. and D. K. Dey (2010). Generalized extreme value regression for binary response data: An application to b2b electronic payments system adoption. *The Annals of Applied Statistics*, 2000–2023.

Wang, Y., Y. Mai, and W. He (2016). A quantitative approach for benefit-risk assessment using stochastic multi-criteria discriminatory method. *Statistics in Biopharmaceutical Research 8*(4), 373–378.

Waters, M. D. (2016). Introduction to predictive toxicogenomics for carcinogenicity. In R. S. Thomas and M. D. Waters (Eds.), *Toxicogenomics in Predictive Carcinogecity*, pp. 1–38. Royal Society of Chemistry.

Webb, A. R. (2003). *Statistical Pattern Recognition*. John Wiley & Sons.

Wechsler, J. (2007). FDAAA empowers FDA to have greater control over drug safety. *Formulary Journal – Clinical Pharmacology*.

Weinstein, M. C., G. Torrance, and A. McGuire (2009). QALYs: the basics. *Value in Health 12*(s1), S5–S9.

Weir, D. L., F. A. McAlister, A. Senthilselvan, J. K. Minhas-Sandhu, and D. T. Eurich (2014). Sitagliptin use in patients with diabetes and heart failure: a population-based retrospective cohort study. *JACC: Heart Failure 2*(6), 573–582.

West, B. T. and R. J. Little (2013). Non-response adjustment of survey estimates based on auxiliary variables subject to error. *Journal of the Royal Statistical Society: Series C (Applied Statistics) 62*(2), 213–231.

West, S., B. Strom, and C. Poole (2014). Validity of pharmacoepidemiologic drug and diagnosis data. In B. Strom, S. Kimmel, and S. Hennessy (Eds.), *Pharmacoepidemiology, 5th Edition*, Chapter 45, pp. 757–786. Chichester, UK: John Wiley & Sons, Ltd.

Wexler, P. (2001). TOXNET: an evolving web resource for toxicology and environmental health information. *Toxicology 157*(1), 3–10.

Whitaker, H. J., C. Paddy Farrington, B. Spiessens, and P. Musonda (2006). Tutorial in biostatistics: the self-controlled case series method. *Statistics in Medicine 25*(10), 1768–1797.

White, R. W., N. P. Tatonetti, N. H. Shah, R. B. Altman, and E. Horvitz (2013). Web-scale pharmacovigilance: listening to signals from the crowd. *Journal of the American Medical Informatics Association 20*(3), 404–408.

Whitehead, A. (2002). *Meta-Analysis of Controlled Clinical Trials.* John Wiley & Sons.

Whitehead, J. and H. Brunier (1995). Bayesian decision procedures for dose determining experiments. *Statistics in Medicine 14*(9), 885–893.

Whitehead, J., H. Thygesen, and A. Whitehead (2010). A Bayesian dose-finding procedure for phase I clinical trials based only on the assumption of monotonicity. *Statistics in Medicine 29*(17), 1808–1824.

WHO (1992). *International Monitoring of Adverse Reactions to Drugs: Adverse Reaction Terminology.* WHO Collaborating Centre for International Drug Monitoring, Uppsala, Sweden.

WHO (2012a). *International Classification of Diseases (ICD).* World Health Organization, Geneva, Switzerland.

WHO (2012b). *WHO Drug Information, 2010.* World Health Organization, Oslo, Norway.

WHO (2013). *Guidelines for ATC classification and DDD assignment.* WHO Collaborating Centre for Drug Statistics Methodology, World Health Organization, Oslo, Norway.

WHO (2014). *VigiBase.* The Uppsala Monitoring Centre, WHO (http://www.umc-products.com/).

Wians, F. H. (2009). Clinical laboratory tests: which, why, and what do the results mean? *Laboratory Medicine 40*(2), 105–113.

Willan, A. R. (2004). Incremental net benefit in the analysis of economic data from clinical trials, with application to the cadet-hp trial. *European Journal of Gastroenterology & Hepatology 16*(6), 543–549.

Willett, C., J. Caverly Rae, K. O. Goyak, B. Landesmann, G. Minsavage, and C. Westmoreland (2014). Pathway-based toxicity: history, current approaches and liver fibrosis and steatosis as prototypes. *Altex 31*(4), 407–421.

Williams, D. (1975). The analysis of binary responses from toxicological experiments involving reproduction and teratogenicity. *Biometrics 31*(4), 949–952.

Williams, R. J., T. Tse, K. DiPiazza, and D. A. Zarin (2015). Terminated trials in the clinicaltrials.gov results database: evaluation of availability of primary outcome data and reasons for termination. *PLoS One 10*(5), 1–12.

Willis, C. D., J. J. McNeil, P. A. Cameron, and L. E. Phillips (2012). Monitoring drug safety with registries: useful components of postmarketing pharmacovigilance systems. *Journal of Clinical Epidemiology 65*(2), 121–125.

Wilson, A. G. (2011). *New Horizons in Predictive Toxicology: Current Status and Application*. Royal Society of Chemistry.

Wilson, K. and S. Hawken (2013). Drug safety studies and measures of effect using the self-controlled case series design. *Pharmacoepidemiology and Drug Safety 22*(1), 108–110.

Wittwehr, C., H. Aladjov, G. Ankley, H. J. Byrne, J. de Knecht, E. Heinzle, G. Klambauer, B. Landesmann, M. Luijten, and C. MacKay (2017). How adverse outcome pathways can aid the development and use of computational prediction models for regulatory toxicology. *Toxicological Sciences 155*(2), 326–336.

Wold, S., M. Sjöström, and L. Eriksson (2001). PLS-regression: a basic tool of chemometrics. *Chemometrics and Intelligent Laboratory Systems 58*(2), 109–130.

Wright, S. (1921). Systems of mating. *Genetics 6*, 111–178.

Xia, A., H. Ma, and B. Carlin (2011). Bayesian hierarchal modeling for detecting safety signals in clinical trials. *Journal of Biopharmaceutical Statistics 21*, 1006–29.

Xu, J., G. Yin, D. Ohlssen, and F. Bretz (2016). Bayesian two-stage dose finding for cytostatic agents via model adaptation. *Journal of the Royal Statistical Society: Series C 65*(3), 465–482.

Yao, B., L. Zhu, Q. Jiang, and H. A. Xia (2013). Safety monitoring in clinical trials. *Pharmaceutics 5*(1), 94–106.

Yao, Y., L. Rosasco, and A. Caponnetto (2007). On early stopping in gradient descent learning. *Constructive Approximation 26*(2), 289–315.

Yap, C., C. Cai, Y. Xue, and Y. Chen (2004). Prediction of torsade-causing potential of drugs by support vector machine approach. *Toxicological Sciences 79*(1), 170–177.

Yee, L. C. and Y. C. Wei (2012). Current modeling methods used in QSAR/QSPR. In M. Dehmer, K. Varmuza, and D. Bonchev (Eds.), *Statistical Modelling of Molecular Descriptors in QSAR/QSPR*, pp. 1–31. Wiley-VCH, Weinheim, Germany.

Yeh, E. T., E. Salvatorelli, P. Menna, and G. Minotti (2014). What is cardiotoxicity? *Progress in Pediatric Cardiology 36*(1), 3–6.

Yih, W. K., M. Kulldorff, B. H. Fireman, I. M. Shui, E. M. Lewis, N. P.
Klein, J. Baggs, E. S. Weintraub, E. A. Belongia, and A. Naleway (2011).
Active surveillance for adverse events: the experience of the vaccine
safety datalink project. *Pediatrics*, peds–2010.

Yih, W. K., J. C. Maro, M. Nguyen, M. A. Baker, C. Balsbaugh, D. V.
Cole, I. Dashevsky, A. Mba-Jonas, and M. Kulldorff (2015). Mini-
sentinel cber/prism methods–pilot of self-controlled tree-temporal scan
analysis of gardasil vaccine. Technical report, The Sentinel System.
https://www.sentinelinitiative.org/sites/default/files/Methods/Mini-
Sentinel_PRISM_Pilot-Self-Controlled-Tree-Temporal-Scan-Analysis-
Gardasil-Vaccine-Report.pdf.

Yih, W. K., J. C. Maro, M. Nguyen, M. A. Baker, C. Balsbaugh, D. V.
Cole, I. Dashevsky, A. Mba-Jonas, and M. Kulldorff (2018). Assessment of quadrivalent human papillomavirus vaccine safety using the
self-controlled tree-temporal scan statistic signal-detection method in
the sentinel system. *American Journal Epidemiology* (000), 000–000.

Yih, W. K., J. D. Nordin, M. Kulldorff, E. Lewis, T. A. Lieu, P. Shi, and
E. S. Weintraub (2009). An assessment of the safety of adolescent and
adult tetanus–diphtheria–acellular pertussis (tdap) vaccine, using active surveillance for adverse events in the vaccine safety datalink. *Vaccine 27*(32), 4257–4262.

Yin, G. and Y. Yuan (2009). Bayesian dose finding in oncology for drug
combinations by copula regression. *Journal of the Royal Statistical Society: Series C 58*(2), 211–224.

Yousefinejad, S. and B. Hemmateenejad (2015). Chemometrics tools in
QSAR/QSPR studies: A historical perspective. *Chemometrics and Intelligent Laboratory Systems 149*, 177–204.

Yuan, Y. and G. Yin (2011). Bayesian phase I/II adaptively randomized
oncology trials with combined drugs. *The Annals of Applied Statistics 5*(2A), 924.

Yuan, Z., G. Chen, and Q. Huang (2016). Adaptive strategies in designing
the simultaneous global drug development program. *Journal of Biopharmaceutical Statistics 26*(3), 590–597.

Yusuf, S., R. Peto, J. Lewis, R. Collins, and P. Sleight (1985). Beta blockade
during and after myocardial infarction: an overview of the randomized
trials. *Progress in Cardiovascular Diseases 27*(5), 335–371.

Zeger, S. L., K.-Y. Liang, and P. S. Albert (1988). Models for longitudinal data: a generalized estimating equation approach. *Biometrics 44*(4), 1049–1060.

Zhang, C., Y. Zhou, S. Gu, Z. Wu, W. Wu, C. Liu, K. Wang, G. Liu, W. Li, and P. W. Lee (2016). *In silico* prediction of hERG potassium channel blockage by chemical category approaches. *Toxicology Research 5*(2), 570–582.

Zhang, G. and R. Little (2009). Extensions of the penalized spline of propensity prediction method of imputation. *Biometrics 65*(3), 911–918.

Zhang, G. and R. Little (2011). A comparative study of doubly robust estimators of the mean with missing data. *Journal of Statistical Computation and Simulation 81*(12), 2039–2058.

Zhang, J., H. Chen, Y. Tsong, and N. Stockbridge (2015). Lessons learned from hundreds of thorough qt studies. *Therapeutic Innovation & Regulatory Science 49*(3), 392–397.

Zhang, L., C. M. McHale, N. Greene, R. D. Snyder, I. N. Rich, M. J. Aardema, S. Roy, S. Pfuhler, and S. Venkatactahalam (2014). Emerging approaches in predictive toxicology. *Environmental and Molecular Mutagenesis 55*(9), 679–688.

Zhang, L., Y. D. Zhang, P. Zhao, and S.-M. Huang (2009). Predicting drug–drug interactions: an FDA perspective. *The AAPS Journal 11*(2), 300–306.

Zhang, T. and B. Yu (2005). Boosting with early stopping: Convergence and consistency. *The Annals of Statistics 33*(4), 1538–1579.

Zhang, W., Y. Chen, F. Liu, F. Luo, G. Tian, and X. Li (2017). Predicting potential drug-drug interactions by integrating chemical, biological, phenotypic and network data. *BMC Bioinformatics 18*(1), 18.

Zhang, Y., Y. S. Wong, J. Deng, C. Anton, S. Gabos, W. Zhang, D. Y. Huang, and C. Jin (2016). Machine learning algorithms for mode-of-action classification in toxicity assessment. *BioData Mining 9*(1), 19.

Zhao, H. and A. A. Tsiatis (1997). A consistent estimator for the distribution of quality adjusted survival time. *Biometrika 84*(2), 339–348.

Zhao, H. and A. A. Tsiatis (1999). Efficient estimation of the distribution of quality-adjusted survival time. *Biometrics 55*(4), 1101–1107.

Zhao, H. and A. A. Tsiatis (2001). Testing equality of survival functions of quality-adjusted lifetime. *Biometrics 57*(3), 861–867.

Zhao, L., B. Claggett, L. Tian, H. Uno, M. A. Pfeffer, S. D. Solomon, L. Trippa, and L. Wei (2016). On the restricted mean survival time curve in survival analysis. *Biometrics 72*(1), 215–221.

Zhao, S., A. Cook, L. Jackson, and J. Nelson (2012). Statistical performance of group sequential methods for observational post-licensure medical product safety surveillance: a simulation study. *Statistics and Its Interface 5*, 381–390.

Zhao, Y., J. Zalkikar, R. C. Tiwari, and L. M. LaVange (2014). A Bayesian approach for benefit-risk assessment. *Statistics in Biopharmaceutical Research 6*(4), 326–337.

Zou, H. and T. Hastie (2005). Regularization and variable selection via the elastic net. *Journal of the Royal Statistical Society: Series B 67*(2), 301–320.

Index